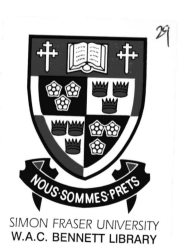

Bill Rawling

DEATH THEIR ENEMY

Canadian Medical Practitioners
and War

Ce livre a été publié simultanément en français sous le titre:
La mort pour ennemi. La médecine militaire canadienne
ISBN 2-922865-01-2

Design   *Zéro Faute*, Outremont

Cover photography   NA C 3453, ISC 91-60-72-2,
                                NA PA 000549

Page-setting and printing thanks to a grant
from the DND Millenium Coordinator.

ISBN 2-922865-01-0

Legal Deposit   first quarter 2001
Bibliothèque nationale du Canada
Bibliothèque nationale du Québec

Printed in Canada

Contents

Introduction

The Practice of Medicine in War

Many years after the end of the Second World War, Doctor A.L. Chute, Dean of Medicine of the University of Toronto, recalled the story of a soldier who had been wounded in battle, but who, thanks to penicillin, recovered quickly and returned to the fighting; within three weeks, he was back in hospital with new wounds. "We took a look at him and decided among ourselves, no penicillin for you chappie. We let him heal the old slow way, figuring he deserved a little holiday."[1] Chute's decision apparently went against hundreds of years of military medical practice, which was supposed to focus on getting sick and wounded soldiers ready for the next battle—the needs or will of the patient being quite secondary. But if military institutions placed their own requirements first, medical practitioners did not always share that perspective. As we shall see, in the nineteenth century surgeons often worked to save a man's life through amputation, the very act rendering him unable to continue soldiering; in the First World War hospitals in England came under severe criticism, not for incompetence but for expending resources on men who would never recover sufficiently to return to the trenches; when Norman Bethune joined Mao's forces in China in the late 1930s, he also relied on amputation on many occasions, saving men's lives but removing them from military rosters in the process. To be fair, there are many counter-examples, and we shall also see how soldiers diagnosed with cholera in the nineteenth century would have refused treatment—if the military hierarchy had allowed; of how those deemed to be hysterics in the First World War underwent painful shock therapy to get them back to the front all the quicker; and of how aircrew in the

---

1. G.W.L. Nicholson, *Seventy Years of Service* (Ottawa, 1977), 186.

Second World War saw their courage denigrated by being diagnosed as "lacking in moral fibre" rather than suffering from battle exhaustion.

Still, a fact that will become evident in the pages that follow is that the concept of treating a soldier so that he (later, he or she) could return to the fighting was more cliché than policy, and there was no real mechanism for enforcing it. In the main, medical practioners operated with no little autonomy, military institutions rarely interfering with how they went about their business, going so far as to leave in doctors' hands the decision as to whether a soldier would return to the fighting or be sent home—possibly with a pension. Deserving or not, medical practitioners were held in some respect, and were simply trusted to carry out their duties to the best of their abilities. One reason for this is that on the battlefield, where most of this study will be focussed, there is little time to sort out administrative or logistical priorities unless such has been done in advance. A First World War surgeon might find himself with hundreds of patients awaiting treatment, or a Second World War nurse could have to deal with dozens of burn victims from a torpedoed tanker, or a medical assistant in the 1990s face thousands of refugees suffering from dehydration. There were no hospital board meetings to determine how these practitioners should proceed, and they were left with their training and instincts to see them through. Furthermore, as for other specialists, they found that war is a different world entirely, where an enemy is actively engaged in interfering with one's operations, sometimes with deadly force; only in peacekeeping operations, and even then not always, have soldiers been able to work without that reality hanging over them. Given the nature of modern conflict, doctors, nurses, NCOs, and soldiers, though well-versed in the medical arts and sciences before they arrived at the front or in a ship, gained most of their tactical knowledge while on the job—along with everyone else. Under such circumstances, people were far more concerned with the needs of the moment—such as a soldier with a severe abdominal wound—than with any sweeping policies military institutions may have promulgated.

That is not to say that military medical practitioners were staunch individualists bent on promoting their patients' best interest, but one should be careful not to bend too far in the other direction. After a hundred years or so of veneration, doctors have come in for severe criticism in recent decades, one academic reading a previous version of this manuscript suggesting the author study the career of Josef Mengele to get a proper perspective on the medical profession, but the approach this narrative will adopt is more anthropological, seeking to study and understand rather than worship or denounce. It must be understood that since this is a study of Canadian medical practitioners, underlying the narrative that follows is a collection of western values that none of these men and women ever questioned—or if so, extremely rarely. The purpose of medicine was to cure, and though that was also the case in China, India, Africa, and among aboriginal communities, in these societies there was not—and is not—the obsession with putting off physical demise that one finds in Europe, North America, and some European-colonized areas. Treatment was aggressive, sometimes with catastrophic results for the patient, and herein lies another clue to how medical practitioners balanced the demands of the military with those of their profession; from their point of view, when all was said and done death was their main enemy.

Chapter One

Early Military Medicine in Canada

Dealing with the casualties of war may well be as old as war itself; those who have the abilities to defend the community can contribute to it in other ways, so it is well worth while attempting to repair their injuries and return them to productive health. Furthermore, humans being social animals develop relationships with one another that encourage them to relieve the pain of friend or family; Neanderthal groups of 30,000 years ago supported those among them who suffered from injury or disabling diseases such as spina bifida. Sources are too scanty to determine when soldiers could first rely on some organized form of medical succour, but as early as 1200 BCE, in Egypt, management systems required for large-scale irrigation and construction projects "encouraged governments to recognize the economy of saving the lives of career soldiers, who represented a costly investment in a state's military armamentaria."[1] The goal of military medicine, if one could call it such, was thus to profit society, not the soldier, which did not exclude his benefiting from the practice. When in 480 BCE the Roman consul Manlius defeated the Etruscans in battle, he ensured the wounded of both sides were billeted in private homes, and within three centuries the *valetudinaria* had evolved on the frontiers of the empire; consisting of single rooms around a rectangular courtyard, the latter had originally been used as sick quarters for slaves but eventually accommodated ill and wounded soldiers—prototype hospitals in effect.[2] As for battlefield casualties, by the time the Romans invaded Britain in 43 CE they had developed a medical organization which saw a surgeon for each cohort

---

1. John S. Haller, *Farmcarts to Fords* (Carbondale, 1992), 8.
2. John S. Haller, *Farmcarts to Fords* (Carbondale, 1992), 8.

(of which there ten to a legion)[3], or one medical practitioner for every 500-600 soldiers, a ratio that would not be improved upon until the twentieth century.

In the two millennia that followed the founding of the Roman Empire, the importance of medical staffs mirrored attitudes towards the common soldiery. When William the Bastard carved out a kingdom for himself in England, hence becoming William the Conqueror, he and his nobles relied on their personal physicians to tend to them in case of injury or illness, but the rest of the army had to fend for itself. It being easier to replace wounded men than maintain a medical organization, when Henry V fought his epic battle at Agincourt in 1415 his army of 30,000 comprised only 20 surgeons and a physician, and these were deemed of lesser rank than shoemakers and tailors. In the early seventeenth century a military manual listed them among "other meane offices," along with fifes and drums.[4]

The army was not alone in holding surgeons in low regard—so did European society as a whole, which perhaps had something to do with patients' survival rates; though statistics were not kept at the time, anecdotal evidence seems to indicate that recovery from battlefield wounds was far from assured. By the early sixteenth century the practice had developed of using boiling oil or water to stop bleeding through cauterization, hence creating burn or scald injuries that were ripe for infection. According to legend—which may not be too far from the truth—the practice began to change after a serendipitous discovery by a surgeon in the army of Francis I of France. In the latter's campaign against Turin in 1536-37, Ambroise Paré ran out of the oil he had been using to cauterize the stumps of amputees, and fell back on using a mixture of herbs and similar plants. Though guilt-ridden at having provided these patients with second-rate treatment, in the days that followed he found that they did better than those who had been ministered to in the traditional manner. As a result ligature, suturing veins and arteries to halt bleeding, eventually became the norm,[5] and with such changes, and the resultant increase in soldier survival, surgeons experienced a marginal rise in status.

So it was that when European armies came to what is now Canada in the seventeenth and eighteenth centuries, each regiment had its surgeon and the necessary supplies to set up a small hospital, though military surgery had changed little since the days of Paré. The people they encountered in what they called the New World (the original

3. G.W.L. Nicholson, *Seventy Years of Service* (Ottawa, 1977), 2.
4. G.W.L. Nicholson, *Seventy Years of Service* (Ottawa, 1977), 2.
5. John S. Haller, *Farmcarts to Fords* (Carbondale, 1992), 10-11.

inhabitants considered it to be rather old) also had their military traditions—and methods to treat the resulting wounds and injuries. Joseph-François Lafitau, who travelled through New France and Aboriginal lands in the early eighteenth century, witnessed the procedure and commented on it at some length, calling it a "masterpiece" of medical art. He related the case of a warrior shot in the shoulder, whose wound was considered sufficiently life-threatening to be ministered the last rites. All was not lost, however, and a mixture of clean water, herbs, roots, bark, and dried animal tissue was applied after the practitioner had "sucked" poison from the injury site. The whole was then wrapped in a dressing treated with herbs to protect the wound from foreign bodies, and in the days that followed the procedure was repeated, the patient recovering.[6] In many ways, such treatment was identical to Paré's, and in fact there had been a fair amount of cross-cultural exchange in the previous century, but Lafitau also pointed out that cauterization on a small scale was still practised by Europeans, but not by their aboriginal allies.

There is no evidence that the Amerindian approach was adopted by the newcomers, and in the early nineteenth century military medical practice in Canada was based almost exclusively on the European model, which meant, in fact, the civilian model. There being nothing to distinguish one from the other, as refugees from the American Revolution moved to Canada in large numbers their health problems could be made the responsibility of army surgeons. As William Canniff explained in the 1890s, "At Kingston, Niagara and Detroit were garrisons with a limited number of soldiers and one or two surgeons. For many years, the pioneers were dependent upon these army surgeons, who were rarely willing to go any distance from the garrison. Some of the settlements were made by disbanded soldiers, and those who settled along the St. Lawrence had as fellow-pioneers a few surgeons who had been attached to their respective corps, and continued to enjoy their medical services."[7]

In time of war, where military medicine differed from that of civilians was in the realm of evacuation. If injured or ill, someone living on a farm or in town was expected to either make his or her way to a doctor, wait for the latter to come to them, or treat the problem themselves. It was at about the same time as American refugees made their way to Upper Canada that European armies looked to devising a different system for their soldiers, perhaps the first being France's Army of the

---

6. Joseph-François Lafitau, *Moeurs des sauvages américains, v.II* (Paris, 1983), 117-119.
7. William Canniff, *The Medical Profession in Upper Canada, 1783-1850* (Toronto, 1894 and 1980), 13.

Rhine in the 1790s. Dominique-Jean Larrey, a young surgeon, noted that many soldiers died of shock on the battlefield because they could not make their way to the usual casualty collecting points at the baggage train, or whose friends were too busy—or themselves wounded— to do so. Procuring several two- and four-wheeled light wagons, Larrey organized them into an *ambulance volante,* or flying ambulance, which carried medical officers and their assistants right into the front line if necessary. Wounds being dressed on the battlefield, the wagons could then be used to transport patients to a field hospital. In the Italian campaign of 1796 one such flying ambulance, with 340 all ranks, was provided for each division of about ten thousand troops.

Such was the state of the art when the United States of America and the United Kingdom went to war against each other in 1812. Typical of the time, and of previous millennia, illness and disease were of more concern to medical practitioners than battle wounds—for good reason. Combat was the exception rather than the rule, and an army could be seriously reduced in numbers by a host of water-borne, flea-transmitted, and human-communicative ailments. According to Charles G. Roland, who has studied the medicine of that time in great detail, "Disease killed or disabled far more men than did wounds. Typhus, dysentery, smallpox, malaria, and syphilis were rampant and often epidemic. Excepting cinchona for malaria, treatment was non-specific and was pursued with a vigour that often finished the job that disease had begun,"[8] leading to a high death rate.

One consequence of such a state of affairs may have been the reliance on Canadian part-time troops; for though these were far less-well trained than British regulars, they were readily available and capable of carrying out line of communication duties. Also, according to John Douglas, in his *Medical Topography of Upper Canada,* "The provincial militia were generally healthy, when employed on active duty, and were more exempted from sickness that the British troops. Their services, though severe, were not always long continued. Some corps being embodied during the war, were constantly employed, either in the field, or in garrison duty; others being called out only on particular emergencies, often enjoyed through winter the tranquillity of their homes,"[9] where they avoided the diseases of the barracks.

Another threat to health offered by garrison life, according to John Douglas, was alcohol, "The young soldier being often addicted to intemperance, his constitutional symptoms of inflammation are generally of

8. Charles G. Roland, "Medical Aspects of War in the West in 1812," K.G. Pryke and L.L. Kusilek, eds, *The Western District: Papers from the Western District Conference* (Windsor, 1983), 50.
9. John Douglas, *Medical Topography of Upper Canada* (Canton, reprinted 1985), 35.

a violent kind."[10] James Mann, serving with American forces, agreed, though reporting that the British were far better off than their opponents in that regard.

> Deserters from the British Army, of whom some hundreds came to our posts, exhibited marks of high health; while those of our soldiers were pallid and emaciated. The difference was too obvious to have escaped the observation of the officers of the army. It led me to seek the cause. Upon enquiry it was learnt, that spirits were no part of the ration of the British soldier; that these liquors could not be procured in the upper province of Canada for money. While, in addition to their daily rations, our soldiers, when they had money in their pockets, had free access to spirits at the stores of the sutlers. Diseases and mortality generally, but not necessarily, followed the pay-masters of the army. With means to make themselves comfortable, soldiers frequently render their lives wretched.[11]

Though there was in truth little difference between the two armies when it came to the consumption of drink, the two doctors had a point—alcohol consumed in the quantities soldiers preferred was not healthy. James Mann suggested, though he knew his proposal would be received as heresy, that spirits should not be used as a common beverage.

Another of his suggestions was that soldiers try to keep as clean as possible, for "Cleanliness is the life of an army; while filth and dirt are among its disease-generating causes,"[12] and Douglas, again, would have agreed. Idleness could also be a factor, for when an army was in action, "Under these strong excitements, with a due proportion of nutriment, disease seldom assails the body. During long intervals of inactivity, the system becomes enervated. Then it is that the deleterious agents exhibit their influences upon animal life. Then it is that an army sickens from causes connected with their local positions. The soldiers are attacked with diseases in the field, which originate from their own filth and imprudence."[13] Mann's pronouncements were in accordance with a common theory of the time, the body becoming susceptible to certain diseases if overly excited (irritability), to others if insufficiently stimulated (debility), the former being countered by bloodletting, blistering, enemas, and a low diet, among others, while the latter was treated by such things as cathartics, enemas (again, though with different ingredients), stimulants such as alcohol, and a nourishing diet.[14] To strike a balance between irritation and debility during active service, "intervals of repose are necessary; but they should be short, and, during rest,

10. John Douglas, *Medical Topography of Upper Canada* (Canton, reprinted 1985), 16.
11. James Mann, *Medical Sketches of the Campaigns of 1812, 13, 14* (Dedham, 1816), 37.
12. James Mann, *Medical Sketches of the Campaigns of 1812, 13, 14* (Dedham, 1816), 38.
13. James Mann, 175.
14. C. Keith Wilbur, *Revolutionary Medicine, 1700-1800* (Old Saybrook, 1980), 17.

unexposed to rain or snow. Profound sleep is increased by fatigue; during this state, the powers of life are either weakened or suspended." The solution was mild exercise, and it was "therefore favourable to the soldier"s health, after a hard march, to be obliged to seek or cut his wood, to make a fire, and cook his provisions. By this gentle exercise a suitable action is preserved upon the several organs, while the perspiration on the surface is gradually evaporated, without the too sudden waste of heat; the powers of life do not sink, and are further supported by his soup, and a short period of rest. He rises refreshed, and is prepared to obey commands."[15]

When such prophylactic measures were impossible to enforce, or if soldiers fell ill anyway, the case was usually dealt with according to current theory as discussed above. One course of treatment was to remove blood to re-establish a healthy equilibrium, a process which modern medicine would consider hazardous, but which no doubt arose from the fact that patients did indeed feel better after being bled. According to John Douglas, "Few diseases, indeed, require a more prompt and decisive treatment than pneumonia. Before congestion and effusion have taken place in important organs, the abstraction of blood from the patient should be immediate and copious. In pneumonia, sparing and untimely bleedings endanger life,"[16] and in one case sixteen pounds of blood had to be taken in the space of four days to treat one patient. Whether the young soldier succumbed to the illness—or the treatment— we do not know.

Ophthalmia, an eye condition, could also force the surgeon "to carry blood-letting to a great length,"[17] but more surprising to the modern reader, no doubt, was the widespread use of the technique in the treatment of such diseases as dysentery and such conditions as diarrhoea, which blood-letting would have worsened. Mann, however, insisted that the treatment was "advantageously employed" in such cases, perhaps in those not yet weak enough to be finished off by the conscientious application of medical theory. The latter is not a facetious conclusion, as Douglas noted that "The acute form of this disease," that is to say, diarrhoea, "which in other countries has often proved distressing to an army, was not much to be dreaded in Upper Canada. In those cases which came under my care the symptoms of inflamation were not very urgent... Gentle bleedings, a few purgatives, and attention to diet, generally overcame the complaint. It terminated in the chronic form, in those men whose viscera were enlarged, or in those who were debilitated

15. James Mann, 175-176.
16. John Douglas, 16.
17. *Ibid*, 27.

from frequent attacks of intermittent fever. Dysentery seemed so blended with that disease, that, in a number of instances, it alternated with the paroxysms of the fever."[18]

The latter, then, was perhaps of greater concern, and the subject of much sophisticated medical investigation—even if the conclusions then were somewhat different from what they would be today. Modern science describes fever as a symptom brought on by the body's attempts to fight off disease inflicted by a virus or bacterium, but prior to the discovery of these small creatures medical theory described fever as a disease brought on by miasma, or bad air, so that practitioners were in fact pretty close to the mark. The medical profession had arrived at such conclusions through observation often confirmed, Douglas pointing out that "Such exhalations have often proved noxious to an army, when encamped within the sphere of their malignant influence."[19] Admitting that "chemical analysis" was unable to determine the precise substance that caused disease—or vector of transmission—practitioners nonetheless rightly made the link between swampy conditions and illness.

> The effect of marsh-miasmata on the human body, is sometimes instantaneous. When marching through an unhealthy tract of the province, I have seen men, who had recently joined the army, suddenly seized with the symptoms of fever. Nausea, lassitude, giddiness, and confused vision, were the precursors of the disease. Others I have seen attacked with difficult respiration, fainting, and immobility of the limbs. Those affections were not, like the former, premonition of fever; but seemed referable to the scorching heat of the sun, and, in a few instances, preceded by an attack of cholera morbus.

> For the most part the human body appears to be insensibly impregnated with marsh-miasmata, and it may be filled with a certain quantity of the poison for a considerable time without producing the symptoms of disease. Under such circumstances, fatigue, the depressing passions, great exposure to cold, or to the heat of the sun, are causes sufficient to call the morbid movements of the system into action. It is well known, that both remittent and intermittent fevers have invaded individuals in places remote from those unhealthy situations in which the seeds of these diseases had been at first generated,[20]

recognizing that the illness could have an incubation period.

As knowledgeable as contemporary medical practitioners might have been, fever could still devastate an army on the Canadian frontier of 1812 or 1814, or just across the border in the nascent United States. When Brigadier William Hull and his army arrived at Detroit in July of

18. John Douglas, 25.
19. John Douglas, 22.
20. John Douglas, 22.

1812, there were already large numbers of sick men within its ranks, and the general himself admitted to 600 of them being out of action due to disease. He may, in fact, have considered the impact illness was having on his forces when he surrendered later in the summer, but that is speculation.[21] Nor were the British immune, as Douglas could attest. "When quartered with my regiment in the unhealthy village of Chippawa, during the summer of 1814, intermittent fever became remarkably prevalent in the battalion. Within the short space of six weeks, one half of the corps was admitted into hospital, labouring under the disease... The sickness at last became so pressing, that we were under the necessity of evacuating the position, and of retiring to the rear of the army to a more salubrious situation."[22]

Circumstances, typical of the time, had developed as a result of a siege; after seesaw battles across the Niagara Peninsula in the summer of 1814, the Americans set up defensive positions in and around Fort Erie. After a 15 August attack against the American positions, Lieutenant-General Gordon Drummond was able to call up two fresh regiments to make up his losses, but by 8 September was advising his superiors of the "possibility of my being compelled by sickness or suffering of the troops, exposed as they will be to the effects of the wet and unhealthy Season which is fast approaching, to withdraw them from their present Position to one which may afford them the means of cover. Sickness has, I am sorry to say, already made its appearance in several of the Corps, particularly the 82nd."[23] Nine days later, after a sortie by the Americans, Drummond again brought up the issue of disease, which had obviously worsened.

> Within the last few days ... the sickness of the troops has increased to such an alarming degree, and their situation has really become one of such extreme wretchedness from the torrents of rain which have continued to fall for the last 13 days, and from the circumstance of the Division being entirely destitute of camp equipage, that I feel it my duty no longer to persevere in a vain attempt to maintain the blockade of so vastly superior and increasing a force of the enemy under such circumstances. I have therefore given orders for the troops to fall back toward the Chippawa, and shall commence my movement at eight o'clock this evening.[24]

The Americans were no doubt in similar shape, deciding to withdraw to their side of the Niagara frontier soon after.

21. Charles G. Roland, "Medical Aspects of War in the West in 1812," K.G. Pryke and L.L. Kusilek, eds, *The Western District: Papers from the Western District Conference* (Windsor, 1983), 55-56.
22. John Douglas, 21.
23. Quoted in J. Mackay Hitsman, *The Incredible War of 1812: A Military History* (Toronto, 1965), 202.
24. *Ibid*, 203-204.

Disease could also have a negative impact on a wounded man's chances of recovery. In the Niagara Peninsula campaign of 1814, which saw some of the more brutal battles of the war, Douglas noted that "Many of the wounded were debilitate from severe service, and had also suffered from the endemic diseases of the country. Their constitutions were not, therefore, in a state well adapted to make reparation for the loss of substance, occasioned by serious injuries. Neither were they in a favourable condition to undergo those formidable operations which are too often the last resort of surgical interference,"[25] notably amputation. The main consequence was not, however, to postpone the desperate act of surgery, but to carry it out all the sooner. Fever often finishing off the patient while awaiting treatment

> tended to convince the surgeon how dangerous it was in a number of cases to postpone amputation, even for a short time after the infliction of a severe injury. They taught him, that in a country, where the wounded are liable to be attacked by those diseases which are endemic to the soil, and to suffer from the impure air of a crowded hospital, there are certain kinds of injuries which it would be improper to trust to the fortuitous efforts of nature. And that, should he allow the first seasonable period of amputation to pass away, he would ultimately witness with painful accusation, the fatal consequence of his ill-timed humanity.[26]

The fever in question, resulting from bacterial infection introduced by the very act of being wounded, was caused by a different agent than that of malaria or swamp fever, but practitioners of the day had a point; removing a badly-lacerated limb did in fact reduce the area in which an opportunistic infection could take hold.

There were other good reasons to rely on amputation, referred to by Adrianne Noe, a recent author on the subject, as "the prototypical act of nineteenth century military surgery."[27] Drastic it may have been, but it was undoubtedly a life-saving technique, and most surgeons would have agreed with a certain Monsieur Larrey, chief surgeon of the French imperial guard and inspector general of the medical staff of the French armies. First was the fact, demonstrated by observation and experience, that an amputee's stump healed more quickly than a large, ragged gunshot wound, and was less likely to develop gangrene. Second, it was subsequently easier to dress, a not unimportant consideration when medical facilities were overwhelmed in the immediate aftermath of a battle. Third, tying in with the above observations, it might be some time before a wounded man was conveyed to a hospital, where he

25. John Douglas, 29.
26. John Douglas, 33.
27. Adrianne Noe, "Medical History," Susan Pfeiffer and Ronald F. Williamson, eds, *Snake Hill: An Investigation of a Military Cemetery from the War of 1812* (Toronto, 1991), 65.

could recover from his wounds, so it was best to ensure the latter were minimized as much as possible—through amputation if necessary.[28]

One surgeon, however, William "Tiger" Dunlop, though accepting the need for such procedures, was willing to point out their imperfections as he looked after the surgical needs of the 89th Foot. After the October 1813 battle of Chrysler's Farm, in modern day Quebec, he noted that some men died, whom he buried, while others recovered, though whether "by remedies employed, or spite of them," he was unsure. His next combat experience was in July 1814 at Lundy's Lane, in the Niagara Peninsula, where he found himself and his sergeant overwhelmed by 220 wounded (a regiment with an optimum strength of 1100 had but one surgeon).[29] "With all this the charge was too much for us, and many a poor fellow had to submit to amputation whose limb might have been preserved had there been only time to take reasonable care of it."[30] Under the circumstances, then, amputation was a necessary evil rather than a preferred treatment.

Surgery was just one step in the process, and after the battles that took place in the Niagara Peninsula in the summer of 1814, it took two or three days to convey British and Canadian wounded, by water, to York. Even then, the hospitals these men were being taken to were very much ad hoc affairs, little more than buildings convenient to hand in which to concentrate patients for convalescence. "The general hospital at York, though a commodious building, was deficient in size for the accommodation of the sick and wounded. Its apartments being originally intended for family use, were too small for the wards of a hospital, and did not admit of free ventilation," considered of crucial importance given the miasmatic theory of disease. "Neither were the adjoining houses of the hospital, which were fitted up for temporary accommodation, any way suitable for the reception of the wounded. When, in the course of the summer, the wounded became so numerous as not to be contained within the general hospital and its outhouses, the church, a large and well-ventilated building, was dismantled of its seats, and, for the time being, converted into a hospital."[31] The latter, thanks to far superior ventilation, benefited the wounded far more, and those who did poorly in the general building were often transferred there.

Whether in a large establishment or in his own, small, regimental hospital, a soldier could expect more in the way of basic nursing than elaborate treatment. A study of the logistics and administration of the

28. James Mann, 206.
29. J. Mackay Hitsman, *The Incredible War of 1812: A Military History* (Toronto, 1965), 30.
30. Quoted in G.W.L. Nicholson, *Seventy Years of Service* (Ottawa, 1977), 21.
31. John Douglas, 28.

time shows that these facilities called for much in the way of basic household items, such as pots and candlesticks, but very little in the way of medical supplies, the two main exceptions being bedpans and urinals. Each institution was staffed by a nurse, an orderly, and a sergeant, a surgeon determining what medicines the latter would dispense and when; he also ensured the wards were clean, the orderly actually carrying out such work. The nurse's duties were somewhat more vague; she was often the sergeant's wife, or the spouse of one of his soldiers, and her duties were probably little different from those of the untrained orderly.[32] Generally, a hospital was a place where nature was allowed to take its course, its personnel concentrating on seeing to the basic needs, such as nutrition, of its patients.

The Treaty of Ghent put an end to the war in the final days of 1814, but medical practitioners in Canada still had work to do dealing with the long-term effects of the conflict. Many soldiers had been partially or totally disabled by their service, either with British regulars or the militia, and these had to be examined and treated to determine their eligibility for pension. For example, a "Return of all persons entitled to Pensions within the limits of the 1st Regiment Glengarry Militia" listed a lieutenant, a sergeant, and eight privates who suffered from "disability from hard labour." Another, for the limits of the 4th Regiment Lincoln Militia, noted a lieutenant-colonel and nine others "who Died of Sickness contracted whilst performing Militia Duty." Generally, such returns seem to confirm that accident and illness created more casualties than combat, the Second Regiment of Gore Militia carrying on its pension rolls eight widows, six of whose husbands succumbed to disease, one who died in captivity, and the other in an accident while on duty.[33]

The role of the medical doctor in such cases is exemplified by the story of Thomas Barrett, late of His Majesty's 83rd Regiment of Foot, with which he had served from 1808 to 1827. Having been discharged in Canada at that time, he later rejoined the colours, having heard that "there was a call made in Canada in the Year 1837 for assembling the Old Soldiers to assist in keeping down the Rebels and Brigands ... Your Petitioner was embodied in the Queens Marine Artillery under the Command of Captain Clarke RN." Military service, even in what would now be called a low-intensity conflict, had its hazards, however, and "when on duty at Night in the Month of March 1838, while stationed at No 3 Block House at Kingston UC was coming down a ladder he fell (the ladder being damaged some two or three days previous from

32. Charles G. Roland, "Medical Aspects of War in the West in 1812," K.G. Pryke and L.L. Kusilek, eds, *The Western District: Papers from the Western District Conference* (Windsor, 1983).
33. National Archives of Canada (NA), RG 9, IB4, v.3.

lowering a 6 Pdr Gun from the Block House) and received a severe injury which has rendered your Petitioner incapable of contributing by his Manual Labor, to Himself or Wife the least subsistence."[34] Requesting a disability pension, he enclosed a certificate from the surgeon of the corps he had been serving with, and later provided another from a different doctor to the effect that the effects of the injury were permanent. His request was granted.

Illness still was, however, the more important creator of pensioners, though military medical practitioners worked hard to make it otherwise. In 1840 one doctor was sent to Canada "to ascertain as far as possible the effect of the climate of this country on the health of Regiments coming from the West Indies," submitting quarterly reports to the principal medical officer of the colony.[35] Such army practitioners brought with them knowledge that might be used in Canada, especially when diseases were imported from other continents. Cholera was one such, first appearing in Asia earlier in the century, then slowly making its way around the world, threatening North America in 1832. Inflicted by a water-borne parasite, it could kill in less than a day through dehydration brought on by excessive vomiting and diarrhea. As Geoffrey Bilson has explained, however, when it seemed the deadly germ was about to strike in Canada, "laymen and doctors alike had access to information about the disease which was widely published in the press... Some military men had served in India and had seen the disease there and military surgeons were familiar with the recommendations of their colleagues in India."[36]

As he further explained, though, such information did not necessarily prove beneficial for the victims of cholera.

> The treatments which Canadian doctors hurled against a disease they did not understand were as barbarous as any used elsewhere in the world and cannot have reassured the patient. In the 1830s, the favoured treatments were bleeding, calomel in doses large enough to make the gums bleed, opium, and counter irritant therapy by cautery and blistering. Some of the hardier patients survived. Private Patrick Mullany of the 32nd Regiment was one. He was taken ill on duty at Quebec City in 1832. He hid from the doctors until he was seen to be sick and was taken to hospital on 17 July at 9:00 a.m. He was bled thirty ounces, given fifteen grains of calomel and two of opium, given a turpentine enema and rubbed with turpentine to ease his cramps, fed ginger tea, and allowed to rest. At 2:00

---

34. NA, RG 9, IB4, v.7, UC Pensions Petitions 1840, A-L, 1, Thomas Barrett to Sir George Arthur, 24 Sep 38.
35. NA, MG 24, E37, Worthington Papers, Staff Surgeon PMO to Worthington, Act Ast Surgeon, 29 July 1840.
36. Geoffrey Bilson, "Canadian Doctors and the Cholera," S.E.D. Shortt, *Medicine in Canadian Society: Historical Perspectives* (Montreal, 1981), 123.

p.m. he was given another three grains of calomel and put on a course of 1/8 grain of opium every half hour with calomel every third hour. That evening he was dosed with castor oil. 18 and 19 July passed with calomel, opium, castor oil, an enema, but also a glass of port wine every two or three hours. On 20 July he was given an acidulated drink, warm wine, lemonade, beef tea, and had a blister applied to his stomach. On 21 July he was dosed with rhubarb, had twelve leeches applied to his stomach, followed by a second blister and was fed beef tea and arrow-root. By 22 July he was able to eat oatmeal porridge for breakfast, but the mercury had begun to affect his mouth. He was given bicarbonate of soda every three hours and beef and arrowroot teas. On 23 July the medicines were ended and he improved slowly until 30 July and was able to return to duty on 11 August. Perhaps he was right to hide on 17 July; but he was receiving the best treatment of the day.[37]

Thus, in the war against disease, engineers perhaps played a more popular role than doctors as they inspected hospitals and barracks and recommended the necessary repairs "with regard to the due accommo-dation for the health of the Troops."[38] Work was to be evaluated as being either urgent, "from their having occasioned evils of which you have had experience," or capable of being put off to another day.

The need to look after soldiers' health was brought home, with a vengeance, during the Crimean War of 1854-56. In that far-flung con-flict, British deaths from all causes totalled 21,000, of whom 2755 were killed in action and 1761 died of their wounds. Some 16,297 succumb-ed to diseases not associated with wounds, amounting to 80 per cent of the total; of these, over 5900 were killed by various bowel illnesses, 4500 by cholera, 3400 by fever, 640 by lung disease, and 1740 by various miscellaneous scourges such as scurvy and frostbite. The British Army's worst month in the Crimea was January 1855, when deaths total-led 3076, almost a tenth of its entire force.[39] It was in this period that Florence Nightingale took her place on the historical stage in her attempts—rewarded with much success—to reform the British hospital system.

She was a civilian, as were military surgeons at the time, hired on contract by individual units. Relations between officers and these practi-tioners were not always cordial, however, as evidenced by a conflict that arose between a Doctor Woods and a Captain Clark of the 100th Regiment, stationed at Toronto in the early 1860s. It would seem that the good doctor had accused the officer, in a letter to the Military

37. Geoffrey Bilson, "Canadian Doctors and the Cholera," S.E.D. Shortt, *Medicine in Canadian Society: Historical Perspectives* (Montreal, 1981), 123.
38. NA, MG 24, E37, Worthington Papers, Inspector General of Hospitals to the Medical Officer in charge of detachment, 50th Regiment, Riviere du Loup, 23 January 1841.
39. Victor Bonham-Carter, *Surgeon in the Crimea* (London, 1968), 115, 117.

Secretary at Montreal, of not taking action when it was brought to his attention that his men were clothed in "very light and imperfect manner."[40] In his defence, the captain, also addressing himself to the Military Secretary, stated that "I do not remember Dr Woods ever having spoken to me *more than once*, upon the subject of Flannels for my men, and that was a short time prior to the date of this letter (12th January), when I told him that a correspondence was then going on about them, and explained to him the purport of my letters in relation thereto, and which letters will be hereafter quoted."

As if that wasn't enough, the doctor also claimed that several men were sick with bronchitis, but again the captain was able to defend himself. "I was not aware of this until the receipt of your letter, of course the Hospital Returns will show the number actually sick, but the only number in my Return as having gone sick during *this month* is *four*, exclusive of two men in Hospital with other diseases, and on *this day*, I have not one man in Hospital, and only one man, to whom the Doctor has given two days convalescence for some slight ailment."[41] He had, in fact, applied for flannels the previous October, but was told to ask for compensatory funding instead, so the men could buy their own. The captain found this unsatisfactory in that "Heretofore the men were furnished with a complete suit of Winter Clothing, and which has in every instance been sanctioned by the Secretary of War."

All-in-all, the issue of warm clothing may seem like a tempest in a teapot today, but no less a personage than the Lieutenant-General Commanding became involved in the controversy. Authorizing the necessary expenditure, he also felt the need to intercede on behalf of the commander of the 100th Regiment's Depot, stating that he was "perfectly satisfied" with his replies in the matter. Communicating to the Inspector General by way of the Acting Military Secretary, he also wished "you to convey to Staff Assistant Surgeon Woods, his entire disapprobation of the course he has seen fit to pursue on this occasion, and further to inform him, that, for the future he must be more careful in bringing such a charge against an officer without foundation, as on repetition of the same, the Lt General will take more serious notice of it."[42] Doctors were supposed to report to unit commanding officers, and it was very bad form to go over their heads.

Which is not to say that they lacked authority or, at least, the courage of their convictions. Some months after the little dust-up described above, the same Doctor Woods presented a scathing report to a Captain

---

40. NA, RG 8, IB, v.1562, Clarke, Capt 100 Regt to Military Secretary Montreal, 19 January 1861.
41. NA, RG 8, IB, v.1562, Clarke, Capt 100 Regt to Military Secretary Montreal, 19 January 1861.
42. NA, RG 8, IB, v.1562, A/Military Secretary to Dy Inspector General, 22 January 1861.

Wilson on the condition of his barracks at Chambly. Among many defects, he found six inches of water in the cellar under the right half of the building, while the back yard was also very wet, all the result of poor drainage. The result was that "The rooms over the wet cellars were, I am given to understand, so unhealthy at one period as not to be habitable, a condition attributable, I have little doubt, to the state of the cellars underneath."[43] Furthermore, ventilating panes in the windows were needed in all rooms, and the latter had not been whitewashed prior to the company's arrival. Worse, "There is no good Water-Supply for the men's barracks, the pump being out of repair. The river received the sewage of the village above. The pump might be easily, and should be at once put in a state of repair. The ground is saturated with springs all around."

The reference to sewage-contaminated water is of particular interest here, as the link between polluted wells and such diseases as cholera had only been established seven years before, in 1854. John Snow, a London doctor, had been arguing since 1849 that cholera was water-borne, but it was not until a particularly violent outbreak five years later that he was able to prove the point, with two different studies. The first mapped out cases in his own neighbourhood, Soho, and linked victims directly to a particular pump; when the handle was removed from the latter, the number of sick diminished dramatically. The second was much larger, comparing those who received their water from downstream as opposed to those who purchased it from up the Thames, different water companies often serving the same city blocks; those drawing from sewer-contaminated water further down were far more likely to fall ill with cholera.[44] Whether Snow's work served to convince practitioners in Canada is doubtful, however, Charles M. Godfrey pointing out in *The Cholera Epidemics in Upper Canada, 1832-1866* that there was a "multiplicity of theories of the the cause of cholera" at this time, and that the proposition that a bacillus was the causative agent had to await the 1880s and the work of Theodor Koch.[45]

Still, there was a certain logic linking dirty water with poor health, though it is unknown whether the necessary work at the Chambly hospital was carried out, for though the army went to some lengths to prevent disease among its troops, it was also very cost-conscious. For example, in the 1866 "Instructions to Commanding Medical and other Officers on the Subject of Cholera," the Director General in England made it clear "that every possible economy should be exercised in the

43. NA, RG 8, IB, v.1562, D Woods MD to Capt Wilson at Chambly, 22 October, 1861.
44. W.F. Bynum, *Science and Practice of Medicine in the Nineteenth Century* (Cambridge, 1994), 79.
45. Charles M Godfrey, *The Cholera Epidemics in Upper Canada, 1832-1866* (Toronto, 1968), 8.

use of disinfectants."[46] When a principal medical officer suggested such prophylactic chemicals be provided to every station in the country, the Director General's reply was adamant. "I would beg to call your attention to the War Department Instructions issued in 1866, which direct the use of unusual disinfectants, only "when the disease has appeared in the vicinity of a military station, or among the military of the station," and to the circumstance that the purchase of quantities of disinfectants to meet a possible contingency which might never arise, if generally practised, would entail a heavy expense which could not be allowed."[47] He concluded with the statement that "I am directed by the authorities at the War Office to point out to you that, in making suggestions, regard should be paid to economy, and that unnecessary extravagance would not fail to be noticed by them."

Cholera epidemics having broken out in Canada six times since 1832, the most recent in 1854, such a policy of economy might seem to entail some risk, but, to be fair, there had not been a serious outbreak in thirteen years. In dealing with another disease, the army was willing to be more aggressive, a memorandum of 1866 warning that "The attention of Medical Officers is called to the first paragraph of the Circular from the Army Medical Department, dated 21st September, 1858, directing that "every Recruit, without exception (whether he bears the marks of natural small pox, of successful vaccination, or otherwise), may be vaccinated on joining the Head Quarters or Depot of the Corps to which he belongs, unless the operation is certified to have been already successfully performed subsequently to his enlistment in the service."[48] Edward Jenner having proven the safety and effectiveness of vaccination with cowpox, at the end of the eighteenth century, as opposed to the risk and complication of inoculation with smallpox, the procedure had become an integral part of the army's medical prevention apparatus by the 1860s or before.

Preventive medicine thus had an important role to play in Canada even though there was no major conflict in the colony between the War of 1812 and the Riel Rebellion of 1885. Medical personnel thus never had to handle the kind of mass casualties that had caused such horrendous conditions to arise in the Crimea, though they did on occasion deal with the odd emergency. One such came to the attention of Assistant Surgeon Alex Kirkmund in September, 1862, when a soldier "on the evening of the 11th was brought into Hospital, in a state of insensibility—his comrades who brought him in informing me that it had come

46. NA, RG 8, IB, v.1560, Director General to PMO Canada, 14 August 1866.
47. NA, RG 8, IB, v.1561, Director General to PMO, 25 July 1867.
48. NA, RG 8, IB, v.1561, Circular Memorandum of Army Medical Department, 21 April, 1868.

on about 3 hours before, without any apparent cause whilst he was on guard."[49] The Assistant Surgeon examined the patient, finding his breathing abnormal, akin to snoring, his pulse intermittent, sometimes strong, sometimes weak, the skin of his arms and legs cold though his body was warm, the eyes fixed and pupils dilated, and lower extremities rigid. There was no smell of alcohol on his breath. Treatment included drawing blood from the upper arm, applying a stomach pump (only to find that that organ was empty) as well as a castor oil and turpentine enema, though the latter was difficult to administer, the physician reporting "that the spasm of the lower extremities was so great that the injection tube was with difficulty introduced into the rectum." Cold water was sprinkled on the soldier's face.

An hour passed, but symptoms persisted, so his temples were cupped, which is to say that hot cups were applied so as to draw blood to that region of his head; further bleeding was performed, but there was still no improvement. Half an hour later he vomited some form of mucous liquid, but aspirated some of it and began to suffocate, and "although tickling the larynx, turning the patient on his face, and pressure on the diaphragm upwards were tried, the face became *gradually* more livid the attempts at breathing occurring at longer intervals."[50] Refusing to relinquish his patient, the assistant surgeon continued to apply heroic methods. "Hoping to ward off the death now threatened, a stomach pump tube was introduced, and artificial respiration kept up for some time with considerable success," but the soldier continued to fade. Performing a laryngotracheotomy, the physician cut a hole in the man's throat through which he could breathe, which seemed to bring an improvement—but it was to no avail, and the soldier died ten minutes later. The incident is noteworthy in what it demonstrates about medicine generally—as well as in the military—in the mid-nineteenth century. Dealing with wounds or trauma was a sophisticated business, involving such apparatus as stomach pumps and such techniques as tracheotomy, though recourse to bleeding might not be considered appropriate today.

As for the practitioner, on paper at least a regimental medical officer like Alex Kirkmund had to meet very exacting standards, and his work was evaluated every year. Among the qualities he had to show were intelligence, self-reliance, and efficiency while performing his duties with "zeal and judgement." He had to attend to the sanitary requirements of his charges, be assiduous in the discharge of his duties, humane and attentive to the sick, be acquainted with the diseases of women and

49. NA, RG 8, IB, v.1562, Alex Kirkmund, Ast Surgeon, Ret, to PMO Montreal, 15 September 1861.
50. NA, RG 8, IB, v.1562, Alex Kirkmund, Ast Surgeon, Ret, to PMO Montreal, 15 September 1861.

children (some soldiers had their families with them), as well as compose and write with facility and clearness. Knowledge of languages other than English, including Hindustani (this was still the British Army, after all) was considered an asset. A catchall question, "Is there any-thing in his conduct, or in the manner in which his duties have been performed, which calls for special remark?" took care of any issues of "character".[51]

Given the nature of a military hierarchy, the annual evaluation had to answer such questions as, "Has he afforded to his Commanding Officer and to his Departmental Superior that support which they are entitled to receive from him?" Another question, number six on the list, asked: "Does he, from age, infirmity, or any other cause, appear to be unfit for his present duties, or for those which would devolve on him on promotion to a higher grade?"[52] It referred to far more than the physical fitness required to carry out military tasks, as one medical officer discovered. In early 1867 the Inspector General related to the Principal Medical Officer for Canada that "A confidential Report having been received in this Department upon the character and capabilities of Assistant Surgeon J.W.A. Tothill, 17th Foot signed by Surgeon Major E.B. Tuson of that Regiment in which it is stated in reply to question 6 that this officer is not rigidly temperate in his habits, I have the honor to direct your attention to the unsatisfactory answer afforded to this question and to request that you will point out to W. Tothill the desirability of self-improvement in this particular."[53]

Tothill exemplified an ever growing centralization within the medical establishments of British, American, and European armies. Whereas in the War of 1812 each regiment was responsible for recruiting its own surgeon, in the American Civil War it soon became clear that while some regimental medical officers were overwhelmed when their units saw hard fighting, their neighbours might not have had any work to perform as the troops they supported remained uncommitted to battle. Thus Jonathan Leterman, the medical director of the Army of the Potomac, which fought mainly against Robert E. Lee in Virginia, replaced the regimental service with one centralized at a higher level. As a result, each division of ten thousand men or so had a large field hospital to support it, as opposed to small regimental establishments dotted about the countryside.[54] The new organization reversed developments of the late eighteenth century, when surgery was performed as close to the

51. NA, RG 8, IB, v.1561, Annual Reports.
52. NA, RG 8, IB, v.1561, Annual Reports.
53. NA, RG 8, IB, v.1560, Inspector General to PMO Canada, 26 February 1867.
54. John S. Haller, *Farmcarts to Fords* (Carbondale, 1992), 35.

battlefield as possible before patients were evacuated; at the battle of Fredericksburg of 13 December 1862, for example, surgeons were kept well back, General Ambrose E. Burnside providing a thousand wagons to clear the wounded from the battlefield. The fighting lasted all day, and the new ambulance corps went to work at nightfall, removing more than nine thousand patients within twelve hours in spite of severe obstacles. Confederate sniper fire made the task of the stretcher-bearers all the more hazardous, while bitter cold threatened frost-bite or worse for the wounded lying on the ground. Forcing the pace was the fact that the Union army was retreating, and though it had suffered defeat at the hands of Robert E. Lee its medical service was able to evacuate its charges across an intervening river by the 15th, and to Washington in time for Christmas. Ulysses S. Grant adopted the system for his Army of the Tennessee in early 1863, and it became a model for British and European forces as well.[55]

The new approach to tending to the victims of war was evident in Canada at the time of the Fenian raids of 1866-1870. These nationalists had as their goal the liberation of Ireland from English rule, their strategy to use Irish veterans of the American Civil War to establish a foothold in British North America, which could then be used to bargain from a position of strength. Military establishments in the colony were increased, and so were medical staff, but it is how the latter operated that is of interest here. The largest confrontation between Fenians and British was at Ridgeway, in southern Ontario, in June 1866. Militia units were heavily involved, including Hamilton's 13th Battalion and the Queen's Own Rifles of Toronto, and though each had its own regimental surgeon, that for the latter unit found himself in charge of all wounded brought to Toronto for a six-month period following the battle, regardless of what regiment they belonged to.[56]

In 1867, while the Fenians were still a threat—or at least a nuisance— some of the British colonies came together under Confederation, and the new federal government set out to acquire the western and northern lands of the Hudson's Bay Company. Some residents, however, led by Louis Riel, balked at the thought of becoming a colony of Ottawa, leading to the outbreak of the Red River Rebellion and a British expedition (Canada still relied on the metropole in such matters) to put it down. Led by a British regular army officer, the force incorporated nonetheless two battalions of volunteers from local militias, including their medical officers. In the end, there were no battles, Riel choosing to go into exile, but the march from central Canada to the plains still

55. John S. Haller, *Farmcarts to Fords* (Carbondale, 1992), 35-37.
56. G.W.L. Nicholson, *Seventy Years of Service* (Ottawa, 1977), 24.

provided medical challenges, some of which would become more familiar in future wars.

First was the recruitment of militia volunteers, not a difficult task when it came to numbers but one which demonstrated the role of military physicians in preventing disease or injury from interfering with a campaign. According to orders, for each of the two units being sent, "A medical inspection of every non commissioned officer and man of the battalion will be made, if possible before the men leave their corps or company head-quarters,"[57] or at brigade rendez-vous if necessary. If fit, the medical officer would report as such through a certificate that stated:

> Also, only men with military experience I have examined the above named man, and find he has no Rupture nor Mark of any old Wound or Ulcer adhering to the Bone; he is free from Varicose Veins of the Legs, and has the full power of Motion of the Joints and Limbs. He is well formed, and has no Scrofulous Affection of the Glands, Scald Head, or other inveterate Cutaneous Eruptions; and he is free from any trace of Corporal Punishment, and not marked as a Deserter with the letter D or the letters BC. His respiration is easy, and his Lungs appear to be sound. He has the perfect use of his Eyes and Ears. His general appearance is healthy, and he possesses strength sufficient to enable him to undergo the fatigue to which Soldiers are liable. He does not bear any marks of medical treatment. I consider him fit for Her Majesty's Service.[58]

Also, only men with military experience were were to be taken, none shorter than 5 feet 4 inches—except where exempted by the medical officer—and all with evidence of having either been vaccinated for or already suffered from smallpox.[59]

The march, to be undertaken on foot, by train, and by boat, would be made by detachments, each of a company or more; it was expected to be brutal, which accounts for the medical examinations above, so procedures had to be established to deal with those who fell out along the way. Most of the trip would be over water, with many a portage to test soldiers' strength, endurance, and patience, and the medical officers were made responsible for determining whether an illness or injury was such as to prevent a man from continuing. If pronounced unfit to work for some time to come, he was to be left behind at the nearest portage, where a non-commissioned officer and private would look after him, with a week's provisions to see them through. As further detachments passed by, they would ensure necessary supplies were maintained, until such time as the casualty could be removed to a hospital at Fort William.

---

57. NA, MG 29, E37, Neilson Papers, f.2, Order of Surgeon Neilson.
58. NA, MG 29, E37, Neilson Papers, f.2, Attestation Paper.
59. NA, MG 29, E37, Neilson Papers, f.2, Senior Medical Officer, Quebec, 27 April 1872.

The commander of the last group to make the voyage, the 12th detachment, would decide as he went along which injured soldiers would accompany him forward, and which would be sent back.[60] Ensuring consistency of treatment as sick and injured men were moved across hundreds of miles of wilderness from one medical practitioner to another was a matter of proper documentation. Each patient was issued a medical certificate, on the reverse of which were detailed instructions in its use and how it was to be filled out. Basic information included the man's regimental number, name, age, and service; medical data consisted of the date he contracted illness or suffered injury, when he was admitted to hospital, and the progress of the condition or cure. If it was deemed necessary to discharge the soldier because he was no longer capable of carrying out his duties, the form was returned to his regiment so it would know of the particulars.[61] Such certification could also, no doubt, be used should the discharged soldier seek a disability pension.

While on expedition, medical officers had far more to do than look after the sick and injured; each was also to keep a daily diary, noting climate and temperature, geography, distances travelled each day, the difficulties of the march, and the impact all this had on men's health. The paperwork expected at headquarters was intimidating (to the author, anyway), including morning hospital states, weekly sick returns, sanitary reports, a return of extras issued (such as brandy), a classified return of wounds and injuries received in action, another classified return of wounds and injuries (all kinds), an admission and discharge book, a medical case book, and—for reference, of course—a copy of medical regulations.[62] In the end, doctors may well have been thankful to have been engaged on a bloodless campaign, not only for the sake of the soldiery but because of the much reduced administrative burden that resulted.

As in previous expeditions, sanitation was a high priority, though basic theories had changed since the War of 1812; many diseases were no longer blamed on "miasmas" from swamps or latrines, but on contaminated water. The result was a more complicated task for the regimental doctor, but one that had to become second nature if an epidemiological disaster was to be avoided.

> Medical officers are requested to take any steps that may seem to them necessary in advising as to sanitary measures, the choice of camping grounds, precautions as to unnecessary exposure, the great desirability that each man be supplied with a cup of hot tea before commencing the daily march, the use of charcoal (which is easily preservable) or of alum

60. NA, MG 29, E37, Neilson Papers, f.2, Standing Orders for the Red River Expeditionary Force, 14 May 1870.
61. NA, MG 29, E37, Neilson Papers, f.2, Medical Certificate, Case No 73.
62. NA, MG 29, E37, Neilson Papers, f.2, Surgeon Major, 60th Rifles, memo, 17 May 1870.

for purification of drinking water when turbid. Latrines should always be placed as far as possible from the camp, and no nuisances suffered to remain in it or its neighbourhood. The men should be enjoined to change their wet clothes for dry on arriving at their encampments, and especially not to sleep in wet shoes and stockings. Sleeping on the bare ground should be avoided, the collection of spruce-sprigs or dry brushwood for lying on is recommended. To vary the monotony of diet, fishing materials have been provided. Several tins of cream of tartar are provided for issue at Fort William, as a protective against scurvy.[63]

Later, having spent some months in the west, the doctor for the 2nd Battalion of Rifles received instructions from the Lieutenant Governor to attend a meeting "on the propriety of adopting steps for preventing the introduction of the Small Pox into the Province and to make the necessary preparations against the spread of the disease in case of its introduction,"[64] military doctors still being considered part of the community in which their units lived.

There being no war to fight in Manitoba, military medicine settled into the routine of camp life, the hospital register for the 2nd Battalion Quebec Rifles, from 1 May to 31 December 1870, listing 251 admissions. There were few fatalities, one of them, Private Michael Donnelly, "found dead cause excessive drink (alcohol),"[65] though his death report stated that he had died while under charge of the guard, diagnosed as having succumbed to "Congestion of brain and lungs."[66] He had probably been sent to the guardhouse for drunkenness. Another victim of alcohol abuse was a Private Thériault, who, having had one (or several) too many, got lost on a February night and was found with both feet frozen.[67] His legs were amputated.[68]

The unfortunate Thériault, and his comrades-in-arms, returned home in the months that followed, neither Riel nor the Fenians proving sufficient threat to keep the militiamen away from their families. They thus returned to their farms, jobs, and businesses, their service limited to the odd evening a month or a summer camp once a year, and it was at these annual gatherings that militia regimental doctors performed their work. By then the research of Louis Pasteur and others had found more specific causes of disease than bad air or contaminated water, blaming them instead on microscopic life forms, which by 1873 were known

63. NA, MG 29, E37, Neilson Papers, f.2, Surgeon Major, 60th Rifles, memo, 17 May 1870.
64. NA, MG 29, E37, Neilson Papers, f.2, Provincial Secretary to Doctor of 2nd Batt. of Rifles, 3 October 1870.
65. NA, MG 29, E37, Neilson Papers, f.2, Hospital of 2nd Battn Quebec Rifles in the Field from 1st May 1870 to 31st December 1870.
66. NA, MG 29, E37, Neilson Papers, f.2, Death Report, 14 September 1870.
67. NA, MG 29, E37, Neilson Papers, f.1, Diary, 16 February 1871.
68. MG 29, E37, Neilson Papers, f.2, Note to Brigade Major, 27 May 1871.

to account for tonsilitis, influenza, dysentery, diarrhoea, cholera, syphilis, gonorrhea, scurvy, scabies, and others.[69] The advantages such knowledge conferred were confined to prevention; for example, water supplies could be tested for contamination by micro-organisms, while men suffering from diseases whose germs were communicated through coughing or sneezing could be quarantined. Treatment was a different matter, sulpha drugs and antibiotics being far in the future, and some viruses proving impossible to defeat even today.

Germ theory was not, however, general knowledge, as evidenced by medical reports from various summer camps in the early 1870s. Various forms of diarrhoea were endemic, as they had been for millennia whenever soldiers congregated, but not all doctors attributed the ailments to bacteria. Of 55 sick and injured in the Prince of Wales Regiment, 24 were such illnesses, as were 43 of 52 in the 51st Battalion, and 10 of 35 in the Hochelaga Light Infantry, all in 1871.[70] "The prevailing diseases in this Regiment," reported the surgeon to the 29th Battalion, "have been diarrhoea & Intermittent Fever," though neither was blamed on germs. Rather, the illnesses were deemed "the result of want of proper foresight at Headquarters whereby this regiment was compelled to sleep the first night upon the damp ground without either blankets or straw."[71] The doctor for the Three Rivers Provisional Battalion also blamed diarrhoea on "the dampness of the ground,"[72] as did the 19th Battalion."[73] An unnamed cavalry regiment may have been closer to the mark when its medical officer suggested the ailment was due to a change in diet (bacteria often multiplying in uncooked or undercooked food),[74] while the 67th Battalion's surgeon was less accurate but more specific. Though generally satisfied with the health of the troops, attributed to "the healthy location of the camp, the good sanitary arrangements and in no small degree to the good quality of rations so liberally supplied to the force," diarrhoea was still prevalent. This the doctor blamed on the issue of fresh meat to "those men from the rural districts who had previously been accustomed principally to the use of salted food. These

---

69. NA, RG 9, IIB2, v.48(2), Return of Sick of the Volunteer Militia Battalion under Canvas for the Annual Drill of 1872-73, 28 July 1873.
70. NA, RG 9, IIB2, v.48(1), Sick Report of the 1st or Prince of Wales Regt during Stay in Camp; Sick Report 51st Batt Hemmingford, Laprairie Camp from 27th June to 12th July 1871; Sick Report of 6th Bat Hochelaga Light Infantry which in Camp at Laprairie June & July 1871.
71. NA, RG 9, IIB2, v.48(2), Weekly Return of Sick of the 29th Battn from 20th June 1872 to 25th June 1872.
72. NA, RG 9, IIB2, v.48(3), Weekly Return of Sick of the Three Rivers Prov. Batt. from 24th June 1872 to 11th July 1872.
73. NA, RG 9, IIB2, v.48(2), Weekly Return of Sick of the Nineteenth Battalion from June 12 1872 to June 27 1872.
74. NA, RG 9, IIB2, v.48(2), Weekly Return of Sick of the Regiment of Cavalry from 22nd June 1872 to 30th June 1872.

cases however proved amenable to ordinary treatment. An allowance of salted meat occasionally would assist in counteracting this tendency to diarrhoea—which the heat and fatigue tends to aggravate."[75]

A certain Surgeon Brown of E Battery, at the end of a divisional camp near Windsor, Ontario, from 19 June to 1 July, 1872, seemed to combine several theories in his report. Noting that 4134 men who attended accounted for 954 sick or injured, of whom 511 suffered from diarrhoea and 246 from other abdominal ailments, he observed that "I have invariably found in all the Camps (Volunteer) in which I have served," such complaints "to have been by far the most common, and to have formed the largest proportion of cases presenting themselves for treatment."

> This is attributable however, in no way whatever to locality, but to the fact, that abdominal derangements consisting either of Diarrhea or its opposite constipation, are invariably produced by the disturbing influence consequent on the excitement incidental always to a change from a home to a Camp life—More especially with Country Battalions, change of water and a fresh instead of a salt meat diet (generally the summer country diet) seeming to affect them, more in this manner, than those Battalions which have been recruited in the Cities—A preponderance of the cases as will be seen by referring to the abstract, occurred during the 1st week, accounted for by the fact of the men settling down and becoming accustomed after this to their new mode of life—most of the cases required but little corrective treatment and went on with their duties.[76]

Experimental doctors such as Pasteur would have insisted it was bacteria in the food and water, without any reference to excitability, that caused these illnesses, but such conclusions had obviously not had time to percolate down to practitioners in the field.

As we shall see, such did not have to be the case, and as some Canadian doctors moved to the forefront in their various fields in the latter part of the 19th century, military practice kept apace. Until then, however, it took some years for the armed services to shift from trying to maintain a balance between humours or between lethargy and excitability, to concentrating on specific agents such as bacteria or viruses. As for the treatment of wounds, there had been little work in that area in Canada after the War of 1812, but the Riel Rebellion of 1885 would demonstrate that the military, in this country at least, tried to keep up with developments such as aseptic surgery. The doctor's main battle continued to be against disease, however, and preventive medicine continued to be a medical practitioner's first priority.

75. NA, RG 9, IIB2, v.48(3), Surgeon 67th Batt to Lt-Col Upton, July 1872.
76. NA, RG 9, IIB2, v.48(2), Surgeon Brown of E Battery to Lt-Col Taylor, Nov 14, 1972.

Chapter Two

Forming the Canadian Army Medical Corps

Canadian Confederation came about in part from a British desire to divest itself of military responsibility for its colonies north of the 49th parallel, though garrisons remained in Halifax and Esquimalt. The new Dominion thus set about the task of forming some kind of armed institution, with George-Etienne Cartier, a father of Confederation, as the country's first minister of militia. There would be no conscription and at first no permanent force, the nation relying instead on reservists who would take the field against the enemy (i.e. the United States) in the hopes of holding the line until help could arrive from Britain—military ties with the centre of empire had not been completely cut. As we have seen, it was the militia that met the Fenians at Ridgeway and made up a large part of the expedition to the Red River, and its first independent effort would be against another Riel enterprise—the Rebellion of 1885. The uprising was the result of a clash between the Métis of the plains, who made their living through hunting and trading, and the central government in Ottawa, seeking to industrialize the new nation; that meant railways, which were paid for in land, which was purchased or otherwise acquired from the Métis. The latter rebelled against a distant and seemingly insensitive regime, and the government of John A. MacDonald organized a militia expedition to re-establish its authority in the west.

In its war against the Métis, Canada was on its own, and since the militia had never been a high priority for government expenditure, when it came time to put together a military force to fight Riel much had to be built up from scratch. The medical service was no exception, and when Doctor Darby Bergin assumed control on 1 April, he found little foundation on which to build an administrative and operational edifice.

Regiments continued to recruit their own civilian surgeons, but there was no departmental medical staff, field hospital, or ambulance service, nor any organized corps of nurses, in spite of the lessons of Crimea and the American Civil War. The situation smacked of the War of 1812, where no one had direct responsibility for evacuating wounded from the battlefield, or getting them to hospital after the regimental surgeon had amputated limbs and otherwise treated their wounds. The whole was thus "inadequate to the requirements of an army in the field when, as almost always happens, the proportion of sick is largely in excess of the capacity of the hospitals."[1]

Bergin recommended that the necessary staff, including purveyors, be recruited or appointed without delay. The latter, though having come under severe criticism in the Crimea and the American Civil War, played an important administrative role in the medical service.

> The Purveyor is to have the sole charge of the Hospital marquee or buildings and their surroundings established there—will be responsible for their condition—will inspect them frequently and secure any defects which he may discover. He will have full charge of all stores for the use of the Field Hospitals and ambulances, of all the Drugs, and Medicines, Medical and Surgical appliances, and, upon requisition duly made, countersigned by the Deputy Surgeon General, will issue such as may be required to fill deficiencies in the Field Hospitals, Ambulances, or Regimental Hospitals.[2]

Past abuses could be avoided by making this a military position, instead of relying on for-profit contractors as had been the case in previous wars.

The purveyor could also play a role in mitigating the ravages of alcohol, which had proven a serious problem on prior campaigns. As Bergin explained,

> I may mention that under no circumstances will permission be given for wine or spirits to be forwarded to troops in the field. All such can only be allowed for hospital use, and, if forwarded to the Purveyor, will be placed in the store of the hospital, and employed for no other purpose than for the sick, and then only upon requisition made by the Surgeon in charge of the hospital, who will be responsible therefor; and in a case where the Purveyor is of opinion that the quantity asked for is in excess of the requirements, he will refuse to issue more than in his opinion is really necessary, reporting his refusal, and reasons therefor, to the Deputy Surgeon General, for the information of the Major General commanding.[3]

---

1. NA, RG 9, III, IIA3, v.13, Bergin to Minister, 11 April 1885.
2. NA, RG 9, IIA3, v.13, Bergin to Minister, 11 April 1885.
3. NA, RG 9, IIA3, v.13, Bergin to Minister, 11 April 1885.

The temperance movement, which was working especially hard in the 1880s, might have approved.

In the hospitals themselves Bergin recommended regulations be framed for the employment of nurses, either voluntary or paid, as well as some fixed method for recognizing such organizations as the St Johns Hospital Aid Society, the Red Cross, and similar charitable associations. Nurses, who would each have no more than 20 patients, would be the responsibility of a Superintendent-General, "specially selected for her qualifications for the office, thoroughly trained to the duties, and of large experience."[4] She would see to discipline and ensure the surgeon's orders were carried out, and be sufficiently knowledgeable of military staff work to be able to communicate directly with the Deputy Surgeon-General accompanying troops in the field. If necessary, she could get in touch with the Director-General in Ottawa.

Bergin himself would not go on campaign, but rely on subordinates such as Doctor Thomas Roddick, the expedition's Principal Medical Officer. The latter's instructions were detailed, including, of course, preventive measures to maintain the troops in good health. "As Principal Medical Officer, upon your arrival at the head quarters of the general commanding, you will, with the sanction of the General, at once, or at such time as may appear to ... be necessary, issue such instructions regarding sanitary precautions to be observed for protecting the health of the troops as he may consider requisite for the guidance of the medical officers."[5] He was to appoint a brigade-surgeon, with the approval of the general, and inspect the camp daily, reporting on the appearance of any communicable disease among the troops. Upon making such a discovery he was to look immediately into its cause, "whether such disease proceed from, or is aggravated by, sanitary defects in the camp, bad or deficient water supply, dampness, marshy ground, insufficient clothing, or from any local cause, or from bad food, intemperance, unwholesome liquors, fruit, or want of shelter, too much exposure, fatigue, or any other cause and report immediately to the Major General commanding."[6]

An important impetus for establishing a sophisticated and competent medical organization was that the troops to be cared for were not regulars from some distant land, but militia soldiers from Canadian families. Bergin referred to them as the "flower of the youth of our country," insisting that "there can be no care too great taken of them by the medical department, nor should any expense be spared in securing for them relief, comfort and safety."[7] For that purpose two field

4. NA, RG 9, IIA3, v.13, Bergin to Minister, 11 April 1885.
5. NA, RG 9, IIA3, v.13, Bergin to Roddick, 6 April 1885.
6. *Ibid.*

hospitals were established, "under the superintendence of first class surgeons," and equipped "with every medical and surgical appliance, and with every known medicine of value likely to be required at any time, with every medical comfort." As for staff, Bergin was receiving applications from "Ladies of the highest standing throughout the country," many of whom had trained under Florence Nightingale, almost the patron saint of military nursing. Others had been educated at hospitals in London and New York. Dressers, who would assist nurses and doctors, were also of the highest calibre, at least in Bergin's estimation, coming from medical schools in Montreal, Kingston, and Toronto. All-in-all it seemed to be an impressive organization.

But would it function at peak efficiency? While Bergin was pulling together the people he thought he needed to see to the medical needs of the troops, the latter were already on their way to the plains after a hurried levy. As a result they were not necessarily fully equipped—or fully clothed, a situation aggravated by "the severity of the weather, the difficulties of transport, exposure of the Troops to the frost and snow in open cars, the long distances to be traversed through the gaps between the finished and unfinished portions of the railway, the difficulties of communication, the distance between this city [Montreal], the base of supply, and the field of operations, the Major-General Commanding having already left Winnipeg for the front with a portion of the Troops,— all conspired to render the task one of unusual difficulty."[8]

Five or six regiments, Bergin was unsure even of the number, as well as two artillery batteries, were thus on the march with "very meagre or ill-regulated medical supplies and very few medical comforts."[9] Equipment for the field hospitals, modern as it might have been, had to come from New York, and it must have been substantial, each establishment comprising 50 beds, the organization as a whole preparing to support an army of 6000 for six months. Field Hospital Number 1 was headed by Campbell Melles Douglas, whose military credentials were certainly in order, the doctor wearing the Victoria Cross on his chest. Field Hospital Number 2 was under Henry Casgrain, and each relied on the skills of five surgeons. The militia, as has been mentioned, had no ambulance corps, but some medical schools had been giving their students lessons in first aid and stretcher drill, and many came forward to volunteer, final selection being made by Doctors Douglas and Casgrain. Their training had, indeed, been near-perfect for the tasks the army expected them to perform, consisting in "lifting up into

7. NA, RG 9, IIA3, v.13, Bergin to Minister, 7 April 1885.
8. *Medical and Surgical History of the Canadian North-West Rebellion of 1885* (Montreal, 1886), 1.
9. *Medical and Surgical History of the Canadian North-West Rebellion of 1885* (Montreal, 1886), 1.

and lifting from the ambulance in such a manner as not to injure or cause discomfort to the wounded, and of placing them on and removing them from the stretchers; the proper method of stretcher-bearing, and of removing them from the stretchers to the beds in the hospitals; they were also instructed in the proper methods of arresting haemorrhage, of bandaging, of setting fractures and of giving temporary relief and assistance until the aid of the Surgeons in the rear or in the hospitals could be obtained."[10]

With help from the Canadian Pacific Railway, the medical organization made its way west to join the troops it was supposed to support. Arriving in Winnipeg, Roddick made a point of checking on the equipment of the various regimental surgeons, confirming Bergin's evaluation. Reporting that "they were all very scantily provided with the medicines, instruments and dressings necessary for the campaign," he concluded that "in the event of an epidemic or an engagement, it would be impossible for them to render the men that service which would be required."[11] Thankfully, the Red Cross corps arrived on 21 April, with Field Hospital Number 2 only three days behind—just in time. The very day Casgrain, his staff, and his supplies pulled into Winnipeg, battle was being joined at Fish Creek, so Roddick loaded up a wagon with the necessary medicines and equipment and made his way to the front.

Fish Creek was soon followed, on 3 May, by an engagement at Cut Knife Hill, which resulted in 35 wounded, Roddick requisitioning three houses in Saskatoon to form a hospital. "It is well situated from a sanitary standpoint, the banks of the river there being high, and the soil naturally porous and dry. In fact, it would be difficult to find a better "sanitarium," and I am convinced that much of the success which followed the treatment of the sick and wounded billeted here was due to the remarkably healthy condition of the place."[12] When filled with wounded, each man would have 1000 cubic feet of air space, considered more than adequate at the time, though some soldiers would need every advantage, Roddick listing the most seriously injured as "Capt. Clark, wounded through the back, not penetrating;... Corp. Code, wounded through both legs; Pte Lethbridge, penetrating wound of chest; Pte Hislop, whose arm had been amputated near the shoulder; and Pte Caniff, shot in the elbow-joint."[13] Corporal Code soon worsened, "having an alarming haemorrhage from one of the wounds in the leg," and died.

10. *Medical and Surgical History of the Canadian North-West Rebellion of 1885* (Montreal, 1886), 4-5, 8.
11. *Medical and Surgical History of the Canadian North-West Rebellion*, 24.
12. *Medical and Surgical History of the Canadian North-West Rebellion*, 27, 29.
13. *Medical and Surgical History of the Canadian North-West Rebellion*, 30.

Thanks to the wonders of the modern telegraph, some families were soon apprised if their loved ones were wounded or fell dangerously ill. Before Fish Creek, even, Bergin had to deal with the case of a Mrs Wiggins, who was applying for a pass to nurse her brother-in-law, sick with fever in Winnipeg. Though insisting that such action "would be to establish a very bad precedent," the doctor was willing to look into the matter, and "if it be found that the case is alarming, it might be done as a special case." The fact of the matter was that "we have not yet appointed a corps of nurses,"[14] the expedition, as we have seen, having set out before Bergin could complete his medical preparations. It is unlikely Wiggins was in any danger, as the great majority of patients at the Winnipeg field hospital in that first month had "colds and other affections incurred owing to the exposure and fatigue during that part of the journey where the soldiers were marched over the uncompleted part of the Canadian Pacific Railway north of Lake Superior."[15]

Surgeon-Major James Kerr, in charge of the hospital, along with an assistant-surgeon and three dressers, remained in Winnipeg for four months, during which time they treated 81 patients. Only two of them are known to have died, one of tonsilitis and the other of cirrhosis of the liver. Three surgical operations were carried out, one to provide drainage in a case of emphysema, another to remove a cyst from a man's neck, and the last—the only one combat related—to extract a bullet from a gunner's knee-joint. Kerr was pleased to report that all three "ran an aseptic course, and resulted in complete cures."[16] That there were no serious cases of post- operative infection was no accident; Doctor Joseph Lister had developed antiseptic surgical techniques 15 years before (using carbolic acid to kill germs), and Thomas Roddick, one of the leading medical practitioners on the expedition, was a devout Listerian convert.

In fact, one of the first accounts of antisepsis published in Canada was by a regimental surgeon, D.S.E. Bain, who in 1868 described the use of the antiseptic carbolic acid for "a case of carbuncle, only remarkable for the method of treatment. It occurred in the ordinary situation, viz, the nape of the neck, free incisions were made, and a pledget of lint saturated with carbolic acid was inserted in the wound, over which a solution of the acid in glycerine ... was used as the ordinary dressing. Within 48 hours the slough separated, leaving a clean healthy surface which healed rapidly under the daily application of the acid in

---

14. NA, RG 9, IIA3, v.12, D.B. to Minister, 21 April 1885.
15. *Medical and Surgical History of the Canadian North-West Rebellion*, 20
16. *Medical and Surgical History of the Canadian North-West Rebellion*, 21

glycerine."[17] Results at the Montreal General Hospital, where Roddick worked, were just as compelling, the death rate after surgery dropping to a little over 3 per cent in the two years ending in September, 1879. When using old techniques, four thigh amputations had all been fatal, as had four of six amputations of the leg; in the two years that followed the adoption of Listerism, however, there was not a single death from post-operative infection in the Montreal General.[18] Upon returning from the Riel campaign, Roddick would relate to a friend, Doctor H.H. Chown of Winnipeg, how his staff had secured "wonderful results" in operations after battle. "Looking back now, this was evidently due to the aseptic atmosphere of the tent hospital."[19]

Meanwhile, in the field, engagements, skirmishes, and ambushes succeeded one another until early May, when a climactic battle at Batoche brought the campaign to an end, Surgeon-Major James Bell subsequently reporting how he and his staff carried out their work in support of government forces.

> May 9th, we left camp at about six o'clock, going in with twenty empty waggons for the wounded, with a bale of hay in each, and our complete hospital equipment. Each man of the Ambulance Corps was equipped with a "haversack" in which he carried iodoform, bandages, and some absorbent cotton, and two of them had Esmarch's rubber bands [a kind of torsion bandage]. We reached Batoche after the fighting began, about half-past eight o'clock. We first located our hospital waggons in a ravine, near the church at Batoche, but subsequently took possession of the church, and had the wounded brought in there to be treated. We had the assistance of two or three nuns, with blankets and utensils, while we remained in the church.[20]

Later, they moved out and set up canvas, though they might have been better off staying in the shelter of a more substantial edifice, as "Several bullets went through the tent that evening, and on subsequent occasions; but owing to the dip of the ground, the wounded men were out of range, the bullets passing through the tent three or four feet from the ground."

The Métis were fighting from trenches, but as government troops made preparations to attack casualties were moderate, amounting to two killed and nine wounded that first day, and even fewer in the days that followed. Then, Canadian militia stormed the rebels' defences, an operation that called upon stretcher-bearers to face heavy fire. "Many

---

17. Charles G. Roland, "The Early Years of Antiseptic Surgery in Canada," S.E.D. Shortt, ed, *Medicine in Canadian Society: Historical Perspectives* (Montreal, 1981).
18. H.E. MacDermot, *Sir Thomas Roddick* (Toronto, 1938), 38.
19. *Ibid*, 83.
20. *Medical and Surgical History of the Canadian North-West Rebellion*, 31.

of these young men did noble work, regardless of danger. Where the bullets fell thickest, with a heroism that has never been exceeded, they were to be found, removing the wounded and the dying to places of shelter and of safety in the rear... At Batoche I am told that during the fight a flag was thrust from the window of the church, and was observed by a surgeon and a student who were under shelter from the fire at a couple of hundred yards distance. The student immediately he perceived it proposed that a party should at once to the relief of the one demanding succor. No one appeared willing to second his proposal."[21] Between their positions and the church was fire-swept ground, but, the surgeon asking for volunteers, two men from the Grenadiers of Toronto stepped forward. The party of four started out, "crawling upon their bellies—taking advantage of any little inequality of ground to cover them." Arriving at the church, they found a priest wounded in the thigh, to whom they administered first aid.

The battle ended in a government victory, and the rebellion soon ended—Riel was hanged for treason later in the year—but the work of the military medical practitioner was far from over. Casualties among militia members had not been heavy, amounting to 26 dead and 103 wounded of the over 5000 who participated, but many of the sick and injured required long-term care, one example being a Private Wilson of the 10th Royal Grenadiers. In reply to a letter to Prime Minister John A. Macdonald from a Mrs Wilson (whether wife, mother, or other relative is unknown), Roddick reported that "he received a gun shot injury of the chest, engaging the lung. This was followed by acute pleurisy and emphysema, for which latter the usual operation was performed. For several weeks his recovery was very doubtful, but, for some days previous to embarkation at Saskatoon he had sufficiently recovered to justify me in thinking that his case would terminate favorably."[22] He promised further reports as the patient continued to improve.

Another worrisome patient was a certain Mister Malliwell (rank unknown) of the Midland Battalion. Writing to Bergin from his home in Port Hope, Ontario, he reported how since his return from the war two small bone splinters had had to be removed after working their way to the surface of his wound. Since the latter refused to heal and continued to discharge instead, he made his way to see Roddick. "He probed the wound and said their (sic) was a piece of dead bone but that it would require more opening of the wound than he wished to take it out at present. He said it would work nearer the surface in a short time. He gave me full instructions for dressing the wound & exercising the

---

21. *Medical and Surgical History of the Canadian North-West Rebellion*, 5-6.
22. NA, RG 9, IIA3, v.12, Roddick to Bergin, MP, Surgeon-Gen Ottawa, 11 July 1885.

shoulder for the present and as he expected to leave almost immediately for Winnipeg he advised me to report to you and to say that it would be two or three weeks at least before the wound healed."[23]

Military doctors were not just responsible for ministering to members of the militia; they were also under orders to treat wounded and sick rebels as well, especially after the last battle had been fought. One unnamed field surgeon, hearing that many Métis were "lying ill and unattended about the districts of Fish Creek and Batoche," set out to find them. Near the first battlefield, he and two colleagues treated a patient with a lung infection, then moved on to where the climactic engagement had taken place, "where we were warmly welcomed."

> The following morning we visited the priest, and learned from him that the wounded in his parish, numbering in all about ten, were mostly convalescent. He asked me however to see a Half-breed named Gardapuy, who had been wounded through the lung. After some trouble I found him, because he feared arrest, and on examination discovered that he had a chest filled with fluid. I did not feel justified in operating under the circumstances, but gave him a letter to the police surgeon at Prince Albert, assuring him that every attention would be paid him.[24]

One member of the small expedition, a Doctor Boyle, was obviously a man of independent means, as he not only provided Gardapuy with the funds needed for his trip, but distributed "a considerable sum of money" for the sick and destitute of the parish. More in tune with their mission, the medical practitioners also left a stock of dressings, bandages, and other supplies.

As for the militiamen who had been wounded at Batoche, within weeks of the battle military authorities began to move them out of the Saskatoon field hospital. One of the first groups, of 28 sick and wounded, left for Moosejaw on 21 May.

> The voyage up the river on board of this steamer was most satisfactory. The wounded, nearly all of whom were comparatively light cases and convalescent, were well accommodated in cabins, state-rooms or on mattrasses [sic] on the cabin floor for the night, and there were facilities for dressing those cases that required it in the wash-room. On the 23rd we arrived at the "Elbow" of the South Saskatchewan river, and continued our journey to Moosejaw overland, next morning, nine teams having been procured for our conveyance. The journey over the trail was more trying to some of the severer cases of wounds, especially to one of compound fracture of the forearm and to a case of amputation of the

23. NA, RG 9, IIA3, v.12, Halliwell CO A Coy Midland Bn to Bergin Surg-Gen, 21 May 1885.
24. *Medical and Surgical History of the Canadian North-west Rebellion*, 42.

arm... I would suggest that no serious cases of wounds should be sent by this route, the journey overland in suitable vehicles being too trying.[25]

The advice was well taken, and on 4 July the remaining 18 patients in the Saskatoon field hospital were removed by steamer, Roddick having arranged to place them in the Winnipeg General Hospital; the latter had agreed to reduce its daily charges from $1.50 to 1.25, "a very moderate sum."[26]

The last page in a wounded man's journey, from a purely medical point of view, was to look to such patients as Herbert Perrin, who wrote Roddick in July:

Judging that you have influence with the Government I venture to ask you to use that influence in my behalf, in obtaining for me some Government appointment.

I was wounded so severely in the arm at the battle of Fish Creek, that amputation of the same was necessary. I was a trooper in Lt Col Boulton's Mounted Infantry.

Before joining this expedition I was a clerk in a store where I was earning $50.00 per month.

At present I am out of employment and know of no occupation that I can follow.[27]

General Orders were soon promulgated to compensate those who, through illness or wounding while on campaign, were either temporarily or permanently incapable of "following their usual occupation," a board of three or four men being set up in each of seven districts for just that purpose.[28]

Another task awaiting medical practitioners in the months following the suppression of the Riel Rebellion was to derive what lessons they could from the conflict, and one aspect of the campaign that came in for particular criticism was the regimental system as it applied to treating the sick and wounded. As in previous centuries, each unit recruited its own surgeon, a civilian, but there was no guarantee the doctor in question had any military experience or would be able to fit into a military organization. Thus, with one exception—the surgeon for the Halifax battalion—"not one of them ... has made a satisfactory report of the cases treated by him or of the sanitary or unsanitary condition of his regiment." According to Bergin, then, "Surgeons recruited in an emergency without any previous military medical training, are apt to be and as in some instances during the late campaign were found to be,

25. *Medical and Surgical History of the Canadian North-West Rebellion*, 35.
26. NA, RG 9, IIA3, v.12, Roddick to Surgeon-Gen Mil, 21 July 1885.
27. NA, RG 9, IIA3, v.12, Herbert Perrin to Roddick, 10 July 1885.
28. *Medical and Surgical History of the Canadian North-West Rebellion*.

very inefficient and, from their want of discipline and ignorance of military law, were very difficult of control, and gave no adequate service in return for the large amounts of money expended upon them for transport, pay and rations." He recommended the formation of a Medical Staff Corps, complete with administrative and executive personnel, Field Hospital Corps, Ambulance Corps, and even a Military Cadet Corps, from which the necessary surgeons could be drawn. The latter would have to prove proficiency in a variety of subjects, including surgery (of course), transport of the sick and wounded, pathology, therapeutics, hygiene, and staff work.[29]

Thankfully, the campaign had been too short for disease to take a serious toll of Canadian soldiers, but the next conflict to involve Dominion troops on a large scale—in South Africa—would demand a far higher price. The result of a clash between a still-expanding British Empire and descendants of Dutch settlers, the Boer War that began in 1899 would eventually involve a quarter-million regular British soldiers, 100,000 enlisted volunteers (50,000 raised in South Africa) and 30,000 from the self-governing colonies. Some 22,000 would die, only a third of them on the battlefield (a ratio similar to that in Crimea),[30] representing a total death rate of over 50 per 1000. The Canadian volunteers were slightly more fortunate, if the word is appropriate, some 270 dying of the 7000 who served, a fatality rate of less than 40 per 1000, about half of them to disease. One of the latter was Trooper Landsdowne Patton, who on 31 March, 1901, was admitted to hospital with influenza complicated by severe bronchitis; developing pleurisy, he then came down with double pneumonia and began to slip away. "The very greatest efforts were made to save him, and by means of very great stimulation with champagne he was enabled to make a deposition."[31] He died of heart failure soon after; a member of the Third Contingent, Patton had not yet embarked for South Africa.

Illness having struck these volunteers before they even left home, it followed them aboard ship, as Captain Perry Fall related after embarking on 26 March, 1901. "I very much regret to report that from the commencement a great deal of sickness prevailed; due largely to the severe climactic change from a Canadian winter to the heat of the tropics in so short a time. The first diseases to develope [sic] were pleurisy and pneumonia," which killed four. The crossing that followed was reminiscent of the 15th-century voyages of discovery, as

---

29. *Medical and Surgical History of the Canadian North-West Rebellion*, 8.
30. Anne Summers, *Angels and Citizens: British Women as Military Nurses 1854-1914* (London, 1988), 205.
31. NA, RG 9, IIA3, v.25, Capt F.L. Vaux MO Cdn Contingent to OC Cdn Contingent, 7 April 1901.

The day after leaving Cape Verde Islands, Measles and Mumps developed and some 60 or 70 cases were treated, fortunately without a fatality and on the 10th of April the Medical Officer reported that Diphtheria was on board. There would appear to be an element of doubt as to this disease as a microscope was not available to make an absolutely correct diagnosis, but it is certain an epidemic of sore throat of a most virulent kind prevailed which it was necessary to make the most strenuous efforts to counteract. Isolation hospitals were improvised, and everything done that could be done in a crowded troopship to prevent contact. Owing to the great amount of sickness on board and the occurrence of two infectious diseases, and the great strain on the only Medical officer it became necessary in my opinion to secure the services of the Ship's Doctor (Dr. D. Davidson) which was done at an expense of £10 an outlay of which I trust it will be considered was warranted. In addition to this a Board of Officers was appointed to examine the ship from a sanitary point of view and certain alterations were advised and carried out, notably in the removal of false decks which admitted of water, and dirt accumu[l]ating in places inaccessible on account of these decks. There were no further fatalities until Capetown was reached,[32]

where two men succumbed to pneumonia.

By the end of 1901 several Canadian contingents had made their way to South Africa and back home again, the major battles were over, and the war had settled into a series of Boer guerrilla raids (bringing the word "commando" into the English language) and small punitive expeditions by empire troops. Sickness continued to take its toll, as well as the odd injury and gun-shot wound, so British authorities accepted an offer of a Canadian medical unit, the 10th Field Hospital. With a capacity of 100 sick and wounded, it was led by Lieutenant-Colonel A.N. Worthington, with Major G. Carlton Jones as his second-in-command, and was made up of volunteers from militia units across the country.[33] One of the latter was D. Macdougall King, a fourth year medical student, whose application to join the hospital was impressive enough, accompanied as it was by recommendations from an associate professor of surgery at the University of Toronto, a professor of anatomy at the same institution, the secretary of the provincial board of health, the provincial medical inspector, the minister of St Andrew's Church, the medical superintendent of Toronto General Hospital, and others.[34]

Not all candidates came forward with such high-calibre support, but all, even drivers and privates, had to meet very stringent standards. When

32. NA, RG 9, IIA3, v.25, Capt Perry Fall to Chief Staff O SAC Modderfontein, 7 May 1901.
33. NA, RG 9, IIB1, v.252, 5492/01, GOC to Minister, 21 December 1901.
34. NA, RG 9, IIB1, v.252, 5492/01, Army Medical Corps, Recommendations for service therein of D. Macdougall King, 28 December 1901.

in early January, 1902, the Adjutant-General advised that the necessary attestation papers, medical forms, and orders had been sent to recruit such "other ranks" for the unit, he pointed out that privates in the hospital section had to prove not only technical knowledge, but "moral character and antecedents." Also, "sober habits must be ascertained, and none but men able to give proofs of the above should be selected." Similarly, drivers not only had to show that they could manage horses, groom them, and harness double as well as single teams, but also "must be of sober habits and good character."[35] Somehow, enough such men were found to form a ward section of 35, a transport section of 22, and fill various other posts for a total of 62 all ranks.[36]

Embarking on 28 January, these men had spent the previous couple of weeks on company and squad drill, as befit a military organization, on top of training with stretchers and practising other medical skills.[37] They did not have to wait to reach South Africa before their services were needed, one of their own coming down with appendicitis which, with relapse, lasted the entire voyage. Then, "A few mild cases of Small Pox and Measles occurred. The former being of the type prevalent throughout Canada at the time, and occurred among men who had not recently been vaccinated, nor showed signs of successful vaccination. The cases were quarantined in a secluded portion of the Ship and every precaution taken to prevent the general spread of the disease. In this respect were most fortunate as some of the cases were not at once recognized and the vaccine on board (a very limited supply) was marked "good only until the 28th of January." (The day of embarkation)."[38] It seems to have been sufficient, the Director-General of Medical Services in Ottawa receiving a message to the effect that "The Officer Commanding Troops SS Victoria desires to express his great appreciation of the services of Corpl Donaldson and Pte Springford during the Small Pox and Measles Epidemic on the voyage. The excellent work performed by this NCO and Man reflect great credit upon themselves and 10th Canadian Field Hospital."[39]

By 1 March the unit was in theatre and being inspected by no less a personage than General Lord Kitchener, who found it "somewhat large" but "thought he could Utilize it."[40] In fact, the hospital received orders to trek to the Transvall on the 14th, a march that proved "a severe test on men and horses," leading to its first engagement only a few days

35. NA, RG 9, IIB1, v.252, 5492/01, Adj-Gen Memo, 6 January 1902.
36. NA, RG 9, IIB1, 1840/02, Daily Journal, 28 January 1902.
37. NA, RG 9, IIB1, 1840/02, Daily Journal, 28 January 1902.
38. NA, RG 9, IIB1, v.275, 4432/02, OC 10th Fd Hosp to DGMS, 20 August 1902.
39. NA, RG 9, IIB1, 1840/02, CO Troops SS Victoria to DGMS Ottawa, 28 February 1902.
40. NA, RG 9, IIB1, 1840/02, Daily Journal, 1 March 1902.

later. By this time the Boers were relying on hit-and-run raids to try to keep the British off balance, and it was in just such a skirmish that some members of the 10th Field Hospital brought attention to themselves "by their pluck and gallantry in dressing and attending to the wounded under a heavy shell fire in which 8 horses were killed on the ambulances."[41] The hardest-hit unit seems to have been the 2nd Canadian Mounted Rifles, with seven killed, two who died of wounds, three dangerously wounded, seven severely wounded, and eight slightly wounded, the last three categories attesting to the confidence (well-placed or otherwise) surgeons felt in making prognoses. Also severely wounded was Private J. Gunn of the 10th Field Hospital. Among those treating these casualties was a Lieutenant Roberts, who "particularly distinguished himself, and to his skill and energy a great deal of the comfort of the sick was due."[42] He was commended "for gallantry under fire," along with a Private Eccuse,[43] evidence that even small actions could call for much ability and courage.

The war against the commandos consisted of military columns to seek them out or carry out punitive campaigns against their supporters' farms. The 10th Field Hospital, located in a lonely spot called Vaal Bank, thus focussed on treating the wounded from these expeditions, tending to over a thousand patients from 28 March to 18 June. As the Principal Medical Officer at Kleeksdorp reported, "The work was most difficult as they had to receive great rushes of sick & wounded from columns operating in their neighbourhood & on every occasion these were met to the comfort of the patients & the credit of the Canadian Field Hosp' l." Indeed, the PMO went so far as to state that "Col Worthington & his staff have carried out their duties, in that isolated position, in an exemplary manner,"[44] and this was not an exaggeration to encourage dominion help. As Worthington himself reported, "Situated within a few hundred yards of several block houses the experience was most trying," the British positions drawing much enemy fire. Thus, "hardly a night passed without continued sniping; at times the firing being quite heavy, and on a few occasions bullets fell within the hospital lines among the tents. This necessitated entrenchments, and stone fortifications being thrown up around the Hospital and the avoidance of fires and lights at night."[45]

If the enemy was not annoying enough, simple logistics could create severe difficulties. As Worthington related, "frequently two Medical

41. NA, RG 9, IIB1, v.275, 4432/02, OC 10th Fd Hosp to DGMS, 20 August 1902.
42. NA, RG 9, IIB1, v.275, 4432/02, OC 10th Fd Hosp to DGMS, 20 August 1902.
43. NA, RG 9, IIB1, v.275, 4432/02, Report of Major Jones, 25 May 1902.
44. NA, RG 9, IIB1, 1840/02, PMO Kleeksdorp to DAAG Kleeksdorp, 17 June 1902.
45. NA, RG 9, IIB1, v.275, 4432/02, OC 10th Fd Hosp to DGMS, 20 August 1902.

Officers were on the road to Klerksdorp with sick convoys at the same time, and as many as 60 and 70 sick being removed at once, it necessitated the sending of many orderlies, leaving the Hospital continually short handed, as three days were generally allowed for the 80 mile trip."[46] Sometimes they were absent even longer, on one occasion because they had fallen into the hands of the Boers. On 7 May Lieutenant Roberts and his section had begun their trip when they saw brush fires on the veld; deviating from their route to avoid them, they encountered the enemy and were taken prisoner. "Nothing was taken," however, and "they met with every consideration and assistance,"[47] though whether this was because of their status as medical practitioners is unknown—certainly future wars of this type would see guerrillas operating with far more ruthlessness. Roberts and his men soon returned to their duties, the Boers not having the facilities to hold prisoners.

On 31 May the Boers, their crops destroyed and their families in concentration camps, signed articles of peace in which they acknowledged allegiance to the British crown. The 10th Field Hospital thus began sending its patients to hospitals in the cities, and by 6 June could report that it was empty, embarking for home on the 27th.[48] Obviously thinking of the future, Worthington reported that "Though no orders were received from the Imperial Authorities, after consultation with the OC Troops, and on his authorization a Board was held to report on all Officers, Non-Commissioned Officers and Men, likely to claim compensation for disability, the result of injuries and sickness received or experienced on active service... The Board had no authority to assess damages, and its report was intended simply as a primary record of all injuries and sickness."[49] Thirteen men had, in fact, been left in South Africa as too ill for the trip home. Medical practitioners could only go so far in helping a patient get a pension, however, as criteria other than the nature of a soldier's wound or illness came into play; the medical history of Private Charles Roy Laird, for example, includes a list of questions concerning his "conduct", "habits", and "temperance", all rated as "good" in his case. Having been diagnosed with rheumatism as a result of the climate, it was then determined that his condition had not been aggravated by intemperance, vice, or misconduct.[50]

46. NA, RG 9, IIB1, v.275, 4432/02, OC 10th Fd Hosp to DGMS, 20 August 1902.
47. NA, RG 9, IIB1, v.275, 4432/02, Report of Major Jones, 25 May 1902.
48. NA, RG 9, IIB1, 1840/02, Copy of Daily Journal of the 10th Canadian Field Hospital, 6, 27 June, 1902.
49. NA, RG 9, IIB1, v.275, 4432/02, OC 10th Fd Hosp to DGMS, 20 August 1902.
50. NA, RG 9, IIA3, v.25, Medical History of an Invalid, No C44 Private Charles Roy Laird, 4 May 1901.

While Canadian medical practitioners were dealing with sickness and injury in South Africa, their profession continued to evolve back home. As Lieutenant-Colonel J.T. Fotheringham explained in 1905, the militia then comprised several branches: cavalry, artillery, engineers, infantry, army service corps, and medical corps, the latter thus being recognized as an integral part of the country's armed services, as Bergin had suggested in the days following the Riel Rebellion. The corps was made up of permanent detachments, needed to look after the health of Canada's career soldiers, and members of the active militia, the latter working part-time. Each infantry or cavalry regiment also had the right to its own medical officer, though he was no longer a contracted civilian. Rather, as Fotheringham explained, he wore "the uniform of his regiment," was "a member of his regiment and its mess, with substantive rank, attained by length of service according to Regulations, and not eligible for staff or other than regimental duty. The system is one which in a Militia Force, organized upon county lines, is far too useful to be given up. Each year's experience in Annual Training as Principal Medical Officer of the District confirms me more strongly in this view."[51] That these doctors wore the uniforms of soldiers and underwent military training might allay the problems Bergin had complained about twenty years before.

The army medical corps, with a paper strength of 1500, was formed into bearer companies and field ambulances, but as the former were eventually merged with the latter, it is the organization of the field ambulance that will interest us here. With an establishment of 90 all ranks, eight of whom were officers (one of them the quartermaster, who looked after stores and equipment), it was broken down into three sections. The first was the bearer section (which previously had been an independent bearer company), responsible for clearing the wounded from the battlefield; the second was the tent section (previously the field hospital), which treated the wounded and sick; and the third was the transport section, which ensured the entire organization was sufficiently mobile to carry out its tasks and keep up with an army column.[52]

The militia's main purpose was to ensure trained troops were available in times of emergency or to form an expeditionary force to support imperial interests. When in early 1906 Colonel W.G. Gwatkin, the militia's chief of the general staff, asked the director-general of medical services how many units he could mobilize if necessary, the latter was

51. NA, MG 30, E53, Fotheringham Papers, v.6, f.30, "The Present Status of Military Medical Arrangements in Canada."
52. NA, MG 30, E53, Fotheringham Papers, v.6, f.30, "The Present Status of Military Medical Arrangements in Canada."

able to reply that 16 field ambulances could be made available, complete with equipment, though only "if my estimates for 1906 are authorized." Mobilization plans were sophisticated, calling for ten field ambulances to support five infantry divisions, as well as five others to look after corps troops (such as engineers and drivers) and various small field forces. Thus, according to plans developed in 1907 the 10th Field Ambulance would mobilize in Toronto for the 1st Cavalry Brigade, the 2nd and 7th at Ottawa and Québec for the 1st Division, the 4th and 5th at Montreal for the 2nd Division, the 1st and 9th at Halifax and Charlottetown for the 3rd, the 3rd and 15th at Hamilton and London for the 4th, the 11th and 13th at Toronto for the 5th, the 14th at Sarnia for the 6th, the 8th at St John for the New Brunswick Field Force, and so on. (Not all formations were the same size, so they did not all get the same allocation of medical support.)[53]

The peacetime medical service was administered by a director-general in Ottawa, with an administrative medical officer (or AMO) in each division or district to command permanent force and active militia alike; to assist him, he had a staff officer and sanitary officer. All told, the service maintained nine hospitals at various military stations to treat the sick and injured of the permanent force, or of the active militia when the latter was on manoeuvres. Each district or division kept medical stores at its headquarters for the standing hospitals as well as for field medical units when they were training; supplies could be replenished from central stores in Ottawa. A central military hygiene laboratory looked after public health work in the nation's capital, while a divisional laboratory resided in Halifax, each under the charge of a specialist sanitary officer, disease continuing to pose a greater threat to the soldier than battle.[54]

Guiding the various headquarters, units, and individual practitioners was a philosophy of operations, or doctrine, one of the best presentations of which was by Lieutenant-Colonel J.T. Fotheringham in a lecture at the University of Toronto. "It will already appear to you that the duties of the Medical Department of an Army must differ radically from those ordinarily associated in the public mind with the medical profession in civil life. War is not made with rose water; it is necessarily accompanied by much suffering, sometimes by what looks like hideous cruelty..." He then quoted military regulations to the effect that "The Army Medical Corps is maintained firstly, with a view to the prevention of disease, and secondly, for the care and treatment of the sick and

---

53. NA, RG 24, v.2406, HQC-357, Gwatkin to DGMS, 31 January 1906; DGMS to Gwatkin; DO&SD to CGS, 10 February 1906; DO&SD to DGMS, 5 June 1907.
54. NA, RG 24, v.6519, HQ 393-8-24, Major Lorne Drum, The Army Medical Service, May 1911.

wounded. The efficient performance of these duties demands a thorough knowledge of medical science, which must be acquired and kept up by deep and continuous study; and any instruction in purely military questions, beyond what is required for the performance of his proper functions, must be regarded as superfluous for an Officer of the AMC."[55] Putting on a uniform thus did nothing to alter a doctor's primary duty, though we shall see how important his military education could be.

By the time Fotheringham made the above presentation, it had been determined that a cavalry field ambulance should have a wartime establishment of 131 all ranks with a capacity for 50 patients, while a field ambulance for infantry formations would be even larger, with 242 all ranks to take care of 150 sick and wounded. Other units included the stationary hospital, with 88 all ranks, among them a matron and 16 nursing sisters to see to 200 beds; the general hospital with 128 people (with matron and 90 nursing sisters) and 520 beds, a convalescent depot with six staff and 520 beds, and an ambulance train with 20 men and two sisters for 100 beds. Thus "the Medical Officer is not simply a Doctor. The administration of this complicated organization lies in his hands. It is the result of experience painfully gained in war, and represents the best modern thought on the subject,"[56] a statement that would be put to a most severe test in a few short years.

In the decade following the Boer War, however, it is doubtful if many members of either the permanent force or the active militia thought in terms of the industrialized warfare that awaited them in 1914. Rather, they joined the service and carried out their training out of sense of duty or adventure—or both—expecting perhaps to have the opportunity to work on some campaign such as the one against Riel in 1885. War was more exciting than catastrophic, and the army, though hierarchical, was not necessarily an institution to which one gave up the rights and privileges of a citizen. For example, in October 1901 several officers of Military District 9 sent a "round-robin" or petition to the director-general of the army medical service pointing out "certain features" of their service "which are objectionable and unfair, but which may be rectified on being noticed," mainly the fact that some had been asked to take the places of others at the last moment, even at pay below their rank, while others had been given assignments not to their liking.[57]

55. NA, MG 30, E53, Fotheringham Papers, v.7, f.31, "Lecture Given by Lt-Colonel J.T. Fotheringham, at Toronto University," 15 November 1911.
56. NA, MG 30, E53, Fotheringham Papers, v.7, f.31, "Lecture Given by Lt-Colonel J.T. Fotheringham, at Toronto University," 15 November 1911.
57. NA, RG 9, IIB1, v.246, 4318/01, Officers AMS MD 9 to DG Army MS, 8 October 1901.

Their timing could only be rated as poor, to say the least, their complaint coming at a time when the army's medical services were undergoing a complex reorganization; the Army Medical Service was subsequently made up of infantry and cavalry regiments' medical officers, while the Army Medical Corps comprised field ambulances and similar units. The Adjutant-General, for one, was far from pleased, writing that

> These officers appear to have forgotten that they are in the Force in the interest of the Militia and not for personal gratification only, and that the AMS and the AMC exist for the same purpose, and they should not forget that both these organizations are still in a tentative stage, and that Officers belonging to these services must be prepared to accept the orders or instructions issued in relation to them, in the spirit as well as in the letter, and that cannot be disputed, but should Officers feel disinclined to carry out the orders or instructions as issued from Head-Quarters, they have the privilege of resigning their appointments.[58]

The officers in question apologized for their actions.

Further evidence that such doctors were in the military, Fotheringham's U of T lecture notwithstanding, is provided by the examination questions they were expected to answer at the medical course given in Camp Aldershot. First, the candidate had to name the articles of uniform, medical equipment, accoutrements, and other kit a medical officer needed when proceeding to a summer camp of instruction. Second, he had to state, briefly, the steps to be taken under General Order 99 to organize stretcher sections and see to their syllabus of instruction. Third, he had to state the number of field hospitals normally allocated to an infantry division in wartime, as well as list the personnel, equipment, wagons, tents, and other materiel required for each. Fourth, he had to provide similar information for a field hospital company in peacetime. Fifth, he had to explain the difference between a medical board assembled to report on a cause of injury in camp and that on an invalid injured in war on active service; he was also expected to state the object of each and the proper forms used, while writing out the proceedings of an imaginary board and filing Form B54. Sixth, the candidate prepared a report to his commanding officer that a case of virulent contagious disease had occurred, suggesting how it should be dealt with. Rounding out the examination was a bit of role-playing, the officer being told that his medical corporal was drunk and being asked what procedure he should adopt.[59]

The Aldershot course was only one way of qualifying for the Army Medical Corps; one could also attend the Volunteer Ambulance School

---

58. NA, RG 9, IIB1, v.246, 4318/01, Adj-Gen to DOC 9, 11 December 1901.
59. NA, RG 9, IIB1, v.251, 5391/01, Camp Aldershot, Examination Questions, Medical Course, 12 September 1901.

of Instruction in London, England, or take Canadian Army Medical Corps courses. Regardless of what route the candidate chose, he had to be a registered medical practitioner by law, be less than 45 years old, as well as qualify in the infantry and in equitation.[60] In 1911 criteria remained pretty much the same, except as concerned age (increased slightly, to 48), and marital status (had to be single), while the candidate was still required to be a graduate of some recognized medical school in the British Empire and, of course, be physically fit.[61] For those interested in joining the permanent force, a school of instruction was formed at Halifax, not only for junior officers but for non-commissioned officers (NCOs) and men as well. Military hospitals also ran courses during the winter, when they were less busy supporting summer camps.[62]

Also by 1911, the distinction between regimental medical officers and members of the medical corps had disappeared entirely. No longer did regiments or batteries choose their own RMOs; rather, qualified doctors appeared on a seniority list, from which they were detailed as administrative medical officers (AMOs) of militia training camps, as staff officers to divisional AMOs, as sanitary officers, for duty with field medical units, or as RMOs, depending on operational requirements. Furthermore, "Officers on the regimental list of the AMC who have not within the 5 preceding years attended 3 Annual Trainings, will be passed over for promotion, but their names will be retained on the regimental list. In this way a large corps reserve of medical officers is maintained available for emergencies and mobilisation without impeding the promotion of officers actively engaged in militia work."[63] Thus the centralization of military medicine was complete, the medical corps being responsible for the training and appointment of each and every practitioner in Canada's armed services.

Also part of this centralized organization were nursing sisters, who since 1900 had had commissions and rank equivalent to lieutenant in the army; in the 1905-06 establishment, there were positions for 25 of them, parallelling the number of male majors, captains, and lieutenants.[64] Many nurses had served in South Africa (though none with 10th Field Hospital), including Miss G.F. Pope of Ottawa, M.E. Affleck of Winnipeg, Elizabeth Russell of Hamilton, and M. Macdonald of Halifax, thus representing most of the major medical institutions in

60. NA, MG 30, E53, Fotheringham Papers, v.6, f.30, "The Present Status of Military Medical Arrangements in Canada."
61. NA, RG 24, v.6519, HQ 393-8-24, Major Lorne Drum, The Army Medical Service, 1 May 1911.
62. NA, RG 24, v.6519, HQ 393-8-24, Major Lorne Drum, The Army Medical Service, May 1911.
63. NA, RG 24, v.6519, HQ 393-8-24, Major Lorne Drum, The Army Medical Service, May 1911.
64. NA, MG 30, E53, Fotheringham Papers, v.6, f.30, "The Present Status of Military Medical Arrangements in Canada."

Canada.[65] One prospective military nurse, writing to the Surgeon-General Medical Services in 1901, explained that "In view of another Contingent being sent to South Africa I beg to again offer my services as a nurse to our Canadian Soldiers and would like to go to South Africa with them. I was one of the nursing sisters of the 2nd Canadian Contingent and was out there from Feb 18th to Dec 13th—1900, during which time I was never ill."[66] Her offer was accepted.

All 25 military nursing sisters were members of the permanent force, working in its many hospitals, but in 1907 the director-general medical services (or DGMS) suggested to the minister of militia that an Army Nursing Reserve be formed. Its members would only be called upon in time of war or similar emergency,[67] and would help complete an organization that already had doctors on a reserve regimental list. Finding volunteers would be no trouble, Dr Helen MacMurchy writing to the DGMS, Lieutenant-Colonel G. Carleton Jones (whom we met in South Africa), that "I have the honor to inform you that at a special meeting of the Editorial Board of "The Canadian Nurse" it was unanimously agreed that the Editorial Board should volunteer in a body for the Canadian Army Nursing Service Reserve," a total of about thirty practitioners. Though some might not be eligible for military service, "still it was thought well to volunteer in a body, in order to show the earnest desire of the profession to strengthen in any time of need, the Army Nursing Service Reserve."[68] By January 1908 the deputy-minister could report that he had a list of 57 such volunteers, including two from the US and another from Mexico.[69]

It was, however, two years before regulations were drawn up, reflecting the usual pace of administrative change in a peacetime army. When prepared, they called for women between the ages of 23 and 45 to be appointed to the reserves for five years, "renewable at the desire of the member and the discretion of the committee" set up to select qualified volunteers. Furthermore, "A candidate will sign a declaration of her willingness, in case of war, to accept service in Canada or any other part of the Empire, in the former case under the regulations governing the Nursing Service of the Militia of Canada in the latter under the Regulations of the Queen Alexandra's Imperial Nursing Service,"[70] a British body. Reservists were eligible to join the permanent force should

65. NA, RG 24, v.6309, HQ 63-16-4, Dy Min to Great West Townsite, 10 April 1909.
66. NA, RG 9, IIB1, v.254, 50/02, D. Hurcomb to Surg-Gen MS, 20 November 1901.
67. NA, RG 24, v.109, 5883-7, DGMS to Sir Frederick, 24 July 1907.
68. NA, RG 24, v.109, 5883-7, Dr Helen MacMurchy to Lt-Col Jones, DGMS, 21 September 1907.
69. NA, RG 24, v.109, 5883-7, Dy Min to Mil Secy Gov Gen, 29 January 1908.
70. NA, RG 24, v.109, 5883-7, Regulations of the Canadian Branch of the Army Nursing Reserve, 6 September 1910.

vacancies occur, or could be detailed as required for duty in hospitals and similar institutions. Courses were held yearly at the Halifax Military Hospital as well as at annual training camps so nurses could earn the necessary military qualifications.[71] As with doctors, nursing sisters had to have their medical certificates in hand before joining either the reserves or the permanent force.

Doctors, nurses, non-commissioned officers, and private soldiers of the permanent army medical corps (or PAMC) and its reserve counterpart had as one of their first duties to prepare for war, which for the permanent force meant dividing training into two seasons. Winter, extending from October to April, was dedicated to educating NCOs and orderlies as well as setting up courses for reservist doctors who had just joined or wanted to qualify for promotion. In the summer, from May to September, the PAMC focussed on field training and sanitation, though much of its personnel was assigned to militia camps as instructors or support staff; a large detachment usually made its way to Petawawa at this time to take part in the permanent force's summer camp there. Reservists followed a similar schedule, getting together at their local headquarters occasionally through the winter to learn their duties, first aid, and drill. Their main training, however, was carried out in summer at various camps, where they were inculcated with "a practical knowledge of the nature and functions of the various field and line of communication units which would have to be organized, equipped and manned by the medical service on mobilization."[72]

Though responsible for looking after the infantrymen, gunners, sappers, troopers, and other soldiers who attended summer training, this in itself did not provide much in the way of preparing for a military campaign. As Fotheringham admitted,

> The work of the Corps has of course been so far confined to the care of the Troops in Camp for Annual Training. This is of course practically Active Service, but under specially easy and favorable conditions. The real problem of Camp Sanitation and Control of Infectious Diseases can scarcely be said to come before us at all in so short a time as a fortnight in a Standing Camp. Still there are invariably a few cases such as Measles, Diphtheria, or Smallpox brought to Camp in incubation, and it speaks well for the promptness and discipline of both the Regimental and the Corps Medical Officers that in the two years during which I have had the medical charge of the Camp at Niagara, of 5000 men or more, not a case has arisen of any contagious disease contracted in camp.[73]

---

71. NA, RG 24, v.6519, HQ 393-8-24, Major Lorne Drum, The Army Medical Service, May 1911.
72. NA, RG 24, v.6519, HQ 393-8-24, Major Lorne Drum, The Army Medical Service, May 1911.
73. NA, MG 30, E53, Fotheringham Papers, v.6, f.30, "The Present Status of Military Medical Arrangements in Canada."

In a very real sense, then, medical units would not know if they were ready for war until it was thrust upon them.

Which is not so say that summer camps did not provide them with work—quite the opposite. Medical developments of the previous century, especially the germ theory of disease, had done much to provide medical practitioners with the knowledge they needed to fight their main foe, but the latter was never completely defeated. Thus at one training camp in 1901, as if in keeping with Fotheringham's report, the Surgeon-Major of the 92nd Regiment had to relate to his commanding officer "that a case of Small Pox has occurred in No 3 tent No 5 Co of this Regiment, and would respectfully recommend that for the patient a tent be pitched quarter of a mile north of the encampment out of the line of travel and that this be a nucleus for an infectuous hospital & that volunteers of one medical officer one corporal medical orderly & two privates be asked to take charge of it be completely isolated supplies & communication being exchanged at a given point. The remainder of those in the tent to be isolated in another tent in the same locality. The remainder of the company also be isolated in some other suitable place."[74] There is no record of the disease having caused any further trouble.

Even typhoid, transmitted through polluted water and hence a disease preventable through good hygiene, could break out at one of these annual gatherings. When Sergeant-Major F.W. McCusker of the 2nd Dragoons took ill at Niagara camp in 1903, he was ordered to the Grace Hospital in Toronto, where he remained from 15 June to 8 August. That he was paid for the time he spent under care (though not for the convalescence that followed) is evidence that the military hierarchy felt the illness was duty-related.[75] One of his comrades was less fortunate, Corporal M.W. McDonald of the 7th Hussars dying in the Montreal General Hospital the following summer. Since "it was during training that he developed such high temperature," having been certified fit on his arrival in camp, the militia paid for his hospital stay, the undertakers, and his father's train fare.[76] Appendicitis, on the other hand, was not deemed to be service (or perhaps we should say sanitation) related, and when Private Arthur Plouffe requested pay for time he spent sick, a Pension and Claims Board concluded that "There is no evidence and there is no suggestion that the claimant's illness was caused by the

---

74. NA, RG 9, IIB1, v.251, 5391/01, Surg-Maj 92nd Regt to OC 92nd Regt, 1901.
75. NA, RG 24, v.236, 2-4-13, Synopsis, Illness of Sgt Maj F.W. McCusker, 2nd Drgs, Niagara Camp, 1903.
76. NA, RG 24, v.245, 2-9-31, DOC MD 6 to Adj-Gen, 3 November 1904; DGMS to QMG, 3 November 1904.

performance of his Military duties, or that the cause was incident to Military service."[77]

Injuries might seem to be more straightforward, such as that of Private J.J. Forrester of the 71st Regiment, who suffered a fracture of the clavicle while wrestling (sport being an important part of military training). It was decided to send him home, but that the principal medical officer in the district in which he resided would see him from time to time until he recovered, expected to take about eight weeks.[78] Another injured hero, however, a Trooper Tucker of the 1st Hussars, had to prove his case through detailed evidence. "My injury was sustained 16/6/04 at about 12.30 P.M. I had just tied my horse to the line previous to being dismissed from morning parade. The horse next to me on parade had his right fore-leg tangled in the line and I endeavoured to extricate it. In doing this the horse kicked forward with both feet striking me with one in the face and other on my right foot."[79] Two other witnesses concurring, it was decided the injury was not the result of negligence on his part. Similarly, when Corporal A. Stevenson "was accidentally struck on the head by a piece of broken china, thrown away by a comrade,"[80] the militia endeavoured to pay his medical expenses.

MOs, NCOs, stretcher bearers, and other members of the Army Medical Corps were not kept so busy with such cases as to preclude their own training. In the first years of the twentieth century such indoctrination could often be rather basic, consisting in "a course of lectures of theoretical instruction in First Aid" for city units, "carried out during the ensuing winter,"[81] perhaps in cooperation with St John's Ambulance. Units were inspected once a year, though these brief annual reports could be dominated by matters other than training. Militia Form Number 142 for 1904, for example, provided space for discussing the commanding officer, dress and deportment, books, the application of regulations, and paperwork.[82] Thus 6th Field Hospital, inspected in June 1903, saw its CO, Major A.N. Hayes, rated a "good executive," though "a little lax in discipline," while privates were evaluated as being "Good material and well instructed."[83] There was no mention, however, of what they were learning. The 1903 annual report for Number 5 Field

77. NA, RG 24, v.243, 2-8-26, Proceedings of a Medical Board for the Purpose of Inquiring into the Case of Pte Arthur Plouffe, 23 September 1904.
78. NA, RG 9, IIB2, v.48(1), Proceedings of a Board of Officers assembled at Field Hospital, 25 September 1903 (?).
79. NA, RG 24, v.235, 2-3-16, Proceedings of a Board of Officers for the Purpose of Enquiring into and Reporting upon the Injuries Received by Trooper Tucker, 24 June 1904.
80. NA, RG 24, v.5884, HQ 7-97-15, DOC MD 10 to Secy Mil Counc, 17 January 1910.
81. NA, RG 9, IIB1, v.479, HQ-GOC, Meeting of Officers Commanding Military Districts, 15 November 1898.
82. NA, RG 24, v.6405, HQ 105, Militia Form 142, 1904.
83. NA, RG 24, v.6405, HQ 105, Annual Inspection Report of the 6th Field Hospital, June 1903.

Hospital was different, not only noting that its commander "is an active young officer... He is a good organizer and a fair horseman," but also relating that hospital duties were well carried out, especially nursing the sick. The following year the inspecting officer went so far as to state that "This unit is one of the best of the Medical Service. Their organization, equipment, esprit de corps—and training—are perfect." With an establishment of only a major, a captain, a lieutenant, five staff sergeants or sergeants, two corporals, and fourteen privates to service the requirements of half an infantry division, the unit would have its work cut out for it in case of emergency, but next year its organization was increased to 42 all ranks.[84] Before such units were merged with field hospitals, Number 6 Bearer Company seemed to set high standards of its own, the annual report relating that "Recruits are easily obtained but much importance is attached to character and intelligence and careful inquiry made before swearing them in."[85]

As we have seen, after amalgamation two types of field ambulance were formed, one to support infantry and the other, smaller unit to provide care for mounted troops. One of the latter was No VI (or 6, the militia never standardized its use of numerals), with headquarters at Sherbrooke, in Quebec's Eastern Townships. In 1907 the principal medical officer for the militia in that province was led to believe that a Major Farwell of the 53rd Regiment was willing to take on the duties of commanding officer. The unit must have been in the process of forming, as its prospective CO was asked to submit recommendations for medical officers to fill out its establishment, even if these were civilians who would have to undergo the necessary courses of military instruction. Farwell, however, bowed out for reasons unknown, and suggested Lieutenant W.W. Lynch, already a member of the Army Medical Corps, be given the job instead.[86] The unit was organized in 1908, and "The officers were chosen from widely separated districts in the Eastern Townships in order to stimulate a wide spread interest in matters military in the Eastern Townships." Taking part in summer manoeuvres with a cavalry brigade, its members learned to construct emergency dressing stations, to provide first aid treatment, to choose water supply points for troopers and their horses, to transport wounded using improvised travois as well as horses, to construct and locate kitchens and latrines, to load and unload ambulance wagons, and of course, the saddling and harnessing of horses as well as their general

84. NA, RG 24, v.6402, HQ 96, Annual Inspection Report of the No 5 Field Hospital, 1903, 1904, 1905.
85. NA, RG 24, v.6405, HQ 106, Annual Inspection Report of the No 6 Bearer Co, 1903; 1904.
86. NA, RG 24, v.4464, 9-6-1, CSO,Q to OC 53rd Regt, 5 December 1907., and subsequent correspondence.

care.[87] The unit thus focussed on several aspects of its role: sanitation and other means of preventing disease; evacuating casualties after a battle or while on a march; the actual treatment of the sick and injured; and ensuring it could keep up with the formation it supported. It seems, however, that some years passed before a cavalry field ambulance was able "to train as such, complete with its transport,"[88] if a 1911 report by Military District 10's commanding officer is to be believed.

Outnumbering the cavalry field ambulances were the field ambulances *tout court*, though these were not always easy to establish. As the commander of the Western Ontario District, which included the city of Hamilton, admitted when it was recommended two medical units be formed there, "I fear the population from which the Militia is drawn is already taxed to its utmost, consequently I am not prepared to recommend this step at present, desirable and all as it certainly is. The accommodation required for each unit is not to be had in any of the present Armouries. To bring these or any other units into existence would only lead to dissatisfaction under present conditions."[89] Months of negotiation and staff work followed, most of the problems nagging the district commander being resolved, but then fiscal realities intervened, the Adjutant-General informing several commanding officers that "it is regretted, the appropriation voted by Parliament for this purpose having been exhausted, no funds are available, and, therefore, it is not the intention to proceed further with this matter until fresh supplies are voted."[90] Infantry, cavalry, and other units having been formed decades before, it was difficult, in peacetime, to get the necessary moneys to establish supporting corps.

One that managed to see the light of day was the 18th Field Ambulance of Vancouver, and its early history can shed much light on the difficulties and challenges such units faced in the years leading up to the First World War. With an establishment of a captain, six lieutenants, a quarter-master, a sergeant-major, ten sergeants and staff sergeants, eight corporals, a bugler, 62 privates, and 11 horses, it was a substantial organization for a peacetime unit. In its first annual inspection it did well, its commander, Captain C. MacTavish, characterized as efficient, and a keen officer with good "Power of Command". His subalterns were found to be efficient and zealous. "This being the first annual inspection the Corps is everything considered in a most satisfactory condition. The

87. NA, RG 24, v.6569, HQ 1135-56-2, 15 July 1908.
88. NA, RG 24, v.6569, HQ 1135-26-1, CO MD 10 to Secy Mil Council, 15 April 1911
89. NA, RG 24, v.6569, HQ 1135-1-14, CO Western Ontario to Secy Militia Council, 12 October 1908.
90. NA, RG 24, v.6569, HQ 1135-1-14, Adj-Gen to OCs E.Ont, W.Ont, Maritime, and Qc, 2 December 1908.

keenness of all ranks being very marked. Particularly as the quarters allotted to the Corps are most unsatisfactory being damp unlighted and unventilated."[91] The next year brought similar praise, the inspecting officer stating that "This ambulance is capable of being made a most serviceable unit—It has, in its limited sphere, done excellent work," though it needed to attend summer camp to gain some experience of field conditions.[92] The unit in fact did so in 1911, the principal medical officer reporting that "In general the state of the unit is satisfactory," though it had sent fewer men than desirable, and the site chosen for training, at Kamloops, was not very suitable.[93] Other problems were more disturbing, MacTavish accused of being "Somewhat "casual" in manner" while the unit "did not impress one in the matter of smartness or spirit" even though "its technical duties were reported as satisfactorily performed."[94] The reviewer was General William Otter, the same inspector-general who had been more than satisfied two years earlier, so one could not blame the criticism on a change in standards.

Rather, according to Otter, "This was its first experience in Camp which may have caused a change in the personnel which I inspected two years ago at its Headquarters,"[95] a speculation confirmed by the Adjutant-General. "The large number wanting to complete, 56 all ranks, interfered very materially with its efficiency," he suggested, which made perfect sense if 34 men were trying to do the work of 90. However, it was a problem that "it is hoped will be remedied before next training... Your attention is particularly drawn to the remarks of the Inspector General concerning the dress of the officers, NCOs and men. There does not seem to be any apparent reason for all ranks being untidy... This being the first year, the unit has been in camp, allowance is made for the falling off in personnel, but better results are looked for next training";[96] in vain, as it turned out, a 1912 report written by the Chief of the General Staff (or CGS) relating that

> For two days this unit was upside down, the CO, Major McTavish, having no idea whatever of how to organize it. The ADMS eventually managed to get it into some order. The men of the 5th Regt RGA [Royal

91. NA, RG 24, v.6221, HQ 9-12-5, Report of the Annual Inspection of the XVIII Field Ambulance, 24 July 1909.
92. NA, RG 24, v.6221, HQ 9-12-5, Report of the Annual Inspection of the No XVIII Field Ambulance, 4 July 1910.
93. NA, RG 24, v.6221, HQ 9-12-5, Report of the Annual Inspection of the XVIII Field Ambulance Unit, 15 June 1911.
94. NA, RG 24, v.6221, HQ 9-12-5, Abridged Annual Report upon No XVIII Field Ambulance on 10th June—1911.
95. NA, RG 24, v.6221, HQ 9-12-5, Abridged Annual Report upon No XVIII Field Ambulance on 10th June—1911.
96. NA, RG 24, v.6221, HQ 9-12-5, Adj-Gen to DOCMD 11, 10 October 1911.

Garrison Artillery] when requiring treatment preferred going to their homes. Major McTavish complained of this, but perhaps there was some reason for it as the CGS found that the only sick man in the ambulance, admitted about 6 p.m. one evening, and suffering from fever, biliousness or such not well defined illness, had not even had his temperature taken when visited by CGS at 9 a.m. the following morning. A number of boys were noticed among the ranks. They belonged to the bugle band in which the OC is much interested, though its value to the ambulance, or its appreciation by the sick, is doubtful. The ambulance brought no horses, and unless they could be provided the unit could do no field ambulance training outside the Camp. The reason given was that horses had been supplied at Kamloops by the DOC [District Officer Commanding] the previous year. The CO did not strike the CGS as being competent.[97]

The unit had been short 36 officers and men, an improvement over the previous year, but still leaving it 40 per cent under establishment.

It was not all bad, and "It is satisfactory to note that this Field Ambulance is reported as being quite efficient in first aid work, ceremonial and shelter drill,"[98] but it proved a shaky foundation on which to build an operational medical unit. In 1913 Number 18 was rated "very unsatisfactory", though "as satisfactory and efficient as was possible with the limited numbers."[99] Discipline was only fair, while "It is noted that 4 Captains and 4 Lieutenants were reported as being absent without leave; they should be called upon for an explanation, and, if necessary, censured for this breach of discipline,"[100] though it was the commanding officer who became the focus of blame. After some backroom negotiation, MacTavish agreed to take leave (he soon resigned) so Captain K.D. Panton could take the unit in hand. Thus, as reported on 27 May, 1914, "This Unit allowed to take one section only to camp as it is in process of re-organization."[101]

Less than a hundred days later, Canada was at war.

97. NA, RG 24, v.6221, HQ 9-12-5, Abridged Annual Report upon No XVIII Field Ambulance, 1 July 1912, Appendix.
98. NA, RG 24, v.6221, HQ 9-12-5, Adg-Gen to DOCMD 11, 23 October 1912.
99. NA, RG 24, v.6221, HQ 9-12-5, Report of the Annual Inspection of the 18th F.A. Unit, 7 June 1913.
100. NA, RG 24, v.6221, HQ 9-12-5, Adj-Gen to OC 11 MD, 29 October 1913.
101. NA, RG 24, v.4625, 2-3-38, Abridged Annual Report upon "A" Section XVIII Field Ambulance, 27 May 1914.

Chapter Three

Medical Practice
and Industrialized Warfare

When in August, 1914, Canada found itself at war with the empires of Germany and Austria-Hungary, there was no shortage of volunteers, and recruiting officers faced not the problem of enticing people to join, but the challenge of testing, examining, and processing the thousands who showed up at their doors. No doubt most of those electing to wear a uniform were influenced by the nature of Canada's wars of the previous three decades, the campaign against Riel and the conflict in South Africa, which were characterized more by challenge, service, and adventure than by death and misery—or so the popular conception went. The battles they were about to engage in were, however, more akin to the American Civil War, with its severe casualties in dead and wounded, though disease would prove far less devastating in 1914-18 than in 1861-65. Medical practitioners thus did not have the viruses and bacteria of the camps as their main enemies; rather, it was the infection following wounding that would prove their most important challenge.

All this was unknown to the volunteers of 1914, among whom were many nursing sisters—certified or still in training—who were coming forward to enlist; in fact, there were too many of them to be immediately absorbed into the military hospital system being mobilized along with the rest of the Canadian Expeditionary Force. As a Mrs James related some fifty years later, "I went right off the wards, went to Kingston and there we were trained in any kind of training such as infantry drill, why I'll never know. There was no place to put us and there were fifty of us nursing sisters descended on Kingston, you see, and the hospital there, the General, was not big enough to take us so we had infantry drill and we were the amusement of the whole of Kingston."[1] They were, however, among the first Canadian medical practitioners to practise their trade near the battlefield, serving not only in Britain and France, in support of the Canadian Corps, but in North Africa and the Mediterranean as well. For example, when in 1915 Britain tried to force Turkey out of the war by landing in the Gallipoli peninsula, supporting the expedition was Number 1 Canadian Stationary Hospital, which set up on the island of Lemnos. According to Constance Bruce, one of the nursing sisters there, operations could be difficult. "Shortly after its arrival the hospital received a convoy of dysentery cases. Provisions were short and there was a scarcity of water, which fell especially hard on these men. One hesitated, to gather courage, before passing down the long rows of tightly packed beds, where sunken eyes were focussed on every one who went by, or parched tongues held out in silent entreaty, yet for hours at a time there was not a drop of water to be had."[2] Mary Darling, on the mainland, related that "we had a terrific amount of Malaria," as well as dysentery, the two forming the main medical complaints in that theatre, though almost unheard-of in Britain and France.[3]

Hospital staff thus had to possess as varied an experience as possible—or have the intelligence and flexibility to be ready for almost anything, and Number 7 (Queen's) Canadian General Hospital was fortunate in gaining someone of such abilities before embarking for Egypt. "It was at this juncture that Nursing Sister B. Willoughby joined the unit as Matron, after an extensive experience in Military Nursing, both prior and subsequent to the outbreak of war. As Matron of a Civil Hospital, possessing the additional qualification of service for six months in War Hospitals in France, our new Matron brought to her duties a knowledge that has always been of advantage in the management and disposition of her Staff."[4] Which was all to the good, as during their stay in Egypt the members of Number 7 would treat over 10,000 patients, including not only the usual sick and injured, but such novel problems as camel bites.[5]

Even when serving on the western front, Canadian hospitals did not necessarily support their compatriots in the Canadian Corps, many serving with the French Army, at least for a time. Integrating them into France's huge medical system was not always easy, however, and Number

1. NA, RG 41, v.20, RCAMC, Mrs James.
2. Constance Bruce, *Humour in Tragedy* (London, n.d.), 23.
3. RG 41, v.20, RCAMC, Miss Mary Darling.
4. *A History of No 7 (Queen's) Canadian General Hospital* (1917), 10.
5. *A History of No 7 (Queen's) Canadian General Hospital* (1917), 10.

6 Canadian General found that "discipline is beginning to suffer owing to continued enforced idleness," after five months with little to do. Its companion, Number 8 Canadian General, did much better, being designated "Class A" by its French hosts, which meant that it could be trusted with the most serious cases. According to a court of enquiry sent to investigate the units Canada sent to support its French ally, "The theatre and annexes were quite up to modern requirements. The work being done was in the opinion of the Court very good and many excellent surgical results had been obtained. The patients appear to be well looked after and comfortable."[6] Later, the Director of Medical Services would report to the Deputy Minister of Overseas Military Forces that "it is thought they will reflect much credit on the French Canadians that had to do with their organization, upon the Province of Quebec and upon the Dominion of Canada," though it is the nature of their operations that is mainly of interest here. Number 6, originally formed of volunteers from Laval's medical school, eventually saw its problems resolved and took over a 1400-bed hospital in early 1917, with a strength of 37 officers, 204 other ranks, and 37 nursing sisters. In its first three months it dealt with 2350 medical cases, 1450 surgeries, and 11,948 treatments and dressings.[7] Installed in a lyceum for young girls, in the course of 1917 it admitted 12,426 patients, returning 8301 to duty; 15 died. The others were transferred to other hospitals, most likely for convalescence.[8]

As the war wore on Canadian hospitals diversified not only in their geographical locations but in their essential roles, and they began to specialize. On 20 October, 1915, for example, the West Cliff Canadian Eye and Ear Hospital opened in Folkestone, with a staff of three administration officers, four medical officers, ten nursing sisters, and 27 other ranks.[9] In early 1916 the Canadian Red Cross Special Hospital opened, "The name 'Special' Hospital implies the class of work carried on in this Hospital, which is for Rheumatism, and all kindred cases of this nature," including using the water of St Ann's Well in Buxton, "for which the place has become so famous." Of note is the fact that the hospital also undertook to take care of shell shock cases, claiming that the "Special Treatment" is particularly beneficial."[10] The institution returned about 70 per cent of its patients to duty, which could not be said of the Canadian Special Hospital at Lenham, in Kent; authorized for a capacity

6. NA, RG 9, III, v.3501, 17-4-13, Proceedings of a Court of Enquiry, 10 November 1916.
7. RG 9, III, v.3501, 17-4-13, DMS Canadians to Dy Min OMF, 16 April 1917.
8. NA, RG 37, D358, v.XII, 1 December 1917.
9. NA, RG 37, D357, v.X, 20 October 1915.
10. NA, RG 37, D357, v.X, February 1916.

of 150, its role was to treat cases of pulmonary tuberculosis[11] which, at the time, was a process requiring months or years of rest and fresh air. The need for such a special institution is of some interest here; TB was endemic throughout the industrialized world, but worsened in those countries of western Europe that were directly affected by the war. Further, though in Canada the incidence of tuberculosis remained stable among civilians, in Ontario it increased among soldiers so that the rate of infection in military camps was noticeably higher than in cities and towns. As George Jasper Wherrett has speculated in *The Miracle of the Empty Beds*, such rise may have been the result of the close physical association of young men in barracks, some of whom had undetected infections. Soldiers were at further risk in the trenches, for very much the same reason, but also because the regions they fought in had a high incidence of the disease within the civilian population,[12] hence the need for the special hospital at Lenham. As we shall see, TB would continue to be a problem into the post-war era.

The far and wide distribution of military hospitals described above contributed to the Canadian Army Medical Corps' biggest controversy of the war, a report prepared by Doctor Herbert A. Bruce in September of 1916. Sent overseas by Sir Sam Hughes, the Minister of Militia, to investigate the hospital system, his criticism was scathing. One of his 23 main complaints was that "The present method of having Canadian hospitals scattered over such a large area is very objectionable," while "There is unnecessary detention in hospitals. There has been no medical inspection by the Canadian Medical Service of Canadian soldiers in Imperial hospitals, and there has been no efficient medical inspection of Canadian hospitals, in consequence of which Canadian soldiers are retained in hospitals in Great Britain, many of whom should have been returned to duty, and others should have been returned to Canada, where they could have been more economically and efficiently treated. The lack of system permits of the aimless moving of patients from hospital to hospital."[13]

Another criticism, that "No attempt has been made to restrict surgical operations which produce no increased military efficiency,"[14] is of great interest here, as it indicates that medical practitioners were not only focussing on the army's needs, but on those of their patients as well. Also of interest is how the statement (criticism number 10 in the

---

11. NA, RG 37, D357, v.X, 11 October 1917.
12. George Jasper Wherrett, *The Miracle of the Empty Beds: A History of Tuberculosis in Canada* (Toronto, 1977), 121.
13. NA, MG 30, E3, Babtie Papers, v.1, Report on the Canadian Army Medical Service, 9.
14. NA, MG 30, E3, Babtie Papers, v.1, Report on the Canadian Army Medical Service, 9.

report) reflects the entire tone of the investigation; at no time did Doctor Bruce suggest that patients were not getting adequate treatment; quite the contrary, the issue of cost often arose, as if the medical corps was too intent on taking care of its charges and not paying enough attention to the demands being made on the public purse. The hospital at Buxton was a case in point, Bruce suggesting that the establishment of a special facility there for the treatment of rheumatics "is ill-advised, as the majority of rheumatics will not be fit again for active service, and could be better and more cheaply treated in Canada,"[15] this in spite of some 60 to 70 per cent of its patients being returned to some form of duty.

To condemn the doctor as a penny-pinching government bureaucrat would be grossly unfair—even in war a nation's resources are limited, and victory will only come with the appropriate application of those resources. His report is important, however, not just for its charges against the medical system, but for the personal experiences that had a part in its making. For Doctor Bruce had no reason to be supportive of the CAMC; when in July, 1915, he volunteered to be a consulting surgeon to the Canadian Expeditionary Force, he wrote that "I might point out that the majority of the Medical Officers, who have gone with the CEF are not competent surgeons,"[16] which was probably true, most of the pre-war corps being made up of general practitioners. The following month he was authorized to join Number 2 General Hospital, serving in France, where he asked to make his way to the front to observe surgical practices there. Being turned down because he lacked military experience, he tendered his resignation on 24 September.

Doctor Bruce's odyssey was evidence that—for good or ill—the CAMC was a military organization, and its members were expected to fit into a martial system as well as be able to fulfill their purely medical duties. Doctors could no longer make their way to the scene of conflict and offer their services to a regiment, formation, or mobile column; they had to be part of an organic whole. No doubt an important impetus to such bureaucratization (or socialization) was the vast scope of the Canadian medical effort in the First World War. On 10 September, 1917, for example, Major-General Sir R.E.W. Turner, commanding Canadian soldiers in England, issued routine orders to the effect that several new hospitals would be formed: Number 4 Canadian General at Basingstoke, with 2500 beds; Number 5 at Kirdale with 1300; and several of 1040-bed capacity, Number 9 at Shorncliffe, Number 10 at Brighton, Number 11 at Moore Barracks, Number 12 at Bramshott, and Number

15. NA, MG 30, E3, Babtie Papers, v.1, Report on the Canadian Army Medical Service, 9.
16. NA, MG 30, E3, Babtie Papers, v.4, Col Herbert Bruce and the CAMC, 1916.

15 at Taplow. Number 13 at Hastings would have 520 beds, as would Number 14 at Eastborne; Number 16 at Orpington would be established with a numerically impressive 2080.[17] Thus, with a stroke of a pen, General Turner was authorizing the creation of 10 institutions, each with the population equivalent of a small Canadian town.

The above units were formed to take care of the large patient population that—tragically—continued to grow in Britain throughout the Canadians' participation in the European War. Number 1 Canadian General Hospital, on the other hand, operated on the continent, often in support of the Canadian Corps. Working closer to the front, it received a wide variety of patients and so could not specialize—that was for institutions further to the rear; accepting its first sick and wounded as early as 21 October, 1914, within four months it had looked at 2896 soldiers for such widely disparate problems as venereal disease, pneumonia, hernia, appendicitis, and tonsilitis.[18] Sophie Hoerner, a nursing sister with the institution, related how its role changed in June, 1915, when it became "The busiest place you ever saw," mainly because it was "really a clearing hospital; don't keep the patients longer than three days, if possible, send them to England to a base hospital."[19]

By July Hoerner had spent enough time in France to be able to describe the medical scene in some detail, explaining in a letter home that

> For days I have been trying to write you but there has not been a minute. We have been dreadfully busy, seven hundred patients. As I sit here in my little hut, ambulance after ambulance bringing in the wounded, it's too terrible to watch and hear, and it goes on all night, too. Convoys coming all the time. Boulogne is having a rest, we hear, and we are getting all the patients. The wounds caused by the bursting shrapnel are most severe. It rips, tears, lacerates and penetrates the tissues in a horrible manner. The doctor tries to repair and make good the best he can, but our best is often of little avail. One man completely blind, another with a knee joint blown open. I am witnessing dreadful suffering. A weary road these men have trod. Some of them go right to pieces. Their nerve has gone and they cry like babies. Others just stare and say nothing, have such a vacant look. Some with stern looks and lots of fight in them still.[20]

As for her previous experience, Hoerner explained that "It's so different from a civil hospital and our training in Quebec we were told to forget," the sheer scale of effort required making the western front a different medical world altogether.

---

17. NA, RG 9, III, v.4716, 109-27, Routine Orders by Maj-Gen Sir R.E.W. Turner, 10 September 1917.
18. NA, RG 9, III, v.4563, 3-3, Synopsis of Work Done by No 1 General Hospital, CEF, from 9 AM October 21st, 1914, to 6 PM Feb 12th, 1915.
19. NA, MG 30, E290, Sophie Hoerner Papers, Letter of 31 May 1915.
20. NA, MG 30, E290, Sophie Hoerner Papers, Letter Home, 4 July 1915.

No civilian hospital, for example, would have had to deal with the arrival of 276 emergency cases in a single convoy, but such is how one 33-day period began for Number 2 Canadian General (according to the matron's war diary). Such pressures could not have allowed time for surgeons to learn much while operating at the front, as a biographer of Sir Frederick Banting has suggested.

> ... the speed which is often necessitated by pressure of work and unfavourable circumstances tend inevitably to produce careless work. Life is despairingly cheap and death is ever present however well the work be done, and the atmosphere is therefore unlikely to generate that watchful solicitude which is seen in times of peace. Scrupulous niceties of technique are often impossible. This in itself constitutes a challenge to the conscientious medical officer; without the resources of a well-equipped hospital to back his efforts, he must frequently rely on self-discovered ingenuity. Without consultants, pressed for time, for basic necessities, for life itself, he must learn to trust his own judgement, to do what he feels must be done, and to do it quickly.[21]

In the realm of surgery, it would thus seem that doctors brought to the front lines techniques they had learned in civilian life, but had little opportunity to add to their knowledge.

As for No 2 Canadian General as a whole, complicating work there was the fact that the institution was short eleven nursing sisters. The day after the arrival of the 276 wounded noted above, another convoy of 120 unfortunates brought the place up to its maximum capacity of 1040, and though some were fit to be evacuated further to the rear "A terrible night" of very high wind, rain, hail, and lightning made this impossible. On the 17th a dozen new nurses arrived, but they were still ill from crossing the Channel and would need a day or two to recover. Six days after the rush began, the matron could report that "Hospital work continues busy though we haven't any serious cases," further convoys keeping staff on their toes: 302 on the 22nd, 352 on 4 March, 230 three days later, 184 on the 10th. On 18 March the war diary noted, somewhat ironically, that "Though we still have over 500 patients, the Hospital seems empty compared with a week ago."[22]

It was into this maelstrom that Number 7 (Queen's) Canadian General Hospital entered in April 1916; after moving from Egypt, it began setting up about twelve miles outside of Le Havre.

> Through the Medical Authorities of this area the order was conveyed to us to proceed with the establishment of a tent hospital of 1,040 beds. In our possession at the time was equipment for 400 beds, which had been

---

21. Lloyd Stevenson, *Sir Frederick Banting* (Toronto, 1946), 41.
22. NA, RG 9, III, v.5034, War Diary of Matron, No 2 Cdn Gen Hosp, 13 February-18 March 1916.

transported from Egypt. The work that laid next our hand was the acquisition of equipment to meet the needs of our new expansion. This was accomplished in due course, and the associated task of the pitching of hospital marquees was undertaken. The work was carried out with skill and zest by our men. Within the period of a week, a city of canvas, with prospective paths and roadways staked, had sprung into existence on the site.

And thus, by work from day to day, the Tent Hospital, which was to be our first charge in France, came to completion. It was not our first-born; but the pleasure of creation was common to every member of the unit. Experience gained in the establishment of our two former Hospitals proved of the greatest value in carrying out our latest task. But many new considerations had to be met in France that were not present in England or Egypt. The ground on which the Hospital was situated had to be surveyed and prepared for erection of tents. Much levelling and road construction proved necessary. There were no permanent buildings that could be utilized, beyond an iron-covered cookhouse. Not only had the Hospital to be established and provision made for carrying on administrative activities, but preparation of quarters for personnel of all ranks constituted a considerable extension of labours.[23]

The site covered twenty acres, with twenty-seven wards, each of 36 beds; there were also tents to be used as offices, with large marquees for dining hall and stores, the whole complex ready to receive patients in June. They were just in time, the British Commander-in-Chief, Sir Douglas Haig, having decided to launch a huge offensive on 1 July, whose impact will be discussed later in this chapter.

By the summer of 1916 Canadian hospitals in France, whether recently arrived like Number 7 or long-time western front veterans like Number 1, had some idea of what to expect after nearly two years of war; for what President Aristide Briand of France referred to as an industrial enterprise had produced the necessary "wastage" statistics for planning purposes. In early 1915 the French Army had determined that "3 per cent losses per day can be counted on for an organization on the march or quartered. Ofttimes the sickness is only temporary and the men rejoin the ranks. With troops under heavy fire, 50 per cent of losses are estimated for a small military formation (company or battalion); 20 per cent for a large unit (division); and 15 per cent for an army corps."[24] In the early part of the war, up to 30 November 1914, the French had dealt with almost 500,000 wounded, of whom over half returned to duty soon after treatment, a quarter required convalescent furlough, 17 per

23. *A History of No 7 (Queen's) Canadian General Hospital* (1917), 13-15.
24. A.M. Fauntleroy, *Report on the Medico-Military Aspects of the European War* (Washington DC, 1915), 39.

cent needed long hospital stays, less than two per cent were unfit for further duty, and 2.5 per cent died while under care.[25]

The emphasis on the western front, then, was on treating the wounded rather than the sick, though the latter were still plentiful, as many conditions, though they failed to kill their victims (at least not in large numbers) still forced tens of thousands to seek treatment. Among them were influenza, with some 65,000 ill in 1917-18, gonorrhea with over 45,000 ill in the course of the war, tonsilitis and sore throat with about 20,000 ill, syphilis with approximately 18,000, trench fever (caused by a bacterium transmitted by fleas—there were no known fatalities) with about the same number of victims, myalgia (muscle pain) with some 15,000 ill, and intestinal disease with approximately the same number of sick.[26] The Canadian Expeditionary Force, however, was free of the kinds of epidemic diseases that had caused such ravages in the Crimea, the Spanish-American War, and South Africa. It was not an easy battle to win, however, as Lieutenant-Colonel J.T. Fotheringham, then a junior officer, recalled in a 1927 presentation. While at Shorncliffe, he had much difficulty

> in getting my battalion all inoculated against typhoid. Our own Adjutant was on leave, and the Acting Adjutant, a Royal Military College Graduate, was inclined to regard the Medical Corps as a bit of a nuisance, and Medical Officers not soldiers in any real sense of the term, and not, therefore, inclined to regard the Medical Officers requests as serious. I had had two reminders from my Assistant Director of Medical Services, and a visit from the Deputy Assistant Director of Medical Services about it, sort of felt myself in a helpless sort of position, and was much too indignant (for a junior officer). In that mood I sat down and wrote the Assistant Director of Medical Services an epistle explaining the situation and rather vigorously stating that I was not the Regimental Sergeant Major,[27]

and hence lacked the authority to enforce regulations.

Fotheringham vented his spleen in his letter, no doubt hoping his superiors, who were in much better positions to ensure that health regulations were adhered to, would sort things out. "Then one evening, when I entered the Officers' Mess of the 27th Battalion, there was thunder in the air. The Officer Commanding was storming and consigning the Canadian Army Medical Corps, and especially the Canadian Army

---

25. A.M. Fauntleroy, *Report on the Medico-Military Aspects of the European War* (Washington DC, 1915), 49.
26. Desmond Morton and Glenn Wright, *Winning the Second Battle: Canadian Veterans and the Return to Civilian Life, 1915-1930* (Toronto, 1987), 231.
27. NA, MG 30, E53, Fotheringham Papers, v.7, f.32, The Present Organization of the Medical Service in the Field, 15 March 1927.

Medical Corps personnel of the 2nd Division to the depths. Being the only member of that long suffering service present, the storm descended upon my bewildered head."[28] He went to see the adjutant, responsible for the unit's administration, to enquire as to the reasons for the outburst (he had forgotten about his own letter of complaint—or so he claimed). Fotheringham was then shown a communication from the brigade commander to the battalion commander, his immediate subordinate, "giving him the very d—l and instructing him that everything else in the Battalion was to stand still until the Anti-typhoid Inoculation was complete." Also on file was a letter from General Steele, responsible for Canadian soldiers in England, along the same lines. Thus, like Doctor Woods we met a few chapters ago, Fotheringham had gone over his commanding officer's head, but now he was part of a medical system with its own chain of command; he and his battalion commander eventually learned to get along nonetheless.

The germ theory of disease, having been elaborated by researchers such as Pasteur and Koch in the late nineteenth century, was thus a part of military science by the First World War, so much so that vaccination was considered more important than a commander's dignity; with the full force of the military hierarchy behind them health measures were thus easy enough for medical practitioners to enforce. Water supplies, for example, were checked for purity, and no less a personage than the Director of Medical Services for a British Army could intercede if necessary, as the Deputy Director Medical Services for the Canadian Corps discovered in August, 1916. "It is notified for your information that during the past month water has been taken from 286 water carts carrying water to units for distribution for drinking and cooking purposes; the water was then examined to determine whether it had been chlorinated, and it was found that in no fewer than 121 cases or 42% the water had not been effectively treated. It is unnecessary to point out the grave danger to the health of the troops that may arise from the neglect to ensure the efficient treatment of water for issue to the troops and it is requested that steps may be taken to enforce the instructions which have already been issued on the subject."[29] The necessary orders were subsequently passed along to every medical officer of the formation, and by spring of 1917 regulations dictated that each one should have the necessary testing equipment and chemicals to carry out his own checks.[30]

28. NA, MG 30, E53, Fotheringham Papers, v.7, f.32, The Present Organization of the Medical Service in the Field, 15 March 1927.
29. NA, RG 9, III, v.4553, 5-8, DMS 2nd Army to DDMS Cdn Corps, 5 August 1916.
30. NA, RG 9, III, v.4553, ADMS 2 Div to RMOs, 17 April 1917.

Equally important was the disposal of that source of so many diseases—human waste—the best means of doing so being described in a late 1916 circular. "It is desirable—nearly necessary—that human faeces in the Canadian Corps area be incinerated. Burial of large quantities involved the digging of holes dangerous to wandering horses, the limitation to movement over the ground, scattering by shell explosion, the fouling of already overcrowded ground, the possible pollution of wells and water courses, and exposure of this dangerous material to the attraction and visitation of flies and then to food. In any large group of men there are bound to be "carriers" or men sick with diseases thus communicable."[31] Burning was not always possible, however, and the necessary equipment difficult to procure or construct, so it was necessary to rely on soldiers, specially assigned to the task, to keep their defensive positions clear of "nuisances". One of the duties of a battalion medical officer was to carry out inspections, every 48 hours, to ensure there was no laxity in that regard,[32] while further to the rear mobile laboratories were available to carry out more sophisticated testing.[33]

Such precautions could not, of course, eliminate sickness entirely—quite the contrary—but disease had nothing of the impact on the Canadian Corps of 1914-1918 as it had in previous conflicts. In the month of March 1917, to give just one example, 2969 men were evacuated as sick, while 1435 were wounded in the trench raids and other operations leading to the storming of Vimy Ridge on 9 April. The assault itself, which lasted three days, obviously reversed the relative importance of sick and wounded, with 8119 of the latter being evacuated, though there were still 1564 sent back due to illness that week.[34] Where hygienic and other precautions really had an impact was on fatalities, some 1906 members of the Canadian Corps dying of disease in France and Belgium in the course of the war, compared to 34,887 killed in battle, 4429 missing (presumed dead), and 11,994 who died of wounds, or a total of 51,310 battlefield deaths.[35] The ratio of those who died of illness as opposed to those killed by the enemy was thus on the order of 1:27, and though one could argue that the lethality of industrial warfare had something to do with the lopsided figures, the American Civil War had also seen myriad battles devastating whole

31. NA, RG 9, III, v.4553, 5-3, The Incineration of Faeces, 12 September 1916.
32. NA, RG 9, III, v.4553, 5-3, ADMS 2 Div to Fd Ambs and MOs, 20 February 1917.
33. NA, MG 40, E4, Adami Papers, Record of Inspections of Canadian Hospitals in France, 1915, 30 August 1915.
34. NA, RG 9, III, v.4555, 4-5, Comparative Statement by Divisions of Canadian Corps, 3 April 1917; Return of Sick and Wounded, Admitted and Evacuated, by Field Ambulances, for Week Ending April 14th, 1917.
35. G.W.L. Nicholson, *Canadian Expeditionary Force* (Ottawa, 1964), Appx C.

armies, and still had a death rate due to sickness not far short of that on the battlefield.

For those who survived their illnesses, statistics are less trustworthy. While all soldiers suffering from particular types of wounds were evacuated, triage in such cases being reasonably objective, the same could not be said of the sick. Many who were ill remained at their posts, while some who presented themselves to the medical officer for evacuation may have been seeking leave from the hazards, boredom, routine, and discomfort of the trenches. As R.J. Manion, leader of the Conservative Party later in life, explained in his retrospective on the war, "The handling of the sick is not so easy a matter as the caring for the wounded in the lines, for the reason that it is not what disease the man has that the medical officer must decide as much as whether he has any disease, or has simply joined the Independent Workers of the World," a syndicalist union movement seeking to reform capitalism through a general strike. "In other words, is he really ill, or is he just suffering from ennui, has he at last become so "fed up" with it all that he has decided to go sick, running the gauntlet of an irate MO with the hope of receiving a few hours or days of rest at the transport or in the hospital?"[36]

The phenomenon could add complexity to an already complicated medical practice, so that, generally speaking, regimental medical officers thoroughly disliked sick parade, that morning ritual when soldiers came forward to present their ills—or their fabrications. To the RMO "It is a thorn in his side that makes itself felt daily. And the reason is that he is between three fires,- the Assistant Director of Medical Services who expects a low sick rate in the different units; the battalion and company commanders who expect the men on parade, which means fit and on duty, while at the same time insisting, quite rightly, that the men get every attention at the hands of the medical department; and a certain small percentage of the men for whom the novelty and glamour of the war has worn off and who have become tired of the food, and find the work arduous and monotonous."[37]

Medical officers thus had to be on the lookout for malingerers, though they were not the only ones to arouse emotions other than sympathy. Venereal disease, though entirely preventable, was a serious problem among troops who had few other ways to relieve the stress of trench warfare. Its victims were certainly numerous, Desmond Morton reminding us that it struck 66,346 times,[38] which amounted to 40% of the

---

36. R.J. Manion, *A Surgeon in Arms* (Toronto, 1918), 104.
37. R.J. Manion, *A Surgeon in Arms*, 106-107.
38. Desmond Morton, *When Your Number's Up* (Toronto, 1993), 200.

159,472 Canadians wounded and gassed on the western front. Put another way, VD claimed as many victims as almost two years of campaigning, which may account for the harshness with which military doctors approached the problem. In 3rd Canadian Infantry Division, for example, officers struck by the disease were immediately segregated, and orders were issued to the effect that they were "on no account to remain with, and be treated by, the Medical Officer in charge of their Units."[39] Further, according to army instructions handed down in 1916, officers admitted to hospital would pay a stoppage of two shillings sixpence a day.[40]

In early 1917, as the Canadian Contingent prepared to spend its third year on the western front, and with the rate of venereal disease refusing to diminish, disciplinary pressure was increased. According to a circular of 27 January, "An Officer, Warrant Officer, Non-commissioned officer, or man, who is admitted to hospital suffering from venereal disease after the date of this memorandum, is not to be granted leave of absence, whilst serving with the British Armies in France, for a period of one year from the date of discharge from hospital, except with the approval of the General Officer Commanding an Army or Cavalry Corps, or the General Officer Commanding Lines of Communication Area."[41] Further, with medical officers taking on detective duties to ensure hygienic and sanitary regulations were adhered to, they formed an alliance with the military police (or APMs) in the war against VD. According to the Assistant Director of Medical Services (ADMS) for the 3rd Canadian Infantry Division,

> APMs should arrange through the ADMS that all cases of venereal disease are reported to them immediately they occur, and that the patient is not evacuated until the APM has had an opportunity of ascertaining where he contracted the disease.
>
> If the man can give the information necessary, the APM will arrange with the ADMS that he may go in an Ambulance Car with a policeman and a gendarme to the house, in order to try and identify the woman. If he identifies her, he should sign a statement of his case, and that he believes the woman he saw was the one who infected him. He can then be evacuated...
>
> If found to be diseased, she is sent to the Hospital, or evacuated by order of the Gendarmes.
>
> APMs are not to order the examination or the evacuation of prostitutes or women alleged to be suffering from venereal disease.[42]

39. NA, RG 9, III, v.4555, 4-5, ADMS 3 Div to OCs Fd Ambs, 5 April 1916.
40. NA, RG 9, III, v.4555, 4-5, Army Council Instruction No 1288, 29 June 1916.
41. NA, RG 9, III, v.4555, 4-5, Circular Memorandum, Venereal Disease, 27 January 1917.
42. NA, RG 9, III, v.4555, 4-5, ADMS 3 Div to OsC Fd Ambs, 12 March 1917.

It was all to no avail.

Generally speaking, sick soldiers presented themselves to medical officers under their own power, but when industrial war led to the clash of armies, the resulting wounded were often incapable of such physical exertion and had to be evacuated. In doing so, an important medical player on the battlefield was the field ambulance, which we last saw trying to prepare for war in the final years of peace; mobilization of such units beginning at the same time as infantry, cavalry, and others, they suffered from the same growing pains as they tried to put themselves on a war footing. Number 6 Field Ambulance Unit, Canadian Overseas Expeditionary Force, for example, had to contact its superiors at headquarters to ask to be allocated a serial number, "as the Acting Officer Commanding informs me that the men's clothing is being stolen and cannot be traced as there is no Regimental Number to trace it by."[43]

A wartime field ambulance (or FA) was a substantial organization, consisting of ten officers, 14 NCOs, 168 rank and file, as well as 57 members of the Army Service Corps to drive some 28 horse-drawn vehicles; to this total of 249 personnel were 59 horses, as well as a motorcycle and a bicycle.[44] Training was simple and straight-forward at first, W.L. Shirly of the 4th FA recalling how his unit moved to Winnipeg in January 1915, where it remained until April. There, indoctrination consisted of "First aid courses and general "get fit" courses, you know, marching and drilling and all that stuff."[45] The experiences of Number 10 Field Ambulance were similar a year later, and "The days of preparation previous to leaving for Overseas were occupied with squad drill, company formation, stretcher drill under competent instructors and lectures by the Officers on various medical subjects. Occasional route marches and systematic exercise, kept the men in the pink of condition physically."[46]

As each of five divisions (of which four served as the Canadian Corps while the other remained in England) formed and completed a certain minimum level of indoctrination, it crossed the Atlantic to the United Kingdom. There, training continued until the move to France or Belgium, by which time the members of a field ambulance were familiar with at least the theory behind the tasks that awaited them. When a soldier was wounded, the first problem faced by his friends, regimental stretcher-bearers, and members of field ambulances was, of course, to get him to treatment. As A.M. Fauntleroy reported to American policy-makers in

43. NA, RG 24, v.4464, 9-6-1, A/ADMS 4th Div to DGMS, 29 December 1914.
44. NA, RG 24, v.4464, 9-6-1, Adg-Gen to OC 4th Div, 23 March 1915.
45. NA, RG 41, v.20, RCAMC, W.L. Shirley, 4th Field Ambulance.
46. NA, RG 9, III, v.4715, 107-20, No 10 Canadian Field Ambulance, Mobilization, 12 January 1916.

1915, "The evacuation of the sick and wounded has always constituted a problem of the gravest import in every campaign of history. Progress in this direction has not by any means kept pace with the advances made in perfecting the means for destroying human life and property. The history of every war has shown that the implacable working formula, so often quoted, "Ammunition first, food second, and wounded third," has not changed, nor has it received the consideration, in regard to alleviating the condition of the last factor of this formula, that its importance warrants."[47] Sophie Hoerner of 1 Canadian General Hospital would have agreed, relating how "Their one hope is that they may not be wounded till after dark as they can't be picked up till after dark and it is terrible to lie wounded on the battle-field all day. Some of the wounds are so dreadful that one's most vivid imagination couldn't even faintly picture them."[48]

Once picked up by stretcher bearers or comrades, the wounded were carried back to a Regimental Aid Post, or RAP, for quick treatment and evacuation rearwards to a dressing station. Sometimes the trip was directly to the latter, which was part of the field ambulance, and one such has left a vivid description of its operations. In May 1916,

> Maple Copse Dressing Station was a sand bagged structure in a wood of that name. The place held about 6 stretcher cases and was 600 yards from the front line. The stretcher cases were carried by battalion stretcher bearers from the line to the dressing station in the first days of clearance. Later this was changed and ambulance stretcher bearers were sent forward to the battalion aid posts to get the cases and carry them back to the Dressing Station, where their wounds were redressed if necessary. At night the Ambulance stretcher bearers carried the wounded through the wood, across a trench spanned by a double trench mat, famous throughout the Canadian Corps as "Blighty Bridge", to a narrow gauge track [known as a "tramline"]. Here were specially built trucks for the accommodation each of two stretcher cases. The trucks were pushed down the track at night to a dump in the village of Zillebeke. Here the cases were transferred to horse ambulances which were at the dump at an appointed time. These ambulances cleared to Menin Hill Dressing Station, a small shrapnel-proof shelter on the Ypres-Menin Road. At this point a squad stationed there transferred the wounded to Motor Ambulances which carried them to the Main Dressing Station at Brandhoek. From here they were taken to the Casualty Clearing Station beyond Poperinghe.[49]

47. A.M. Fauntleroy, *Report on the Medico-Military Aspects of the European War* (Washington DC, 1915), 30.
48. NA, MG 30, E290, Sophie Hoerner Papers, Letter Home, 7 June 1915.

Dressing stations were close enough to the front line to be within range of German artillery, so field ambulances often found themselves treating the wounds of their own personnel.

Working in such conditions obviously required a certain fortitude—and even demanded acts of outright courage. When the front was relatively static, as in the spring of 1916, such a unit rotated personnel between its headquarters, somewhat to the rear, and the various dressing stations closer to the front. In the course of one such rotation, a party making its way forward to relieve some of the unit's men was caught by enemy shelling. Three were killed and five wounded, and to take care of the latter "Corporal L.H. Mansell, 2nd Canadian Field Ambulance, left a place of comparative safety and ran out fifty yards over open ground swept by shell fire. He dressed the wounds of the injured men, and carried them in."[50] His was not an isolated act.

As hazardous as the routine of trench warfare could be on occasion, combat was much worse, and though to the military historian each battle has its own distinguishing characteristics from which lessons can be learned, to the participants they all tend to be pretty much the same—periods of confusion, excitement, fear, and occasional bravery. By early June of 1916 the Canadian contingent had been in France over a year, first arriving in March 1915. Taking over a portion of the British line near Ypres, in Belgium, it found itself defending part of a salient that jutted into the German lines, which the enemy sought to reduce or destroy. It was here that poison gas had first been used in a major attack on the western front, in April and May 1915, and it would be here that the muddy battle of Passchendaele would be fought in mid to late 1917.

The Canadian line incorporated a copse called Sanctuary Wood, and the engagement of interest to us here (later called the Battle of Mount Sorel) opened when the Germans began shelling on 2 June 1916. It soon became obvious that this was no bombardment typical of the routine of trench warfare, but a much heavier attack. According to a report by Number 10 Field Ambulance, "Trees were uprooted or snapped off like matchwood. Great chunks of earth and fragments of dugouts were thrown high in the air. Everywhere was the din of bursting shells and smashing trees and branches."[51] Then the wounded "commenced to pour into the dressing station," where a Captain Wadge was in command, with 31 NCOs and stretcher bearers. The bombard-

49. NA, RG 9, III, v.4715, 107-20, No 10 Canadian Field Ambulance, May 1916.
50. NA, RG 9, III, v.4714, 106-27, Notes from the Front, No 2 Cdn Fd Amb, 1 May 1916.
51. NA, RG 9, III, v.4715, 107-20, Second of June—Strafe.

ment's ferocity soon filled the dressing station to capacity, and then targeted the post itself. "At about 11 o'clock a high explosive shell blew in the middle room of the dugout. There were six stretcher cases in the place as well as several stretcher bearers. One of the wounded was killed and some of the staff buried or hit by flying sand bags." To make matters worse, word came from the front that German infantry had attacked and taken the forward trenches, with the copse possibly their next objective. Captain Wadge decided to move the wounded. "There was no sign of life around the dressing station—nothing but the dead, a travesty of a wood and the breaking shells."

Of the five surviving stretcher cases, one was carried down a communication trench which led to the rear, while the other four were loaded on a tramline. As for the other patients, "There were 20 walking cases which had been entered on the records before the post was blown in, and this number was being constantly added to by men coming back from the line, where furious fighting was in progress. These wounded were divided into small parties, each in charge of a stretcher bearer. Before these men left the rear room and south wall of the dugout were destroyed by direct hits."[52] The captain was in the last group to leave, and the resulting voyage could well have come out of Dante.

> The trench which the party had to take was almost levelled in places by the terrific hammering it was receiving. It was clogged with dead—singly and in agonised heaps—buried under portions of parapet, until only bloody limbs were exposed—in every conceivable attitude. The wounded lay quivering at the bottom of the trench or crawled desperately along, dragging their mutilated bodies to some place of shelter. Soon after the ambulance party commenced the downward journey, a shell burst near a group of men with a stretcher case. Two of the men were killed outright and another wounded. A stretcher was hastily procured, the newly wounded man placed upon it, and the party carried him down. On the way as many wounded were dressed as it was possible to attend to. At the point where the trench crossed another, Corporal Burkett was wounded and had to be assisted. The trip seemed an eternity. The party could not hurry because of the condition of some of the patients. The air was heavy with smoke and shell fumes, and German machine guns sent showers of steel hail through the gaps in the trench, forcing the party almost to crawl.[53]

Patients were turned over to the 42nd Battalion's Regimental Aid Post.

Further back, Number 10 Field Ambulance's headquarters was dealing with the deluge of wounded that people like Captain Wadge were bringing back from the fighting; patients were moved by stretcher

52. NA, RG 9, III, v.4715, 107-20, Second of June—Strafe.
53. NA, RG 9, III, v.4715, 107-20, Second of June—Strafe.

to a place called Transport Farm, where they were loaded onto horse and motor ambulances. The entire area was within range of German artillery, and the road being used to evacuate the wounded was a shambles after a few hours' pounding, as "Dead and terribly mutilated men and horses dotted its length. Great craters were torn in the pavé. Thick clusters of shrapnel smoke spit, unrolled, and drifted away."[54] It was declared impassable, an indication of the scale of fighting those first few days of the battle; also symptomatic of the maelstrom the Canadians now found themselves in was the fact that of Number 10 Field Ambulance's 11 casualties, two were for shell shock.

Communications soon began to break down, and on the 4th one of the unit's officers received word that large numbers of wounded were still in the trenches, but there were no details as to their location. A rescue operation was launched with personnel of the 5th, 8th, and 9th Field Ambulances, helped by 200 men of the 7th Infantry Brigade, the front line, such as it was in the midst of this confusing battle, being divided into sectors and combed for wounded. Thankfully, the German attack petered out in the days that followed, allowing time for such operations and to piece together the events of the battle. Number 10 Field Ambulance found the bodies of three of its own, including its commanding officer, and brought official recognition to those of the living who had particularly distinguished themselves. For example, Major T.M. Leask related to the new officer commanding how "Staff Sergeant Cameron carried several patients out of the Dugouts at Zillebeke Village under heavy shell fire and his work on the Road at Transport Farm where he stood directing Ambulances and giving great assistance in loading same under continuous shell fire was magnificent. His work during this strenuous time was wonderful and I consider if any honour is coming to any man, it is coming to Staff Sergeant Cameron."[55] There were others.

The attack, though brutal, was directed against a single Canadian division, so casualties were easily taken into the British hospital system behind the front, which as we have seen included many Canadian units. These would face a far more severe test a month later, when the British Expeditionary Force launched a major offensive on the Somme beginning 1 July, that first day being one of the worst in the history of the British Army, with 59,000 losses, a third of them dead, including the bulk of Newfoundland's contribution. One of the Canadian hospitals facing the deluge was No 7 (Queen's), which as we have seen had only established itself on the western front on 5 June. At first, "The

54. NA, RG 9, III, v.4715, 107-20, Second of June—Strafe.
55. NA, RG 9, III, v.4715, 107-20, Major T.M. Leask of 10 Fd Amb to OC 10 Fd Amb, n.d

amount of work that fell to us increased gradually, affording opportunity for testing all points of the system of management that had been inaugurated,"[56] but that changed on 2 July, the day after the British catastrophe, "when all our previous figures of admission were eclipsed."

They were not alone, as the matron for 2 Canadian General Hospital could attest. With little or no knowledge of the disaster that had befallen the BEF, the first convoy to arrive on 2 July, of 235 victims, was not much different from those of previous battles, though the matron noted that they were "mostly stretcher cases and all very badly wounded."[57] Then, "Another bad convoy came in at 6:30 mostly surgical and a great many serious cases," and nursing sisters were busy in the operating room until three in morning. Next day 64 operations were booked, with a third convoy expected to come in. On the 4th, it soon became obvious that the medical system closer to the front was being overwhelmed, as cases came in that still had on the dressings they had received on the battlefield or at Regimental Aid Posts. Field Ambulances, and their dressing stations, only had time to determine, quickly, which could survive a trip further down the line, but lacked the time to change their bandages. Some 130 men were operated on at No 2 General that day, and the last of the 1 July victims was taken care of on the 10th.[58]

Regardless of the number of patients, hospitals attempted to remain true to procedures that had proven themselves in the civilian world as well as on the battlefield.

> The prompt and orderly disposal of patients to the wards, with the acquisition of name, regiment, religion, etc, as he passed the Admitting Officer was the first step in the procedure of admission. Once in the ward where treatment was to be carried on, the removal of the soiled uniform, the bath, the first examination of dressings and wounds were undertaken. The subsequent treatment depended upon the patient's condition. In many cases the use of the X-Ray and operation proved necessary; in others, investigation through the Laboratory; and, just as in a civil hospital, the facilities of the various departments were utilized in any combination required to establish diagnosis and promote treatment. During the busy period in July, fifty operations per day was a common record, with seventy examinations with X-Ray, and a still higher number of investigations in the Laboratory. In the wards innumerable dressings were done, splints applied, various details of treatment and matters of diet arranged. Some patients with trivial wounds would be sent from Hospital to a Convalescent Depot; others, with more severe wounds, were sent to England;

56. *A History of No 7 (Queen's) Canadian General Hospital* (1917), 15.
57. NA, RG 9, III, v.5034, War Diary of Matron, 2 Cdn Gen Hosp, 2 July 1916.
58. NA, RG 9, III, v.5034, War Diary of Matron, 2 Cdn Gen Hosp, 3-10 July 1916.

a large proportion had their treatment continued in Hospital for a period of three or four weeks. By such stages, then, work was carried on. The picture was ever changing. At one time ambulances were stringing in bearing sick and wounded; at another men were being congregated on stretchers at a central point for transfer to England; and always there were the long rows of wards with neatly aligned beds along either side, each with its occupant, with Nurses and Orderlies pursuing their beneficient tasks.[59]

There was no report, however, on the fatality rate, or whether it was any higher due to the pressures of having to treat so many patients in so little time.

Responsibility for the sick, wounded, and injured did not, however, end with the evacuation of the survivors. The main role (in the eyes of military authority) of the medical practitioner in war being to return soldiers to the fighting as soon as possible, doctors in convalescent hospitals and other institutions performed their own form of triage, dividing up their patients into those who could go back to battle, those who could serve in some non-combatant capacity, and those who were no longer capable of carrying out any kind of military duty. In the days of the battle at Mount Sorrel and the Somme offensive, the chief officer tasked for such work was the awkwardly named Assistant Inspector of Drafts and Dentistry, his main instrument a standing board made up of himself and two medical officers, one of them a specialist in eye and ear cases. Operating at Etaples, in France, with a total staff of 21, he not only checked out those who had been evacuated from the front, but reinforcements as well, many of the latter having somehow been accepted as totally fit for military service when the reality of their situation was otherwise.[60] In 1916, 3651 new arrivals from Canada were deemed unfit for the trenches.[61]

The British offensives of 1916 gradually petered out in the mud of the Somme in November, where the 4th Canadian Infantry Division suffered its baptism of fire. It was then time to prepare for the next big push, which for the Canadian Corps meant moving to the base of Vimy Ridge, in France, where it remained during the winter of 1916-1917. In the routine of trench raids, artillery bombardments, and sundry other warlike incidents of the period, casualties were much lighter than during the previous campaigning season, though some of them could be horrific all the same. For even if medical practitioners, sanitary personnel, officers, and NCOs had gone a long way towards mitigating the effects of communicable diseases, there was still much to be done towards defeating the infections that could attack wounds, especially gas gangrene.

59. *A History of No 7 (Queen's) Canadian General Hospital* (1917), 20.
60. NA, RG 37, D357, v.XII, 1916.
61. NA, RG 24, v.1066, HQ 54-21-34-27, Unfit Enlisted for Service Overseas, 1916.

The war on the western front was fought, in a large degree, on farmland that had been well-fertilized with manure, and its accompanying bacteria, for decades or centuries. The result, according to Canada's official medical historian of the conflict, was that nearly all wounds were infected.[62]

The problem was no surprise to Canadian medical practitioners, since as early as 1914 reports from the front emphasized, in technical language that still left room for horror, how "The ordinary pyogenic [or pus-causing] organisms are conspicuous by their absence, or at least by their unexpected rarity, but their place is taken by the deadlier anaerobes [which flourish in the absence of oxygen], such as the bacilli of tetanus, malignant oedema [fluid accumulation in organs], and the aerogenes capsulatus [one of the causes of gas gangrene]. Moreover there would seem to be at least one anareobe which is causing gangrene and which is new to experienced bacteriologists. Certainly it is difficult to identify it with known forms. The explanation offered is the intensive cultivation of the soil in France and Belgium; such a soil everywhere thoroughly manured for centuries past, constitutes a congenial habitat for the anaerobic organisms."[63] Further, as one editorial in the *Canadian Medical Association Journal* noted, "In the present war the wounds that come under treatment in the base hospitals are, in one respect at least, very similar to those met in the American Civil War and the Franco-Prussian War: they are all infected, and for the most part heavily infected,"[64] so that the problem should have had a ring of familiarity about it.

A heavier reliance on artillery aggravated the situation, however, shrapnel and shell fragments creating injuries in which infection was all but inevitable, as H.E. Munroe explained.

> The sinus tract is very irregular, as muscle fibres cut at different levels, retract unevenly. If the sinus is parallel to the muscular fibres the sheath of the muscle may be torn, causing rupture of the muscle into and obliteration of the sinus tract at different points in its course. This interferes with drainage, has a tendency to produce a closed cavity causing the rapid incubation of bacteria. If bone is encountered by the portion of shrapnel you will invariably get cavities leading in various directions from the main sinus. In many cases portions of clothing, varying in size, are carried in with the shrapnel the full length of the sinus. These particles of clothing are covered with the highly-fertilized germ-laden soil found in France, which accounts for every shrapnel wound being septic.[65]

62. Andrew Macphail, *The Medical Services* (Ottawa, 1925), 268.
63. "The Wounded," *Canadian Medical Association Journal* (December, 1914).
64. "War Wounds—The Prevalence of Infection—Treatment," *Canadian Medical Association Journal* (August, 1915).
65. H.E. Munroe, "Remarks on the Character and Treatment of Wounds in War," *Canadian Medical Association Journal* (November, 1915).

A possible, two-fold solution emerged in the course of 1915 and 1916: first, it was necessary to cut away all damaged tissue that might serve as a culture medium for bacteria, in a process call debridement; second, the wound was left open to drain.[66] As the 1914 article in the *Canadian Medical Association Journal* had explained, the enemy thrived in the absence of oxygen, so allowing air access to the wound could only be beneficial.

Thus, though against some micro-organisms, like tetanus, doctors and nurses were armed with the necessary weapons in the form of serum, against gas gangrene there was no such chemical defence, and the symptoms of this affliction were nothing short of horrific. As they broke down human tissue bacteria released gas that caused the area to bloat; huge ulcers could result, in some cases of abdominal injury exposing the entire stomach and digestive tract, killing the patient in a most agonizing manner. If debridement and drainage offered effective countermeasures, just as important was good nursing, which ensured the patient was kept strong enough so his own immune system could then take on the task of destroying the invader.[67] The battle began long before the patient started treatment, however, and whether it was won or lost depended in no small way on how quickly a wounded soldier was evacuated from the scene of infection; for gas gangrene could begin its grim work within hours of entering the body. To give one example, when two Canadians died of the affliction near the end of 1916, Number 2 Field Ambulance, responsible for the sector in which they had been wounded, was called upon to investigate. Its report was to cover the date and hour they were wounded, when they were first admitted to the dressing station, and how and why they were evacuated. The unit's explanation sheds light not only on how quickly the bacterium could begin to cause havoc, but on how patients were triaged, even in quiet periods. One of them, a Private Morby, was wounded before noon on 19 December 1916 and admitted to the main dressing station at about 5 p.m. A Private Wyatt received his wound about 12:30 but did not arrive until 11 a.m. the following day, almost 24 hours later. The medical officer in charge at the time deemed that the condition of the two men "was not such as to justify their removal or their being considered cases for Urgent Operation on the night of 19th & 20th December or forenoon of 20th December as they were at that time moribund."[68]

66. H.E. Munroe, "Remarks on the Character and Treatment of Wounds in War," *Canadian Medical Association Journal* (November, 1915); Edward A. Archibald, "A Brief Survey of Some Experiences in the Surgery of the Present War," *CMAJ* (September, 1916).
67. Woods Hutchinson, *The Doctor in War* (Boston, 1918), 137-139.
68. NA, RG 9, III, v.4546, 1-9, DDMS Cdn Corps to No 2 Fd Amb, 2 January 1917; OC 2 Fd Amb to ADMS 1 Div, 7 January 1917.

Their wounds considered too severe to allow immediate evacuation, they subsequently died of the gas gangrene that then developed.

Perhaps a cure lay with more extreme methods, such as those developed by Docteur Alexis Carrel. As described by an American proponent of the technique, it rid the body of bacteria by "first, depriving them of the food on which they could live; second, poisoning them as fast as they came out of the walls of the wound, before they could begin multiplying or get a first foothold." Like other armies, the French were dealing with a problem not usually faced in civilian life; whereas since the days of Lister surgeons had sought to operate aseptically, keeping germs out of the wounds they created, on the battlefields of France and Belgium patients arrived with injuries already infected, forcing a return to the use of chemicals to cleanse them. To do so, Carrel devised a system of tubing, some of it perforated with small holes, which could be snaked into the various corners and sinuses of a wound to irrigate it with a suspension of chloride of lime (now still used as bleach) in water. To avoid having the chemical pouring out of the wound into the bedding and onto the floor, doctors could simply flush the injury at intervals instead of relying on a constant flow.[69]

The British and Canadians, however, chose not to adopt the method, though it had been successful in trials. Andrew Macphail, Canada's official historian of the medical corps in the First World War, suggested that

> The hardest lesson the medical services had to learn was, that a method of treatment which yielded excellent results in one set of conditions might be a menace where those conditions did not prevail, and that theoretical perfection could easily turn to disaster. The most logically perfect method of dealing with an infected wound is to keep the deeper parts constantly flooded with an antiseptic solution... but it was not generally applicable for English needs, and the British hospital system could not be completely changed to meet the demands of one special form of treatment.
>
> Crowded against the coast, the British Army had not an area sufficient to contain the required hospitals, and there was always the remote fear that even Calais and Boulogne might have to be evacuated. For the wounded there was therefore a long line from field ambulance, to casualty clearing station, through the base in France to the base in England. In ambulance trains and hospital ships it was quite impossible to observe the meticulous routine by which alone a constant irrigation was maintained, and as a result the cases would arrive with foul wounds packed with tubes which were filled with pus. Even at the advanced base in a general hospital there could not be enough nurses devoted to so exacting a system.[70]

69. Woods Hutchinson, *The Doctor in War* (Boston and New York, 1918), 149, 150, 153, 156, 160.
70. Andrew Macphail, *The Medical Services* (Ottawa, 1925), 107, 111-112.

Macphail's explanation is not entirely satisfactory, however, as the British hospital system, once a patient was well behind the lines, was comparable to the French in staffing and sophistication. But whether the variance in techniques made any difference is impossible to determine at this late date, no studies comparing the two having been carried out, and fatality statistics being pretty much the same in both French and British armies.

In treating a different affliction, trench foot (what would now be called immersion foot), there was far greater unanimity. The condition arose from a combination of cold and dampness, and in its most severe form could become gangrenous. Thankfully, the Canadian Contingent missed the first winter of the war, in 1914-15, and was thus able to learn from the BEF without actually having to experience trench foot's worst effects. By the time the Canadians faced their first winter on the western front, much in the way of preventive procedures was already in place, following the recognition that the condition was "brought on much more rapidly when the blood circulation in the feet and legs is interfered with by the use of tight boots, tight puttees, or the wearing of anything calculated to cause constriction of the lower limbs."[71] Prevention could be a matter of improving drainage in trenches so it would be easier to keep feet dry (a measure necessary for better sanitation in any case), reducing the time spent in such defences, "as far as military situation permits," and by providing hot food and facilities for washing and drying feet. Discipline also had a role to play, certain procedures being carried out unremittingly and under the strictest supervision, i.e. "Before entering the trenches, feet and legs will be washed and dried, then well rubbed with whale oil or anti-frostbite grease, and dry socks put on. It is of the utmost importance that whale oil or anti-frostbite grease should not merely be applied, *but thoroughly rubbed in until the skin is dry.* Unless this precaution is systematically carried out the oil and grease become in great measure valueless."[72] By the winter of 1916-17, as the Canadians prepared to storm Vimy Ridge, it was standard for all wounded men to be checked for frost bite or trench foot[73] so the effectiveness of the above procedures could be monitored. Thus by early 1917 it had been reduced from being a major problem to a largely-controllable nuisance, thanks to making everyone responsible for dealing with the condition, from medical officers to infantry NCOs to stretcher bearers.

71. NA, RG 9, III, v.4551, 1-4, GRO 1275, Chilled Feet and Frostbite, Prevention of, 28 November 1915.
72. NA, RG 9, III, v.4551, 1-4, GRO 1275, Chilled Feet and Frostbite, Prevention of, 28 November 1915.
73. NA, RG 9, III, v.4551, 1-4, DMS to DsDMS, 9 February 1917.

The latter have been faceless and voiceless so far in this account, and it is only in discussing the medical arrangements prior to the assault on Vimy that we come across letters penned by one of these soldiers, identified only as R.A.L. Along with the nursing sister, the stretcher bearer has become a legendary figure in Canadian military history, complementing her selfless heroism in the wards with his bravery on the battlefield, but if R.A.L. is to be believed how he was viewed by his comrades at the time is somewhat more ambiguous. In December, 1916, his battalion, unfortunately unidentified, asked for volunteers to train on machine guns, but he admitted that "I want to get a job as Battn stretcher bearer. It's a rotten job, of course, and nobody wants it; but I rather think I would be more use binding up wounds than I would be just carrying a gun in the ordinary way. I got quite a little experience in the ward at Boulogne, which will be a lot of help. Moreover, I think it's interesting—much more so than merely being in the line."[74] The following March, he gave further details on the status of his position. "I particularly hope they make me a stretcher bearer; but they may not. There's no honour in the damn job, and no chance of advancement, or anything but work. But I like the work and I understand it a little, while I hate looking after a beastly gun and forming fours and all that."[75]

Why a stretcher-bearer might be unpopular is subject for conjecture, but probably has to do with the timing of R.A.L's seeking the task; in periods of static warfare his role was more one of returning malingerers to duty than rescuing wounded on the battlefield. It was only in combat that other members of the battalion would be appreciative of his efforts, for his role in ensuring their survival was crucial. As R.J. Manion explained,

> It must be remembered that in actions of a severe nature, such as great advances, the first object of advancing troops is to obtain their objective and to hold it. Therefore care of the wounded may not be possible till the action is over. But during these hours the wounded are by no means without attention. It is here that the battalion stretcher bearers do their finest and most self-sacrificing work. They go over the top with the fighting troops, and as the men are hit it is their duty to give them first aid, while the fight still goes on, with machine-gun bullets whistling by their ears and shells bursting all about them. Their duty it is, and nobly they perform it, to dress the wounded, stop bleeding if possible, and temporarily set fractures. Then they place the wounded men in the most protected side of a shellhole, or in any other sheltered spot, and pass on

74. RAL, *Letters of a Canadian Stretcher Bearer* (Toronto, 1918), December 1916.
75. *Ibid*, 3 March 1917.

to the next needy one, after placing any bit of available rag on a stick or old bayonet to attract the attention of the field clearing parties who come over that area.[76]

In ministering to their comrades, stretcher-bearers had little in the way of supplies, R.A.L. writing that he did not even carry morphine, but only "bandages, dressings (shell and field), iodine which I splash liberally on every wound [ouch!], a pair of scissors,"[77] and little else.

In 1917 it was the battalion medical officer (or regimental medical officer—RMO) at the RAP who gave a dose of morphine if pain was severe; he also stopped any haemorrhaging and made the patient as comfortable as circumstances allowed. The next step was to hand him over to the stretcher bearers of a field ambulance unit, who usually lived in an adjoining dug-out awaiting the doctor's orders. These carried the patient to an advanced dressing station, or, if the distance was too great, to a relay post, where other hands took over. As R.J. Manion later related, "The ADS is usually situated a mile or so in the rear of the trenches, preferably in a large cellar, but at any rate in a fairly well sheltered area where cots are ready to receive fifty or more patients. At the ADS one or two of the medical officers of the field ambulance are stationed with a large staff of men. The patient is here made comfortable; given coffee or cocoa; name, number and battalion recorded; and finally he is inoculated with an anti-tetanic serum."[78]

When convenient and safe, usually after dark, the wounded soldier was moved by ambulance to a main dressing station, a trip of two or three miles. Located in a chateau, group of huts, or in tents if the weather was mild, the MDS accommodated light cases until these could be returned to the front, transferring more serious problems, such as a shattered leg or large flesh wound, to a Casualty Clearing Station, two to four miles further along and outside the Corps' jurisdiction. "The CCS, usually in huts or tents, is the first real hospital behind the firing zone. It may have accommodation for a couple of hundred patients; is supplied with X-Ray equipment, a well-arranged operating room with expert surgical assistance, and is the nearest place to the line that trained nurses are sent."[79] It was also the first institution in a wounded man's odyssey that could perform surgery. Cases requiring such intervention were, in fact, moved from the front line to the operating room as soon as possible, the RMO, if faced with a wound to the abdomen, which might quickly develop life-threatening peritonitis, or injury to the head or chest, marking the case as "Serious" on a tag attached to

76. R.J. Manion, *A Surgeon in Arms*, 138-139.
77. R.A.L, *Letters of a Canadian Stretcher-Bearer*, 24 June 1917.
78. R.J. Manion, *A Surgeon in Arms*, 134-135.
79. R.J. Manion, *A Surgeon in Arms*, 136.

the soldier's clothing. Those identified in such manner were rushed to the ADS, where ambulances picked them up for direct evacuation to the CCS.[80]

Shell shock, or psychological casualties, were not so straight-forward. In fact, according to Tom Brown, who studied the condition within the Canadian Expeditionary Force in some detail, it was "the storm centre of military medicine" at that time.[81] The expression "shell shock" first entered the medical vocabulary, or so it would seem, on 13 February 1915, in a *Lancet* article by Charles S. Myers of the Royal Army Medical Corps. His view fit neatly into a paradigm that might be said to date to 1844, when Wilhelm Griesenger declared that "all mental diseases are brain diseases," so that Myers could refer to the First World War manifestation as "traumatic neurosis." This theory, that insanity and other psychological disorders were the result of organic damage, did not go unchallenged, however, Sigmund Freud and others, in pre-war days, having convinced many of their colleagues that the psychological was a non-physical sphere of human experience.[82]

In the first few years of the war, according to Brown, the British Expeditionary Force did not treat the issue as being of great importance one way or the other, so that "During 1915 and 1916 it was standard procedure in the British Army to move suspected shell-shocked cases rapidly from the Regimental Aid Posts and Casualty Clearing Stations at the front to the Base or Stationary Hospitals on the French coast for sorting, and directly to England for treatment, where a large majority, it appears, were discharged as unfit for further active service."[83] The campaign on the Somme, however, with its 59,000 casualties the first day (20,000 of them dead) and its subsequent losses numbering in the hundreds of thousands, forced a change within the British military hierarchy, of which the Canadian Expeditionary Force was a part. It became crucial for the sake of the war effort to return as many wounded soldiers as possible back to the fighting, including those whose injuries were of the mind.

Advice on how to do so came from many quarters. One who presented his case in the *Canadian Medical Association Journal* was Captain Edward Ryan, of the CAMC, who described in detail the case of an individual of the Canadian Mounted Rifles. Landing in France on 26 May, 1916, on 1 June a shell blew in his dug-out, killing all his

---

80. R.J. Manion, *A Surgeon in Arms*, 136.
81. Tom Brown, "Shell Shock in the Canadian Expeditionary Force, 1914-1918: Canadian Psychiatry in the Great War," Charles G. Roland, ed, *Health, Disease and Medicine: Essays in Canadian History* (Toronto, 1983), 308.
82. *Ibid*, 309, 311-312, 314.
83. Tom Brown, "Shell Shock in the Canadian Expeditionary Force," 315.

companions and rendering him unconscious for a time. "On recovering, his ears were ringing and his voice was very low. He crawled back to a machine gun which he turned on the enemy. Another shell blew him up and he again lost consciousness. When he came to, he was being taken to a dressing station. He had a violent headache and was completely deaf and mute." In the days that followed, his symptoms included weeping, hints of suicide, and continuing deafness, but Ryan, being a member of the psychological rather than the physiological school, refused to attribute these to the original explosion, insisting that "it is now generally conceded that the condition is purely psychic."[84]

There was, of course, still the view that such problems were physical, one practitioner, Lord Sydenham, having conducted extensive studies on the effects of explosive shock waves on the brain. "It is, or may be supposed, that the dendrons of the cerebral cells are temporarily paralyzed and the association tracts are thrown out of adjustment, if only temporarily. It is also suggested that pressure is exerted on the cerebrospinal fluid causing oedema [unusual fluid accumulation] of the cerebral cells with the consequent diminution of function," but Ryan would have none of it. In true Freudian fashion (though it is unknown if he was in fact a Freudian), he insisted that other influences, either inherited from his parents or acquired in the course of his life, determined whether an individual would suffer shell shock or not. In the latter category, he described "lowered resistance due to alcoholism, syphilis, or previous disease or head injury," or "nervous exhaustion due to mental stress, anxiety, insomnia, terrifying dreams, etc," and finally "bodily exhaustion from heat, cold and hunger, etc." Further, "In many of the cases I have seen in the various hospitals the ear marks of degeneracy were observable and the histories of the cases confirmed the observations... In our own wards at present two cases had syphilis, one a serious head injury, for nearly eighteen months two had been free drinkers, and one was a congenital defective. These cases will not stand the strain, they go down and out very early in the game."[85] As for treatment, "It is of course essential that they be taken early... The idea of injury must be removed and all influences that will contribute to that end should be employed... We have used the hot packs, hot baths, continuous baths, alcohol rubs and massage with very good results. Rest in bed with forced feeding is always essential. We have not found that anaesthesia

---

84. Captain Edward Ryan, CAMC, "A Case of Shell Shock," *Canadian Medical Association Journal* (December, 1916).
85. *Ibid.*

has been of any service." The patient he used as a case study reacted well to such a regimen, and regained his hearing.

In the months following the above report, during the spring and summer of 1917, the British established the basic infrastructure for dealing with such casualties, forming five "neurological hospitals" staffed with neurologists or psychiatrists, one for each of their armies fighting on the Western Front.[86] At the same time, the physical theory of brain injury continued to lose influence, the result of reports like that of Captain H.P. Wright of the CAMC. In a July 1917 article, he reported that "Shell shock has been defined as the symptoms produced by exposure to the forces generated by the explosion of high explosives without visible injury. This is the only definition that I have ever heard given to shell shock, and while I have no quarrel with it as far as it goes, my only concern is that it does not go far enough."[87] He recommended four classifications, being shell concussion, shell hysteria, shell neurasthenia, and simple malingering. The first was a straight-forward physical injury caused by an explosion, an admission that such "events" could in fact lead to "traumatic neurosis," while the last was a disciplinary issue where soldiers faked symptoms so as to leave the front line, though diagnosis could be extremely difficult.

Distinguishing between the other two conditions, hysteria and neurasthenia, was no easy matter, however. Both were cases where "the "will" seems to have lost control of the brain" and they shared a common psychic cause. Potential factors in the former were hereditary mental instability, acquired mental instability, and alcoholism, and "seldom occurs in a veteran of some months standing." The latter was "A condition of bodily and psychic asthenia as a result of the exigencies of active service," in an individual who normally kept himself under control.

> However, after months, the struggle is too much for him and he succumbs to nervous and bodily exhaustion, and the result is the typical neurasthenic. Neurasthenia, in a man who has put up a good fight for some months under trying circumstances, is an unreasonable disease with a reasonable cause—and I would go further, and say that shell neurasthenia would almost certainly result in any one of us if we "stood the gaff" long enough. It is only by the judicious withdrawal of battalions, etc, from the front line to billets, where they may rest and recuperate, that the British Army is saved from being an army of neurasthenics.[88]

---

86. Tom Brown, "Shell Shock in the Canadian Expeditionary Force," 316.
87. Captain H.P. Wright, CAMC, "Suggestions for a Further Classification of Cases of So-called Shell Shock," *Canadian Medical Association Journal* (July, 1917).
88. Captain H.P. Wright, CAMC, "Suggestions for a Further Classification of Cases of So-called Shell Shock.".

Thus the neurasthenic put up a fight, while the hysteric gave up at the first opportunity. Wright mused that in the latter case venereal disease might be a contributing factor, "and I suppose no two things age a man more quickly than alcohol and syphilis."

Treatment differed according to the nature of the condition, Tom Brown suggesting that officers tended to be diagnosed as neurasthenics while other ranks were labelled hysterics, the former being dealt with far more sympathetically than the latter. Neurasthenics were sent on what before the war had been called the Weir Mitchell rest cure, consisting of being evacuated to a bucolic setting where rest, good food, mild exercise and diversion, massage, and hot baths were the order of the day. Hysterics fared similarly or not depending on whether they fell into the hands of psychotherapists or disciplinarians; the first relied on talk therapy and similar techniques that are familiar tools of the psychologist today, the second might isolate a soldier in a small room until lack of companionship, loneliness, and boredom forced an improvement in his symptoms. Electric shock might also figure rather prominently in such a regimen.[89]

In the Canadian context claimed cure rates were nothing short of spectacular. Most psychological patients were sent to No 3 Canadian Stationary Hospital in France, where Doctor Frederick Dillon, of the Royal Army Medical Corps, claimed 62.5 per cent were returned to duty. His first approach was bed rest (with sleep induced by drugs if necessary) and hypnosis, though he often relied on "seclusion or faradism," the latter a benign word for electric shock, because "in treating large numbers of patients, saving of time and energy was essential." Those Dillon could not cure, or could not cure quickly, were sent to Colin Russel, who worked at the Granville Hospital at Ramsgate, in Kent. Claiming that he returned 71.4 per cent of his patients to duty, he explained that "The patient must be made to understand the causative factor played by the primitive emotions, and he must be made to rationalize the ideas which have been set up." Electric shock, for example, could prove, in dramatic fashion, that a limb still worked. In total, about 9000 Canadians were treated as hysterics or neurasthenics.[90]

Controversy concerning psychological conditions continued into the post-war era, so that the official history of the medical services in the First World War could be dismissive of efforts to treat them. Macphail, a one-time editor of the *Canadian Medical Association Journal* described the issue in near-scathing terms, describing how "Shell-shock was a

89. Tom Brown, "Shell Shock in the Canadian Expeditionary Force," 318-319.
90. Tom Brown, "Shell Shock in the Canadian Expeditionary Force," 321-322.

term used in the early days to describe a variety of conditions ranging from cowardice to maniacal insanity," but later, "What was once a disease had in 1917 become a stigma, and yet, as one nail drives out one nail and one fire one fire, so fear of the ostracism of contempt for weakness at best and cowardice at worst did much to counteract the emotion of fear of the enemy." Going even further, Macphail suggested that "Hysteria is the most epidemical of all diseases, and too obvious special facilities for treatment encouraged its development. "Shell-shock" is a manifestation of childishness and femininity. Against such there is no remedy."[91] Greater consensus on the treatment of shell shock or battle exhaustion as a medical condition would have to wait until the middle part of the next world war.

Such was the state of the art as the Canadian Corps assaulted Vimy Ridge in April, Hill 70 in August, and Passchendaele in October and November of 1917. From a purely medical point of view, there was little to distinguish these battles from those of 1916, with nodes in the system sometimes almost overwhelmed by the number of casualties they had to treat; the last campaign of the season, however, the capture of the ridge and village of Passchendaele, stands out because of one terrible feature—the mud. As Number 20 Field Ambulance reported,

> Stretcher bearing, heavy work under the best of conditions became a nightmare. Men sank thigh deep in the slime, or a precarious foothold giving way, were precipitated into the filth and water of the shell holes. To cap the adverse weather conditions the rain fell steadily all day, blotting out the distant view and making of the battle ground a chaos of mud, water, and bursting shells.

> The dressing stations in the forward area were, by reason of their position amid batteries and support lines, the objects of constant attention from the German gunners.

> To approach an aid post alone and unencumbered was a task requiring no little muscular effort and courage, yet day and night stretcher squads went through the danger zone, surmounting inconceivable difficulties, but ever returning to the Aid Posts and keeping them cleared of wounded. The total length of carry from the Advanced Posts to Midland House was about three miles.[92]

It thus surprised no one that five men of the unit were awarded the Military Medal for their actions during the campaign.

To add to the problems of naturally-occurring mud was human-invented poison gas. The knowledgeable reader would, of course, point

91. Andrew Macphail, *The Medical Services* (Ottawa, 1925), 276, 278.
92. NA, RG 9, III, v.4715, 107-20, No 20 Canadian Field Ambulance, October 16th to November 16th, 1917.

out that the substance was first used on the western front *en masse* at Second Ypres, in April 1915, but a development two years later, mustard gas, was a major leap in the effectiveness of chemical warfare, so its discussion is appropriate here. Of the 6000 casualties the Canadians suffered in that first major use of airborne poison, few fatalities were actually due to gas; since it entered the body through the respiratory tract and affected mainly the lungs, the substance used in 1915 and 1916, either chlorine or its derivative phosgene, could be defeated with a simple apparatus that filtered out the poison. The respirator in question, admittedly, was uncomfortable, and itself led to casualties among men fatigued by having to wear the device and were unable to defend themselves to the best of their abilities, but it was still an effective countermeasure.

The possibility remained, however, of soldiers being caught by surprise or with respirators whose filtering chemicals had degraded with time, so various treatments were devised to deal with the casualties that could result. Major G.B. Peat, writing in a 1918 issue of the *Canadian Medical Association Journal*, related how his first experience with mass chemical injuries was in April, 1916, exactly a year after they first became a terrible feature on the western front. "At midnight we heard heavy firing and could see shells bursting along a certain section of our line. About 1.30 a.m. we could distinguish the smell of gas at the hospital. At about 4 a.m. our first cases began to arrive and between now and 8.30 a.m., when our tour ended, we received sixty-five cases. Of these two were dead on arrival and three died in the receiving room before any remedial measures could be begun. There were fifteen very bad cases, twenty-five severe ones, and twenty fairly mild ones."[93] One of the worst victims was an officer who had tried to warn his men of the attack before putting on his mask, his violent convulsions a sign of how little time had been available.

The mode of treatment he received exemplifies the variety of approaches available after a year's experience with chemical warfare: he was first given atropine (still used today as an antidote to nerve gas) and morphine, as well as fifteen-minute inhalations of ammonia; then, for ten minutes every hour, he was put on oxygen. When such methods failed to bring about an improvement, oxygen was injected directly into the muscles, caffeine (a stimulant) was administered every three hours, and after he showed healthier colour he was given frequent oxygen inhalations, caffeine, and hydrogen peroxide (the latter substance rich in oxygen). After about 36 hours of such chemical bombardment, he "seemed out

---

93. Major G.B. Peat, CAMC, "The Effects of Gassing as Seen at a Casualty Clearing Station," *Canadian Medical Association Journal* (January, 1918).

of danger," returning to duty about two months later. Other victims were treated in like manner, though strychnine (an extremely toxic stimulant) was also used in some cases, as well as digitalin (known to stimulate the heart). One soldier's circulation proved so poor the doctor turned to a centuries-old technique, removing eight ounces of blood—though slowly—reporting that "In the cases I bled the blood was very dark and clotted very quickly." From such experiences, Major Peat concluded that the main approach to treating gas victims should be four-fold; first, it was necessary to get oxygen into the patient's system; second, he should be kept quiet; third, the heart needed to be relieved from the burden of pumping contaminated blood, which could be achieved through rest; finally, also through resting the patient, the lungs had to be relieved of extra work while being cleared of secretions and detritus; drugs, as mentioned above, were called for to achieve the latter.[94]

Doctors thus seemed to have an appropriate chemical arsenal at their disposal in dealing with gas victims, but as with so much else on the western front even the best treatment systems could be overwhelmed by numbers. The next major attack Major Peat had to deal with was on 17 June, also in 1916, which created an appalling 420 gas victims. One had already succumbed by the time he arrived at the Casualty Clearing Station, while another died while being admitted; the remainder were treated in accordance with the lessons of the previous year, though for many it proved to be insufficient. "We noticed that a number had the lips covered with froth. This was a bad prognostic sign, all of such cases dying, mostly the first day."[95] Seventeen died within 24 hours, though 300 were deemed in good enough condition to be sent further back down the line. For the remainder, "The agony suffered by this group of cases was intense and the scene was the most gruesome one could imagine, whilst the sounds of suffering were horrible, and the evidently hopeless outlook for so many of them made it most discouraging for us. One would be at the end of the ward, give some orders about a patient, go to the other end of the ward, then get called back to the first patient, and get there in time to see a gush of froth and serum followed by death in a moment or two."[96] Twenty more died on the 18th, five the following day, and two on the 20th, for a total of 44 fatalities while under treatment, or almost 15 per cent of those admitted.

As if such statistics were not bad enough, mustard gas was introduced on the Western Front in 1917. It differed from previously-used agents in that it could cause damage even if the intended victim was

94. *Ibid.*
95. Major G.B. Peat, CAMC, "The Effects of Gassing as Seen at a Casualty Clearing Station," *Canadian Medical Association Journal* (January, 1918).
96. *Ibid.*

wearing a protective mask; for it was a blistering agent which attacked not just the lungs but the flesh as well. Counter-measures were thus problematic, and medical practitioners found themselves with far more chemical casualties than in previous years; in the month-and-a-half following 1 February, 1918, for example, a period in which there were no major campaigns on the western front, the matron for Number 2 Field Hospital reported several convoys of such patients. One group of 324 was made up "chiefly" of light chemical casualties, while another of 226 was described simply as "gas cases", in numbers heretofore unheard of.[97] At first, treatment was somewhat hit and miss, but was based on common sense and experience with similar symptoms of blistering such as second degree burns. The Director Medical Services for British First Army, for example, related how "On admission, the patient's clothes are removed, and he is given a bath, plenty of soap being used; the alkali in the soap allays the irritation and prevents subsequent blistering. After this, the whole body should be sponged with a solution of Bicarbonate of Soda, special attention being paid to flexures, and regions where sweating is excessive. The patient is then put into a suit of pajamas."[98] He further suggested that, weather permitting, "Patients should be treated in marquees without side walls, or in the open air."

Mustard gas was not the only danger to be added to the western front in the last year of the war—so was aerial bombing, which prouded further particular hazards to hospital operations. Unlike artillery, gas, machine guns, rifles, or any of the other weapons previously deployed in the conflict, aerial bombs had ranges of hundreds of miles, and even cities like London could become targets. Thus general hospitals far from the front line had to prepare to receive emergency cases resulting from raids, Number 3 instituting procedures by which "At the sounding of the "Alarm", or in the event of a sudden raid without warning, the opening of anti-aircraft gun fire, two medical officers, and two ambulance orderlies will take post ... and will remain on duty until the "All Clear" is sounded."[99] Such precautions were well-advised, and in March the hospital's commander wrote "to report that during the air-raid last night, an ambulance drove up here containing four wounded French Officers, a French woman, civilian, with her baby, and an elderly woman, a friend, who was carrying the baby... The four French officers were wounded about the face, none of them severe."[100] They were treated and—when the all clear was sounded—evacuated.

97. NA, RG 9, III, v.5034, War Diary, Matron, 2 Fd Hosp, 1 February to 15 March, 1918.
98. NA, RG 9, III, v.4547, 1-2, DMS First Army to distribution list, Suggestions regarding the treatment of cases suffering from the new Shell Gas Poisoning, 29 July 1917.
99. NA, RG 9, III, v.4570, 1-8, O i/c Surgery, 3 Cdn Genl Hosp, 6 February 1918.
100. NA, RG 9, III, v.4570, 1-8, OC No 3 Cdn Gen to DDMS Boulogne, 24 March 1918.

The latter raid may have been part of Germany's Operation Michael, which was launched on 21 March in an attempt to end the war before the Americans could bring their full weight to bear. By July these attacks had petered out, and it was the turn of the Allies and Associated Powers to go on the offensive; the Canadian Corps would thus fight a series of battles from Amiens in early August to Valenciennes in the first days of November, with, of course, medical practitioners in support. These continued to carry out their dual role: on the one hand they tried to prevent disease through sanitation inspections, water and food testing, checking clothing and blankets, seeing to the provision of bath houses and delousing stations, vaccinating and inoculating troops, while isolating those who came down with infectious diseases; on the other hand, they also focussed on corrective measures, most of which have been described earlier. A new wrinkle in medical treatment as Canadians prepared to go on the offensive was the Rest Station, where field ambulances sent "Cases of minor disease, where unfitness would extend over but two or three weeks, especially those who could be up and about; cases of skin disease and scabies, cases requiring correction of vision,"[101] so they would not be sent to a CCS or even further to the rear, where they could be lost to the Corps for some time.

Also gaining currency in the middle part of 1918 were attempts to alleviate shock by administering blood products, though such procedures had a history going back several years. As surgeon Norman Guiou later recalled, "Captain D.E. Robertson of the First Canadian Division had done a blood transfusion in the 3rd Field Ambulance Main Dressing Station at Albert on the Somme in the fall of 1916." Adopting civilian techniques then under development, he used an apparatus "sent to him by Dr Gallie of the Toronto General Hospital. The badly wounded man lived and Dr Robertson (then of the Sick Children's Hospital, Toronto) met him eight years later."[102] In May of 1917 the French Army posted some success with transfusions, while O.H. Robertson of the Harvard Medical Unit (whom we shall meet again) attached to the British Third Army, also worked on the problem. "Blood was collected into citrate-dextrose and stored in an improvised refrigerator consisting of a sawdust-insulated box with the blood bottles surrounded with ice brought daily from a nearby village. The blood was used with great success in the treatment of casualties in the battle of

---

101. A.E. Snell, *The CAMC with the Canadian Corps during the Last Hundred Days of the Great War* (Ottawa, 1924), 9.
102. Norman Guiou, *Transfusion: A Canadian Surgeon's Story in War and Peace* (Yarmouth, 1985), 29.

Cambrai,"[103] better known to military historians as the first attempt to use tanks *en masse*, in October 1917. Blood typing was introduced into the British Expeditionary Force, and hence the Canadian Corps, in the last year of the war.

The technique saw greater use after the campaigns of 1917, Norman Guiou recalling how, in January 1918, he was sent to a Royal Army Medical Corps School at No 22 Casualty Clearing Station. "There, lectures on blood transfusion by Major McNee and Captains Gladden and Cowell of the RAMC and Major Harrison of the Canadian Army Medical Corps, convinced me that blood transfusion was distinctly feasible in the forward area."[104] Soon thereafter, "The first opportunity for a transfusion came at a main dressing station. A man was brought in with a shell wound to the chest. It was audibly sucking air and the man was in severe shock. It was an order to close air sucking wounds as soon as possible... The man had lost a lot of blood and was probably bleeding internally." A transfusion was carried out, "The wounded man rallied a bit, we kept him warm for awhile, but he died." It was not cause for celebration: "I was severely reprimanded by a senior officer and was told I had killed a man. This hit me very hard. Sleep deserted me that night."[105]

Obviously, Guiou rallied, for a few months later, in April, he reported how "We had our first opportunity to do several transfusions. The dressing station was set up in a Nissen hut, the stretchers were supported on trestles. There were a number of seriously wounded... One lad was brought in on a blood-soaked stretcher, with a shattered humerus—his upper arm swathed in copious blood-soaked dressings. A flicker of pulse was present. He was pale, "starey-eyed", and tossed about and pulled his wound tag off... We bled a donor about 750cc while the chaplain talked to him. If there is a dramatic procedure in medicine it is the blood transfusion. Color came into that lad's cheeks. He raised himself on his good elbow, drank tea, and ate some YMCA fancy biscuits, then was on to the casualty clearing station."[106]

Such miracles were definitely the exception, however, Guiou noting that "We were able to trace our three cases that were transfused. One died just before reaching the casualty clearing station; another reached there in splendid condition, had a thigh amputation and later died of gas gangrene." There was a lesson to be learned, or perhaps relearned. "These cases had had a long journey before they got to us at the main dressing station. We felt they should be resuscitated closer to the main

103. NA, MG 30, D187, v.35, f.7, Orville F. Densdedt, The Evolution of the Clinical Use of Preserved Blood, Medical Meetings, Montreal Physiological Society.
104. Norman Guiou, 30.
105. Norman Guiou, 31.
106. Norman Guiou, 34-35.

front." As a result, "Blood transfusion was then started in our Advanced Dressing Station." The donor was "Private Bryant of the 6th Field Ambulance," who "gave 850cc of his blood to Private A.J. Hunt of the 32nd Division Machine Gun Company (British), who had a severe shell wound of the back. In five hours he was evacuated to the Main Dressing Station."[107]

While the process was moving closer to the fighting, basic techniques were evolving. Until 1918 transfusion had relied on the syringe method, though there were exceptions (some cited above). Blood was drawn from the donor through tubing, into a syringe, then injected directly, through more tubing, into the recipient. As Guiou explained, "This method required two operators, and necessitated placing the donor close to the patient which was often difficult to accomplish." An alternative was "The citrate method," as "fully described in the British Medical Journal of April 27, 1918, by Captain Oswald Robertson of the American Base Hospital at Boulogne."[108] The essence of the system was a bottle of citrate solution which sterilized the blood stored within it. When on 22 June the CEF's 19th Battalion staged a raid, "The citrate method showed its usefulness. The donors were bled lying on a blanket on the ground in an adjacent dugout. The blood was then carried to the Regimental Aid Post,"[109] where the raid's wounded were being treated.

It was with such procedures in place that the Canadians began a series of assaults, near the railway centre at Amiens, on 8 August 1918. The battle was perhaps their most successful engagement of the war, the formation advancing some eight miles the first day, but victory came at a price, the Main Dressing Station receiving 2622 wounded the first 24 hours, then 1334, 2544, and 1615 on subsequent days, casualties dropping to 702 on the fifth. To evacuate these men, horsed ambulances followed a few hundred yards behind waves of attacking infantry and thirty motor lorries were made available to carry casualties from the MDS to Casualty Clearing Stations. A new feature in procedures was to dispense with Regimental Aid Posts, stretcher cases instead being collected at protected points marked by strips of white bandage, from which ambulances could remove them. Weather allowed the MDS to use an open field for its work on the first day of the campaign, but even it was mobile, a tent section moving up as the Corps made progress to turn an advanced dressing station into an MDS, so the latter would always be within useful range of the fighting.[110]

107. Norman Guiou, 36.
108. Norman Guiou, 36.
109. Norman Guiou, 43.
110. NA, RG 9, III, v.4551, 1-13, Medical Arrangements Canadian Corps during Second Battle of Amiens August 8th to 20th.

The Corps' next battle was at Arras, beginning 26 August, and the first day seemed to indicate that medical treatment would be carried out at peak efficiency. According to Number 10 Field Ambulance, "The wounded began to arrive in steady numbers at about 6.30 a.m. on the morning of the attack and from then onward both dressing stations were kept busy. Everything worked with smooth precision. At one end of the admission room records were kept and anti-tetanus serum administered. The wounded were then carried through a hall into the dressing room. Here 8 stretcher cases could be "dressed" simultaneously, after which they received hot drinks and then loaded into cars of the motor ambulance convoy and were swiftly conveyed to the casualty clearing stations,"[111] though only for the first few days. On 29 August, the unit had to report that

> The continued fire on the roads unfortunately had effect on the ambulances. A shell near the walking wounded post destroyed two cars, wounding some of the drivers of Nos 8 and 9 Field Ambulances, also Pte Phillips of this Unit. At night hostile bombing set an ambulance on fire just near the ADS at Bourlon. The car had a load of 4 stretcher cases and 2 sitting cases aboard. The bomb killed a wounded prisoner who was being conveyed in it, and two of the other stretcher cases died later. Sgt M.E. Markle and Pte J.W. McLean who were driving, were slightly wounded and burned, but the escape of any was miraculous as the car was blown completely over and the hood stripped from its framework. The work of rescuing the patients and extinguishing the fire was rendered more difficult owing to the overturned condition of the car and the congested nature of the road, the same bomb having killed 4 horses and wrecked a wagon, this completely blocking the roadway.[112]

Like the plans of any other military institution, those of the medical corps could begin to unravel once combat was joined.

It was not just the human enemy, however, who could create surprise and uncertainty; so could disease, and while dealing with the injuries of war the medical corps also found itself fighting one of the great pandemics of human history—the influenza scourge of 1918-19. Killing millions, in absolute terms it compared with the plague of Justinian of the sixth century or the Black Death of the fourteenth, but though 30-50,000 Canadians would succumb to the disease the very great majority of them were on the home front and not members of the expeditionary force. (According to Andrew Macphail, 3825 of those who went overseas died of disease—776 of influenza.) The CEF still had a problem on its hands, as the illness "flooded the rest station and camps

---

111. NA, RG 9, III, v.4715, 107-20, The Battle of Arras, August 1918.
112. NA, RG 9, III, v.4715, 107-20, The Battle of Arras, August 1918.

with sick" in the summer of 1918, and "The ailment was peculiar in that, while exhibiting the symptoms of influenza, it ran its course in a week or eight days. It spread rapidly and necessitated the promulgation of extensive and stringent precautionary orders to prevent its spread. All public places such as Unit Entertainments, YMCA Cinema Shows, Estaminets &c were closed for a time. In the latter places it was permitted to serve drinks at tables outside the buildings."[113]

This first wave subsided, coincidentally in time for the summer offensives to begin, and does not seem to have struck again until after the Armistice was declared, on 11 November. By then medical practitioners had diagnosed a variety of symptoms, some victims struck by a mild form, exhibiting fever for four to six days before recovering, while others came down with pneumonia and died; the total number of ill soldiers eventually reached over 45,000.[114] Poignantly, some men hid their ailment in an understandable wish to get home after the war, Number 3 General Hospital reporting that "Most of the patients gave a history of having felt poorly while in their forward areas but had not reported sick for fear of having their demobilization delayed." Interestingly, "The same attitude of concealment of illness was noticed amongst the Released Prisoners of War soon after the Armistice."[115] There is no evidence, however, that early detection increased one's chances of survival.

The flu epidemic of 1918-1919 was proof to all medical practitioners, military and civilian alike, that their science had limits. The First World War was, however, the first conflict in millennia where the fatality rate from disease was sufficiently low to have had no appreciable impact on operations—at least where the Canadian Expeditionary Force was concerned. As for the injured, first aid, evacuation procedures, surgery, and basic techniques to fight infection meant that almost four out of five wounded survived, and that includes those who were killed instantly; of those who made it to medical care, the survival rate was more than nine in ten. In the process, 504 members of the army medical corps were killed and a further 127 succumbed to disease,[116] but for the time being the bleeding had ended, allowing doctors, nurses, orderlies, stretcher bearers, and ambulance drivers to return to peacetime pursuits—including preparations for another war.

---

113. NA, RG 9, III, v.4715, 107-20, Passchendaele to Gouy-en-Artois, June 1918.
114. NA, RG 9, III, v.5035, War Diary, No 3 Cdn Gen Hosp McGill, Appx, November 1918; Andrew MacPhail, *Medical Services*, 271.
115. NA, RG 9, III, v.5035, War Diary, No 3 Cdn Gen Hosp McGill, A Report on the Influenza Epidemic January to March, 1919, March 1919.
116. NA, RG 24, v.1872, 13-4.

Chapter Four

The Consequences of War, and Preparing for the Next

The Armistice of 11 November 1918 did not bring the war to an end for everyone. For those who were released from the armed services because of wounds or illness it ended sometime before; for those who were seriously wounded and permanently disabled (over 69,000 qualified for pensions by 31 March 1920),[1] it lasted forever. Thus as early as January 1915 the Department of Militia had to consider its policy towards those disabled by military service, the Adjutant-General informing the commander of Canada's 2nd Division that, "As regards men returned to Canada to be discharged as medically unfit, the amount of compensation or pension to which they may be entitled depends upon the extent of their incapacitation and whether their disabilities are the result of active service, and are not due to their own fault."[2] Six months later, however, it was obvious that military authorities had not completely thought out the consequences of sending men to war, the Paymaster General noting that "It appears that many men returned medically unfit previous to the establishment of a Discharge Depot at Quebec and who have scattered all over the country"[3] were complaining of not getting proper attention even though they could not carry out regular work. As to their ailments, one list of seven men included rheumatic arthritis, rheumatism, pulmonary tuberculosis, paralysis, chronic sciatica (a form of lower back pain), synovitis (joint inflamation), and an abscessed kidney.[4]

1. Desmond Morton and Glenn Wright, *Winning the Second Battle: Canadian Veterans and the Return to Civilian Life, 1915-1930* (Toronto, 1987), 156.
2. NA, RG 24, v.1241, HQ 593-1-55, Adg-Gen to OC 2nd Div, 26 January 1915.
3. NA, RG 24, v.1241, HQ 593-1-55, A&PMG to Paymaster 6 Divs and 3 Districts, 10 June 1915.
4. NA, RG 24, v.1241, HQ 593-1-55, OA 1st Div Area to Secy Mil Council, 31 August 1915.

From this handful, lists soon expanded to several thousand patients, with over 2600 in 1915, 6600 in 1916, and almost 4600 in the first three months of the following year. Of these 14,000 men, 2891 "were entitled to immediate discharge without pension, being either unfit for overseas service and able to take up their previous civilian occupations, or suffering from disabilities not the result of service, and involving no claim as a result of, or aggravated by the result of, military service."[5] Of the remainder, most would, it was thought, benefit from further medical treatment, and so stayed in uniform, though 1975, or about one in seven, suffered from severe disabilities. Given the lesser impact of disease on military operations in the First World War it is of interest that while 177 of these men suffered from major amputations and 180 were insane, 670 were affected by tuberculosis (almost 5 per cent).[6]

Thus, in the spring of 1917, even before the major battles of Vimy, Hill 70, Passchendaele, and the Hundred Days, the General Officer Commanding one of the most urban military districts in the country reported that

> Convalescent Hospital accommodation is urgently needed in Toronto immediately as over five hundred returned invalids are now on pass because of lack of accommodation. Five hundred beds are required at once and to anticipate arrival of others it is estimated that another five hundred will be required in two weeks. These one thousand beds should be provided in Toronto where Medical Service can be carried on to best advantage. Later it may be feasible to recommend accommodation outside of Toronto when situation is in hand. Medical Service cannot reasonably be expected to be held responsible for efficient treatment of invalids without proper Hospital facilities. Four hundred bedsteads are now available in Ordnance Stores if building is provided. It is understood that City of Toronto might materially aid in providing building.[7]

With a House of Commons committee reporting that disabled soldiers were returning to Canada at the rate of 1500 to 2000 per month, Toronto was not alone.[8]

It is now unknown how far into the future medical planners looked in determining the needs of returning soldiers, but the postwar era certainly saw a continuing need for medical care. In January 1921 the Department of Pensions and National Health reported it was responsible for 5804 returned soldiers as in-patients, their numbers declining some-

5. *Preliminary and Second Report of the Special Committee of the House of Commons of Canada on the Care and Treatment of Returned Soldiers* (1917), 8.
6. *Preliminary and Second Report of the Special Committee of the House of Commons of Canada on the Care and Treatment of Returned Soldiers*, (1917), 8.
7. NA, RG 24, v.4269, 15-2-42, GOC MD 2 to Secy Mil Council, 22 March 1917.
8. *Preliminary and Second Report of the Special Committee of the House of Commons of Canada on the Care and Treatment of Returned Soldiers*, (1917), 6.

what, to 3184, by June 1924. From then on the remainder represented a near-permanent responsibility, with 3042 in hospital in January 1926 and 3143 in March 1929.[9] The number of completely blinded soldiers at the end of the war was estimated at 62,[10] a testament either to the short-term effects of mustard gas or the effectiveness of procedures developed to treat the damage it created.

For a definitive treatment of the whole pension issue, the reader is advised to consult Desmond Morton and Glenn Wright's *Winning the Second Battle: Canadian Veterans and the Return to Civilian Life*. As they relate, policy makers had from the beginning determined that local medical boards would first examine claimants, and rely on precise diagnoses, not on vague terms such as "soldiers' heart". Pension categories, however, would be decided by a committee in Ottawa based on doctors' reports, though not exclusively.[11] "Soldiers trapped in a YMCA dugout without their respirators had no recourse for injuries from poison gas; they had disobeyed orders"[12] to the effect that the devices had to be to hand at all times. Another such example was Private Krezanovsky, who "reported that in France he had been knocked on the head and left unconscious near a railway track before a train tore off his arm." His disability was obvious and an army court of enquiry had found no reason to disbelieve his story, but the Board of Pension Commissioners somehow concluded that he had been drunk and hence unworthy of government largesse.[13]

This work, however, is about medical practitioners, and when it came to veterans of the First World war doctors could generally agree on the level of disability and advise pension boards and hospitals accordingly. In dealing with injuries to the human mind, however, there was nothing resembling unanimity, with practitioners at the Department of Soldiers Civil Re-establishment, responsible for getting veterans back to work, taking a different tack from those of the Pension Commissioners trying to determine the level of a man's disability, who themselves might disagree with their colleagues of the Royal Canadian Army Medical Corps (the prefix was authorized for the Permanent Force on 3 November 1919), who continued to take responsibility for anyone still in uniform. As the Commissioner of the Board of Commissioners complained to the Deputy Minister of the Department of Soldiers' Civil Re-establishment,

9.   NA, RG 38, v.288, Department of Pensions and National Health, Week Ending 29 January 1921; 21 June 1924; 9 January 1926; 16 March 1929.
10. NA, RG 24, v.1043, HQ 54-21-34-9, A/DGMS to Dr H.W. Paddell, 7 January 1919.
11. Desmond Morton and Glenn Wright, *Winning the Second Battle* (Toronto, 1987), 55
12. *Ibid*, 158.
13. *Ibid*, 205-206.

In a considerable number of cases it is the opinion of the Medical Examiner and Assistant Medical Advisor which is based on a thorough examination of the pensioner and his papers and only after a complete report has been received from the Neurologist that the pensioner requires treatment at the Neurological Centre. These cases are referred through your Department and come back to our District Office with a statement from the Unit Medical Director that treatment is not required or it is not considered that treatment would be of any benefit to the condition. The result of this, you will agree, is unsatisfactory. The pensioner is told by one set of medical men that he requires treatment and is persuaded to take treatment. He goes to another set and is told that he does not require treatment but should remain on pension.[14]

To complicate matters, unlike wounds to body and limb, or disabilities like deafness and blindness, the number of psychiatric cases could continue to rise even after the war was over. In the course of 1920, according to the Director of Medical Services, the number of such men undergoing treatment increased by almost 40 per cent. "Cases are constantly presenting themselves in which a nervous or mental disability is complained of or has become noticeable after the lapse of periods varying from a few months to several years since discharge from the army,"[15] requiring special vigilance on the part of doctors, the DMS warned.

One practitioner, the unnamed director of the K unit (most likely dealing with psychiatric cases), proposed a clinical explanation for those whose problems had first manifested themselves only after their return home. "From time to time is brought to my attention cases of men who were discharged on Demobilization as apparently fit and who afterwards developed symptoms of Neuropsychiatric disability. This is not unexpected, in so far as a great many men kept up while under Military discipline living on their nerve so to speak, but as soon as the restraining hand of discipline was removed these men collapsed. In other words they were potential neuropsychiatric cases from the first and the Psychosis only became evident subsequent to discharge."[16] He promised, however, that particular care would be taken to weed out undeserving cases, men being taken on strength for treatment only "when it is quite obvious that the disability can be traced to Military Service."

Thus military medicine was a more difficult task than its civilian equivalent; not only did doctors have to diagnose a patient's symptoms and determine a proper course of treatment, they also had to act as

---

14. NA, RG 38, v.215, Treatment Services, Neurasthenia, Comr Board of Pension Commissioners to Dy Min Dpt Soldiers' Civil Re-Establishment, 31 October 1919.
15. NA, RG 38, v.215, Treatment Services, Neurasthenia, DMS to Unit Medical Directors, 15 February 1921.
16. NA, RG 38, v.215, Unit Med Dir, K Unit, to DMS, 21 February 1921.

detectives, determining who was financially responsible for a soldier's illness or disability. Perhaps the most difficult of such cases was tuberculosis; for though its cause, the tubercle virus, had been known since 1882, it was impossible to determine when the agent had entered the body. Certainly a case could be made that life in the military, with its barracks and communal living, would increase an individual's exposure to such an airborne disease, and Doctor Herman M. Biggs of New York, sent to France by the Rockefeller Foundation, found an increased prevalence of TB in all armies on the western front. There was an exception however—the British Expeditionary Force—which muddied the waters somewhat in determining whether a Canadian with the condition had contracted it on active service or before joining the army.[17]

Near the end of 1917 Doctor C.D. Parfitt, of Gravenhurst, conducted a statistical study of TB in the Canadian Expeditionary Force, discovering a total of 2904 cases under the care of the Military Hospitals Commission. With a morbidity rate among soldiers in Canada of 2.7 per thousand, and a higher rate of 6.2 per thousand overseas, the total for the CEF was 4.3, about 20 per cent lower than within the civilian population.[18] There was no doubt, however, that soldiers in France and Belgium were more likely to fall sick than anyone in Canada, whether civilian or military; either members of the Canadian Corps were contracting TB overseas or the conditions of the western front were such as to bring on symptoms more often than the camps or cities of home. In May, 1918, with the war in its last year, the Invalided Soldiers' Commission explained its policy in taking care of these men. "In Canada as in other countries the treatment of tuberculosis and the provision of preventive measures has been left largely to voluntary effort... The Commission early recognized that no half measures would be sufficient and that provision on an ample scale should be made so that those who had broken down with this disease on active service, whether it was present previously or contracted entirely on service, should receive the best treatment modern science could provide."[19] It was an early example of state-run medicine in Canada.

Soldiers thus found themselves in a variety of institutions; one was the Laurentide Inn of Ste-Agathe, along with the nearby Laurentian Sanatorium providing treatment for men from Quebec and the Maritime provinces; Kingston had the Oliver Mowat Sanatorium to take care of those from eastern Ontario, and for the western counties there was the London Health Association. The National Free Sanatorium in

17. NA, RG 38, v.371, *Military Hospitals Commission Bulletin*, 30 September 1917.
18. NA, RG 38, v.371, *Military Hospitals Commission Bulletin* (No 5), 30 October 1917.
19. *Report of the Work of the Invalided Soldiers' Commission* (May, 1918), 26.

Muskoka failed to live up to expectations, so policy makers turned to the Minnewaska Sanatarium at Gravenhurst, but its managers hoped to salvage a failing investment by providing poor food and medical attention; Ottawa had to replace staff with its own appointments until other institutions became available near Kitchener and on Hamilton Mountain. Eventually the Military Hospitals Commission ran institutions "from the highest point on Prince Edward Island (six hundred feet above sea level) to Tranquille outside Kamloops and the Kootenay Lake Hotel at Balfour in British Columbia."[20]

The Ministry of Pensions, however, whose responsibility was limited to determining how much society "owed" those who had served in the Great War, hesitated to provide financial support to men and women who may have been ill before they joined up. The Tuberculous Veterans' Section of the Board of Tuberculosis Consultants had a different view, noting that "a man was enlisted as "fit". He may have had a disability of which he had no knowledge, but this makes no difference. He was passed as "fit" and his intentions were of the best. Only in the case where a man wilfully concealed a disability, or where it was obvious and had not been aggravated by service, would the man's condition not be considered in full."[21] The speaker, unfortunately anonymous, made the case for tuberculous veterans in sometimes moving terms.

> We must clear our minds of the idea that the ex-soldier should be considered in the same category as the civilian sufferer from a chest disability. The law is clear on this point. The law, in effect, agrees that "We needed you in the army. We took you from the civilian life and put you to full use under extraordinary trying conditions. We subjected you to hardships which in civilian life would have been considered sufficient to kill the ordinary man. You had to lie in mud and water. You slept in wet clothes. You worked when you were hardly able to carry on and you were subject to the filth and disease always present under war conditions. If there is any truth in disease and the theory of germs, you were forced to take a terrible risk". The law further says "We knew that most of you will suffer in the future; therefore we are responsible for any disability that "occurred" during service and for any condition that arises as the result of your service." This we consider was the right course to take, and we find today that the public of Canada continues to recognize the justice of this and only from a few quarters do we hear any challenge as to the soundness of the idea.[22]

20. Desmond Morton and Glenn Wright, *Winning the Second Battle* (Toronto, 1987), 26.
21. NA, RG 38, v.221, Conference in Christie Street, June, 1927, Board of Tuberculosis Consultants, Tuberculous Veterans' Section, 15 June 1927.
22. NA, RG 38, v.221, Conference in Christie Street, June, 1927, Board of Tuberculosis Consultants, Tuberculous Veterans' Section, 15 June 1927.

Thus, "if any condition of life predisposes to tuberculosis, weakening the individual and lessening his resistance, it is army life on active service," and given studies that showed markedly different TB rates according to occupation, the speaker had a point.

For pension purposes, therefore, a candidate could only be denied if "the disease existed on entry and has not been aggravated by service." As to the latter, "It would only be possible to deny aggravation if there was definite evidence that the man's condition on discharge was the sane [sic] as on entry, or that, in view of the short duration of his service and the nature of his environment and employment during that service, there were no circumstances that would have accelerated the natural progress of the disease existing on entry."[23] At a conference held in April, 1924, it was announced that the Department of Soldiers' Civil Re-establishment had accepted 407 cases of tuberculosis diagnosed during 1923, bringing the total number of ex-soldiers treated for TB to 10,000, each of whom required long-term care in a sanatorium.[24]

Interestingly, some of the treatments available in these institutions had been developed or gained support as a result of the Great War. As R.Y. Keers has explained in *Pulmonary Tuberculosis: A Journey Down the Centuries*, "Collapse therapy," or artificial pneumothorax, by which air was injected into the chest so the lung would deflate and hence rob the bacterium of the medium it needed to live, "had gained a firm foothold on the therapeutic ladder by 1914 when the outbreak of World War I initiated a startling increase in the incidence of tuberculosis in Europe." Greater numbers of patients "made imperative the mobilization and exploitation of all possible forms of treatment and ushered in an era in which therapy was dominated by the sanatorium, artificial pneumothorax, phrenic paralysis and thoracoplasty,"[25] the latter two achieving the same end as collapse therapy, but by other means. Phrenic paralysis was obtained by cutting or crushing nerves to the diaphragm, while thoracoplasty caused lung collapse by removing ribs. However, "The immediate post-war years saw the beginning of the boom in collapse therapy that was to dominate the treatment of pulmonary tuberculosis for the next quarter of a century,"[26] including Canadian institutions, whether for returned soldiers or civilians.

While the Canadian medical profession dealt with the disabilities and diseases of the conflict of 1914-1918, it also, though only for a short time, had to prepare for yet another war. In early 1917 the monarchy

23. NA, RG 38, v.221, Ministry of Pensions, Attributability of Aggravation, 18 February 1921.
24. NA, RG 38, v.221, Percis of TB Conference, 8-9 April 1924.
25. R.Y. Keers, *Pulmonary Tuberculosis: A Journey Down the Centuries* (London, 1978), 126.
26. *Ibid*, 158.

in Russia had fallen, and later in the year the Bolsheviks took over, subsequently forming the Union of Soviet Socialist Republics. With mixed motives that included trying to keep Russia in the war against Germany and removing the Bolsheviks from power, Great Britain, the United States, Japan, and other countries sent troops to various footholds in Siberia, the Ural mountains, and the Kola peninsula to support anti-Bolshevik forces. The campaign is of interest here mainly in how the medical corps mobilized the necessary forces to support the Canadian effort—a mobilization strangely reminiscent of the Boer War, even though it was carried out in the midst of one of the greatest conflicts in history.

In August, 1918, the Director-General of Mobilization informed the Director-General of Medical Services that a field ambulance would be required for the Siberian Expeditionary Force, and suggested the necessary personnel be gathered in British Columbia, from where they could be transported to Vladivostok. A few days later a stationary hospital and sanitary section were also authorized, requiring hundreds of medical personnel,[27] and the Minister of Militia and Defence, Major-General S.C. Mewburn, went so far as to suggest that "If men are not coming forward voluntarily rapidly enough fill ranks with men obtained under Military Service Act by selections,"[28] one of the first times it was suggested conscripts be used to fight communism. In the case of the field ambulance, stationary hospital, and sanitary section, such would not be necessary, however, many of the needed trained personnel being available in Canada's military districts. As the Assistant Director-General of Medical Services explained, "These men were not sent to Europe for the reason that Reinforcements, AMC other ranks were not required there; and transfer to Infantry Units was withheld as an evidence of good faith—they having enlisted in the CAMC and were not subject to the Military Service Act."[29]

It may seem ironic that military authorities were willing to turn to conscription to make up for horrific losses among infantry units on the western front, but would not retrain those who had volunteered for other services, but such was indeed the case. By the end of August some 55 officers had come forward to serve in Siberia, so that 14 of the necessary 18 doctors were easily found for the stationary hospital, as well as all 12 for the field ambulance. An indication of the variety of expertise necessary for even a small operation was evidenced by the appointment of Captain Joseph Race, of the Canadian Army Hydrolo-

27. NA, RG 24, v.1995, HQ 762-12-2, DG Mob to DGMS, 15 August 1918; DDGMS to A/DGMS, 16 August 1918.
28. NA, RG 24, v.1994, HQ 762-12-2, Mewburn to Gwatkin, 15 August 1918.
29. NA, RG 24, v.1994, HQ 762-12-2, A/DGMS, Circular Letter Med 206, 22 August 1918.

gical Corps, as Special Bacteriologist, and the recall from Europe of Captain A.F. Menzies as Cholera Specialist.[30]

In tracing the letters, memoranda, and other correspondence surrounding such an operation one might get the impression that all went according to plan and that the necessary personnel were gathered without a hiccup. That was not, as the knowledgeable reader might suspect, the case, as the NCOs who volunteered for the expedition soon discovered; they were taken on strength as privates, not with the rank of corporal or sergeant they had earned in the reserves.[31] Further problems cropped up after the end of the war in Europe; the Field Ambulance, for example, had 166 other ranks on strength on 7 December, but the General Officer Commanding in Victoria, responsible for assembling the force, had to report that "This is being reduced by men in hospital," others failing medical boards, and still others likely to be discharged on compassionate grounds. In all he expected the ambulance to end up 33 other ranks under establishment. "As this unit is due to sail in about [a] week may immediate steps be taken to furnish them with personnel needed who should be here by thirteenth instant."[32]

It is not known whether the necessary men were found, but thankfully the force being sent to Siberia was to ensure security of stores and ammunition and was not expected to engage the Bolsheviks directly—that task was left to White Russian forces. Thus the Assistant Director-General Medical Services suggested to the Chief of the General Staff that the chief medical officer "be authorized to make such disposal of the Medical Personnel already available as seems to him best,"[33] such as splitting up the field ambulance and stationary hospital into smaller detachments to serve a wider area. "Of course if it is the intention to have the Medical Resources of the CEF Siberia called upon to care for other troops in addition to Canadians the thinning out of the Personnel along the lines of communication might not be desirable..." In the event, the CAMC treated 2118 sick in Siberia, of whom 466 were not Canadians, in the first six months of 1919.[34]

As history recalls, the Bolsheviks eventually won, though only after a terrible civil war lasting several years and costing the lives of millions (many to typhus). The British, American, Japanese, Canadian, and other troops that had intervened in the conflict were, however, long gone by the time Lenin and his supporters consolidated their grip on power in

30. NA, RG 24, v.2003, HQ 762-17-8, ADMS to DGMS, 31 August 1918; A/ADG-Gen to GOC MD 3, 16 September 1918; DAG Pers Serv to Dept Mil and Def, 5 October 1918.
31. NA, RG 24, v.1994, HQ 762-12-2, ADMS to GOC MD 11, 17 September 1918.
32. NA, RG 24, v.1996, HQ 762-12-2, GOC Victoria to CGS, 7 December 1918.
33. NA, RG 24, v.1998, HQ 762-12-25, A/DGMS to CGS, 12 December 1918.
34. NA, RG 24, v.1872, 13-4, 30 June 1919.

the early 1920s, and with no wars to fight Canada's armed services reverted to their status and organization of summer 1914. With a standing army (if it could be called that) of only a few thousand, of whom no more than a few hundred were replaced in a given year, one might expect military doctors to have little to do in the way of recruit examinations, but physical standards in peacetime, perhaps ironically, were much higher than during the war. Having been put through his paces by a medical officer at a local headquarters a potential recruit also had to be passed by a medical board, of which "one Member should be an Eye and Ear Specialist."[35] The aim of the process was to determine, first, "That the recruit is sufficiently intelligent," which left much room for subjectivity on the part of the examining officer, and also

> That his vision with either eye is up to the required standard. That his hearing is good. That his speech is without impediment. That he has no glandular swellings. That his chest is capacious and well formed and that his heart and lungs are sound. That he is not ruptured in any degree or form. That his limbs are well formed and fully developed. That there is free and perfect motion of all joints. That the feet and toes are well formed. That he has no congenital malformation or defects. That he does not bear traces of previous acute or chronic disease pointing to an impaired constitution. That he is between the ages of 18 and 45 years.[36]

The candidate was then categorized, A for general service, B for service abroad but not general service, C for service in Canada only, and D applying to those who had already been accepted but were undergoing medical treatment. Only those in the first and last categories were deemed physically fit for the permanent force.

The reserves applied the same standards, "with the exception that, where Officers Commanding Militia Units consider that recruits who have seen service in the present War or have had good service in Canada during the present War are found to be in Category "B", these also may be accepted. In no case shall a man lower than Category "B" be accepted for the non- permanent Active Militia unless the authority of Militia Headquarters has been previously obtained."[37] (As we shall see, however, having passed the original entrance examination did not guarantee a soldier would remain healthy his entire career as a reservist.) The Royal Canadian Navy, founded in 1910, and the Royal Canadian Air Force, more recently formed in 1924, used the same standards as the Permanent Active Militia (or army), and even the same doctors to

---

35. NA, RG 24, v.6601, HQ 1982-1-109, v.2, Physical Standards and Instructions for the Medical Examination of Recruits for the Permanent Force of Canada, 1919.
36. NA, RG 24, v.6601, HQ 1982-1-109, v.2, Physical Standards and Instructions for the Medical Examination of Recruits for the Permanent Force of Canada, 1919.
37. NA, RG 24, v.6601, HQ 1982-1-109, v.2, Adj-Gen to Districts, 7 May 1920.

carry out examinations. Procedures seem to have remained in force until 1938[38] when there were some changes, notably to the section on intelligence; whereas before the examiner relied on whatever criteria had been a part of his university training and subsequent experience, new regulations suggested that "Defective intelligence is frequently associated with adenoids (growths in the nasal cavity), nasal obstruction, mouth breathing, evidence of rickets and so-called stigmata of degeneracy. Intelligence should be assessed as alert, average, or dull."[39]

One problem medical officers faced was tuberculosis, a disease which, as we have seen, was endemic in Canadian society, difficult to detect, and very costly and time-consuming to treat. Tuberculin, developed in the late nineteenth century as a possible vaccination against the ailment, failed in its original role but proved of some value as a diagnostic aid. In the mid-thirties, however, the Director-General Medical Services reported that generally accepted medical opinion suspected "The tuberculin test is of no practical value in the initial examination of recruits," because the majority of adults tested positive, having been exposed to the disease at some point in their lives. Further, clinical and X-ray examination indicated presence of the disease only a few months before the victim showed full-blown symptoms.[40] Given the small size of the forces involved, however, just a few cases of TB were cause for concern, and from 1930 to 1936 the RCN had 11 victims, the Permanent Force 26, and the RCAF only two; regionally, 15 of these 39 were from Military District 11 in British Columbia. As in the civilian population the great majority were aged between 25 and 35 years, and given the length of time most of these men had served when diagnosed, "it is very unlikely that a recognizable form of tuberculosis was present at the time of enlistment."[41] Overall, Canada's armed Services suffered tuberculosis at a rate of 120 per 100,000, well above the national average of 79.4, though medical authorities insisted the civilian figures were based on incomplete health returns. They could have added that a group numbering only a few thousand, all of whom were in the age categories most likely to show full-blown symptoms, would have led to higher figures in any case.

Among those taking care of these unfortunates, as well as others who might fall ill or become injured, were the doctors of the small but varied organization of the army medical corps, both permanent and reserve. Many of those serving in the latter, however, found that they

38. NA, RG 24, v.6001, HQ 1982-1-109, v.3, DGMS to AG, 31 January 1938.
39. NA, RG 24, v.6001, HQ 1982-1-109, v.3, Physical Standards and Instructions for the Medical Examination of Recruits for the Naval, Military and Air Services, 1938.
40. NA, RG 24, v.6001, HQ 1982-1-109, v.2, DGMS to AG, 10 December 1935.
41. NA, RG 24, v.6001, HQ 1982-1-109, v.2, Capt K.A. Hunter to DGMS, Survey of Tuberculosis in Navy, Army and Air Force 1930-1936, 19 January 1917.

had volunteered twice; not only were they giving of their free time to don a uniform, they were sometimes expected to give up their pay for doing so. This was a common approach to dealing with financial difficulties, reservists often donating their military pay to a regimental fund which could then be used to purchase uniforms, accoutrements, and equipment. Thus the May, 1921 message from the Director of Organization and Personnel to the commander of Military District 2 should have come as no surprise; dealing with a request for authority to pay medical officers to serve at rifle ranges on Saturdays, he replied that "In pre-war days, militia medical officers, MD No 2, were very glad to allow their names on a roster for duty at the Long Branch Rifle Ranges without pay, and it is suggested that a similar arrangement might now be made."[42] Perhaps in an attempt to ensure the task would not seem too onerous, he added that "If a roster is prepared, it is considered that an MO would not be called upon to attend the ranges more than once or twice during the summer."

By the mid-1920s, perhaps in part because of insufficient remuneration, but most likely because the reserves as a whole were cash-strapped and rarely able to carry out interesting training, qualified medical practitioners were not coming forward in numbers sufficient to fill available vacancies in the part-time militia. As the district medical officer for Montreal complained, "It is noted that many of the Medical Units of the Non-Permanent Active Militia are not up to strength in Officers." So, in a letter to the commander of a militia general hospital, he requested "that an effort be made during the next six months to complete the establishment of officers... Young officers with Overseas service are exceptionally valuable, but it is also desirous that young practitioners, who are just starting up, be encouraged to affiliate themselves with some Militia Unit." These men would come to the reserves with the necessary qualifications in hand, but would still require training and education to take their places in a military establishment, and to that end, "It is the intention to hold a Provisional School of Instruction, next Winter, for the purpose of qualifying Medical Officers as Lieutenants and Captains. It is, therefore, desirous that you make an effort to complete your establishment, before the class opens, in order that the newly appointed Provisional Officers may avail themselves of the opportunity to qualify." Doctors required being five for a cavalry field ambulance, nine for a field ambulance, 32 for a stationary hospital, and two for a general hospital, there was certainly room for those who might wish to volunteer their services.[43]

42. NA, RG 24, v.6255, HQ 18-35-35, Dir Org and Per Ser to GOC MD 2, 26 May 1921.
43. NA, RG 24, v.4464, 9-6-1, Dist MO MD 4 to OC No 6 General Hospital Montreal, 29 April 1925.

For any male doctor who wished to pursue a part- or full-time career in the army, the qualifications were straight forward; he needed to pass the usual recruiting examinations and had to be registered to practise in a province or territory of the Dominion of Canada. But applying civilian standards to potential military officers might not always be in the army's best interests, especially if insufficient numbers of qualified personnel were coming forward to serve. In the province of Quebec, for example, medical education was organized differently than in other regions, so that a staff officer for Military District 4 had to inform headquarters in Ottawa that "There are in Montreal a considerable number of young physicians who are Licentiates of the Medical Council of Canada, but are not yet registered to practise in any of the Provinces, although they have the necessary qualifications to permit registration... They are employed as Internes [sic] in the large hospitals, for a period of from two to three years and will not register in a Province until their interneeships are completed and they have decided where they will start practise."[44] Given that they had the necessary education, but not the paper that went with it, they were allowed to join.

At the opposite end of the scale were those who, in a sense, were over-qualified for the role they had volunteered for. As the interwar period approached its end, the Deputy Officer Commanding Military District No 13, George R. Pearkes (a VC winner of the First World War who would become a divisional commander in the Second), reported in the late 1930s that "A review of the professional and other qualifications of the Medical Officers serving in the Field Ambulances and attached to units of other arms in this District shows that the great majority of these officers are professional men, of middle age, who have become thoroughly established in their communities and have usually specialized in some branch of medicine or surgery,"[45] not the rough-and-tumble medicine that had characterized operations close to the front in 1918. Thus, "In the event of an emergency it is felt that the professional experience of these officers might be used to better advantage in CCS and hospitals than with Field units of the RCAMC." The problem in 1938 was similar to that of 1925, however, as "Difficulty is experienced in obtaining young general practitioners for the Militia. The conditions of civil life usually makes it necessary for the younger men to devote their energies to building up a practice and, consequently, few are prepared to spend the necessary time with the Militia; this applies particularly to camp training." Pearkes suggested Militia Orders be amended so under-

44.   NA, RG 24, v.6519, HQ 393-8-41, DOC MD 4 to Secy DND, 4 November 1938.
45.   NA, RG 24, v.6519, 393-8-41, DOC MD 13 to Secy DND, 4 March 1939.

graduate medical students could join as officers, but it seems war broke out before the issue came up for detailed discussion.

Clearly, maintaining a full-strength medical establishment for the military in time of peace was out of the question—and there was not so much as a hint within the RCAMC that such should be attempted; but if in the opening stages of a conflict the great majority of military practitioners were to be mobilized from civilian life, the groundwork for such an eventuality would have to be laid in advance. Thus in 1930 a group of medical officers in Nova Scotia petitioned the Canadian Medical Association to form a Military Section within the umbrella organization, given "The necessity for some pre-arranged plan for the proper distribution and employment of the members of the profession on mobilization so as to avoid the stripping of localities and institutions of necessary practitioners and specialists; while ensuring at the same time a sufficient supply of Medical Officers to the mobilized forces."[46] Such a section was also called for by the horrors of modern conflict, to ensure "Medical arrangements for civil population during gas attacks in war."

The call for close liaison between the military and the CMA was a lesson of the First World War, when many hospitals were denuded of pathologists, surgeons, or radiologists. A military section could also encourage the study of bacteriological and chemical warfare so members could become instructors, as the DGMS suggested.

> Somebody must then teach the people in a hurry how to improvise gas respirators, and protective clothing, and how to do the decontamination of clothing, articles, and areas which have been splashed by gas, how to give First Aid to those who have been exposed, and what materials should be kept on hand for those purposes. The struggle in the next war will not be confined to the areas where the troops are concentrated, but aeroplanes will carry the offensive directly to the home cities which supply the re-inforcements, and the factory areas which supply the equipment for war.[47]

For the 1932 meeting of the Canadian Medical Association, the Section of Military Medicine called for papers on "the mobilization of the medical profession in event of war," "the use and abuse of lethal gas in warfare and means of defence therefrom," and "the use of pathogenic bacteria in warfare, and means of defence therefrom."[48]

The situation as regarded nursing sisters differed from that of doctors in one respect- peacetime positions were far easier to fill because establish-

46. NA, RG 24, v.6519, HQ 393-8-167, MOs of Nova Scotia to Secy, CMA, 31 October 1930.
47. NA, RG 24, v.6519, HQ 393-8-167, Address by the Director-General Medical Services, Read at the Inauguration of the Military Section, June 1931.
48. NA, RG 24, v.6519, HQ 393-8-167, Resume of Section of Military Medicine, June 1931.

ments were smaller. In the First World War, nurses had served almost exclusively in hospitals that disappeared with the Armistice, while doctors had worked within regiments, in sanitary sections, and with field ambulances which became the backbone of the post-war militia. Thus, while in the interwar period there were attempts on the part of staff officers to change qualifications so more doctors could join, the reverse was the case for nurses; for example, the requirement that they be single women never changed, the Assistant Director for Personnel Services ruling in 1927 that a nursing sister who married had to resign from the militia.[49] Further, in 1937 the age limit was dropped from 45 to 30, while candidates still had to be British subjects, physically fit, and graduates of schools accredited by the Canadian Nurses' Association.[50]

If no more than a few dozen nurses could be enrolled in peacetime, some means of mobilizing them was needed, perhaps through a reserve list. Such was suggested by the Canadian Nurses' Association in 1927, and those whose names figured on the roll would "be known to be ready for emergency service, in the case of war or disaster."[51] The Director-General Medical Services agreed, suggesting to the Adjutant-General that "For sometime [sic] it has been desirable to have a better organization of the Nursing Services in Canada. The want of this was made evident at the outbreak of the late war, and, in a smaller degree, at the Halifax disaster in 1917, when the relief needed was furnished, in great part, by the Organization of the American Red Cross, and Nursing Services. Had the Canadian Service been properly organized at that time, it would not have been necessary for these outside Organizations to have intervened."[52] With a pool of about 7000 registered nurses in Canada, and keeping in mind that 2500 had been needed in the First World War, drawing up and maintaining the proposed reserve list was well-advised.

Administering such a file proved problematic, however, perhaps because neither the Canadian Nurses' Association nor the RCAMC had the necessary clerical personnel to keep track of hundreds of potential volunteers. As the Deputy Officer Commanding Military District 2 complained, "The list of Nursing Sisters of the Reserve General list CAMC, in this District is being reviewed. It has been found extremely difficult to ascertain the present whereabouts of many of these ladies. For the most part their files have not been drawn for ten years or more and letters sent to their last recorded addresses have been returned... It

49. NA, RG 24, v.6603, HQ 5883-13, Asst Dir Per Serv to DCO MD 7, 8 March 1927.
50. NA, RG 24, v.6603, HQ 5883-44, Draft Order, KR&Os, 24 June 1937.
51. NA, RG 24, v.6603, HQ 5883-44, Record of Conference between DGMS et al and Canadian Nurses' Association, 20 January 1927.
52. NA, RG 24, v.6603, HQ 5883-44, DGMS to AG, 21 January 1927.

may be stated that the average age of these ladies is between 45 and 50 years and, no doubt many are married or have died."[53] Resolving the issue was not easy, and when in 1938 it looked as if the DGMS was going to do away with Nursing Sister reservists, the president of the Canadian Nurses' Association protested that "If my understanding of your letter is correct, the Canadian Red Cross Society and the Canadian Nurses" Association must now face the fact that the list which has been prepared from year to year since 1926 may not be used in the event of a necessity arising for the use of nurses in the emergency of war or disaster."[54] The DGMS moved quickly to clarify any misunderstanding; the most recent roll, of February 1938, contained the names of 1883 volunteers, and the army's highest-ranking doctor insisted that it was "filed with the intention they shall be used under the circumstances referred to."[55] Further, though not mentioned in his reply, those nursing sisters carried on Reserve General Lists in their respective military districts (presuming they were better administered than in MD 2), enabled them to attend courses and hence obtain the necessary military qualifications for officer rank.[56]

The operational focus for nursing sisters was the hospital, and though they were recruited exclusively according to their qualifications, that was not necessarily the case for other staff members. Military hospitals were, after all, government institutions, and hence subject to the same harsh laws of patronage as post offices and toll gates. Just a few days after the Armistice, for example, a certain Adam Brown wrote the Minister of Militia and Defence, insisting that

> It is very seldom that I trouble ministers in relation to positions, and I only do so in the present case because the person really deserves anything anyone can do for him. I refer to Julian Boyd, who is now the X-ray operator or expert in the Hamilton City Hospital, where the wages are so low that it is hard to live upon them. He receives $75.00 a month, and I understand he is a most excellent operator. He has spoken to me, and asked me to do what I could for him in the matter of having him appointed as X-ray operator at the Brant House Hospital, where he would get a larger salary. He tells me they have an equipment there, but not set up. Of course, I do not know what arrangements have been made, but if the matter has not been settled, would you please consider him in connection with it, and if it has been disposed of, kindly let me know.[57]

53. NA, RG 24, v.6603, HQ 5883-44, DOC MD 2 to Secy DND, 17 January 1936.
54. NA, RG 24, v.6603, HQ 5883-44, Pres Cdn Nurses' Assoc to DGMS, 26 April 1936.
55. NA, RG 24, v.6603, HQ 5883-44, DGMS to Pres Cdn Nurses' Assoc, 11 May 1938.
56. NA, RG 24, v.6603, HQ 5883-44, AG to DGMS, 24 March 1939.
57. NA, RG 24, v.6573, HQ 1211-2-35, Adam Brown to Min Mil and Def, 15 November 1918.

The letter was passed on to military medical authorities, who recommended Boyd meet with a Lieutenant-Colonel Wilson, the Officer Commanding the School of Orthopaedic Surgery and Physiotherapy at Hart House, in Toronto. It is unknown whether he got a job there, but that his case was dealt with in some detail indicates how a well-connected individual could fare in a small organization like the peace-time RCAMC.

Mind you, hospitals were more than government agencies, they were also military institutions with procedures and traditions of their own; for instance, in 1935 the Deputy Officer Commanding Military District Number 3, with headquarters in Kingston, complained that "At the present time there is no lavatory for officers who are patients at the Kingston Military Hospital. Officers must go through the main ward and along the main corridor of the hospital to the lavatory adjoining the DMOs office,"[58] a situation not in keeping with their rank and status. "An item to cover the cost of installing lavatory accommodation for officers has been included in the annual estimates for some years, but it has not been possible to provide the necessary funds in the Revised Estimates. Proper lavatory accommodation is urgently required." He suggested spending 650 dollars on renovations, which were approved. In a civilian hospital, costs incurred to maintain class divisions could be covered by billing wealthier patients more, but in the army rank divisions had to be financed by the tax-payer, which was perhaps fair enough given that only the highest incomes paid taxes in the interwar period.

Generally-speaking, though, military hospitals were organized pretty much along the lines of their civilian equivalents, but the Militia was also supposed to train for war, requiring some sort of medical establishment in the field to deal with the sick and injured that were the inevitable consequences of such training. Though strapped for funding, in 1930 the Adjutant-General issued orders to the effect that each district would be provided with a Casualty Clearing Station to support summer camps, each CCS made up of four officers and 24 other ranks.[59] For cases requiring longer care in areas where military hospitals were not available, soldiers could be evacuated to civilian institutions or those of the Department of Soldiers' Civil Re-establishment. Military rank would, however, continue to be respected, officers being sent to private wards at a cost of about a third more than for other ranks.[60]

58. NA, RG 24, v.6573, HQ 1211-3-17, DOC MD 3 to Secy DND, 13 August 1934.
59. NA, RG 24, v.6553, HQ 848-8-2, Adj-Gen to CGS and others, 29 March 1930
60. NA, RG 24, v.316, HQ 33-2-245-10, A/DGMS to Dir Trg, 12 May 1921; A/DGMS to Dir Med Serv, Dept Soldiers' Civil Re-est, 6 June 1921; CO MD 1 to Secy Mil Council, 4 June 1921.

Such arrangements could take on an ad hoc quality, and on occasion could even lead to near-tragedy, as was the case with Gunner D.E. Nickerson of the 61st Field Battery, an artillery unit. While in training he was examined and found to be "Undernourished. Very pale and at times livid," with a heart murmur. A medical board opined "that he cannot undergo training without serious risk to his health and that he should be returned to his home." The unfortunate artillerist stated "that he was examined before coming to Camp, but no stethoscope was used... He knew he had a "weak" heart... His father died of "Heart disease"... He had been studying very hard at School and was very much run down,"[61] which begs the question as to why he volunteered for summer camp in the first place. Nonetheless, his statement that the examining doctor had not used a stethoscope suggested that something was not right with the system, and his case was not unique. At Military District Number 13's camp that same summer, three men were found unfit due to heart murmur or similar condition, the officer commanding the Canadian Artillery (or CA) Brigade explaining that

> Capt E.C. Smith, CAMC attached to the 20th Field Brigade, CA as Medical Officer has never really functioned in that capacity, and in spite of the request made by me some time ago, to have him removed, he still appeared as our Medical Officer on paper. When I wished to take advantage of his services for the purpose of having the other ranks of the Brigade medically examined, I found that he was absent from the district, and in fact, travelling abroad, so that another Medical Officer had to be secured at short notice. I arranged with Capt F.H.H. Mewburn, CAMC to conduct the examinations and in the hurry prior to proceeding to camp, it would be quite possible for any Medical Officer to overlook *slight* cases of cardiac trouble.[62]

The District Medical Officer disagreed, pointing out that two of the cases were not, in fact, slight in nature. His impression, "based on interrogations of Personnel coming to Camps and Schools is that medical examinations are not as carefully carried by MOs as they must exercise in their private practice, and it is possible that the paltry fee allowed [35 cents] has some bearing on the situation."[63]

The RCAF faced a similar problem—though one with far different causes. In the same way that non-permanent militia personnel were showing up at camp with previously undiagnosed ailments, pilots could come down with conditions impossible to determine at the time of recruitment. One of these was described in detail in a 1925 publication,

61. NA, RG 24, v.333, HQ 33-1-250-16, Proceedings of a Board of Medical Officers, Sarcee Camp, 17 July 1925.
62. NA, RG 24, v.333, HQ 33-1-250-16, OC 20th Fd Bde CA to HQ MD 13, 24 July 1925.
63. NA, RG 24, v.333, HQ 33-1-250-16, J.L. Potter to AA&QMG MD 13, 28 July 1925.

and can serve to exemplify the medical challenges RCAF doctors (who were members of the RCAMC) faced in the early days of military aviation in Canada. "One of the commonest symptoms which we find associated with flying is "Wind-Up". The word or expression is used to mean a variety of conditions, i.e. the apprehension which the pupil feels before going on his first Solo, the emotion of fear excited by actual danger, and loss of confidence following active service or crashes."[64] Though the statement that "All Pilots suffer more or less apprehension whilst flying" would be contradicted by almost all flyers, occasional loss of confidence was well-documented, with symptoms such as fatigue, insomnia alternating with nightmares, restlessness, and a desire for alcohol. The eventual consequences could be disastrous.

The discipline of psychiatry, which sometimes used drugs to deal with such ailments, was still in its infancy, and doctors relied on chemical-free psychology to keep pilots flying. One approach anticipated the group therapy sessions of decades later, suggesting that "If a pilot comes back to a cheerful sympathetic lot of fellow officers and describes his emotions and finds that the other pilots are passing through similar experiences, he has no objection to confessing his fear and promptly forgets it; conversely, if the fear of ridicule is present he may conceal it and the anxiety becomes cumulative to his physical and mental detriment."[65] On a more mundane level, treatment could consist of relieving strain through frequent breaks from duty, palatable food and drink, comfortable quarters, music, reading material, games, concerts; in short, the same morale builders expounded by the army, navy, lumber camps, and similar organizations. Also, however, "The value of "Religious Instinct" and superstitious beliefs in preventing the onset of anxiety stated is considerable. There is no doubt that many get a great deal of comfort from their belief that they are assisted and protected by a Supreme Being, or from wearing charms and mascots, and the assistance of an intelligent broad minded chaplin (sic) may greatly assist in keeping up the moral of the unit." Finally, the medical officer had to become a member of the team, and fly as often as possible.

Regardless of which service they supported, military health personnel had as a high priority to prepare for war "or disaster," though it is doubtful any of them thought the latter might be economic in nature. In the Great Depression of the 1930s, however, the crisis reached such proportions that the army became involved in government-sponsored

---

64. NA, RG 24, v.333, HQ 33-1-250-16, The Care of Pilots with Special Reference to the Prevention of "Wind-Up", 1925.
65. NA, RG 24, v.333, HQ 33-1-250-16, The Care of Pilots with Special Reference to the Prevention of "Wind-Up", 1925.

social engineering in which its medical practitioners would have no little involvement. As unemployment reached previously unheard-of levels of over twenty per cent, policy makers became ever more worried about what untold thousands of jobless young men might turn to in desperation; perhaps crime—or worse—communism. The solution—or so it seemed—was to gather them together in work camps, pay them for construction, tree planting, or similar tasks, and hence remove them as potential criminals or revolutionaries. The results were problematic to say to the least, climaxing in a violent confrontation in Regina between "the Royal Twenty-Centers' as these men came to refer to themselves (they had an allowance of 20 cents a day) and the Mounted Police on 1 July 1935.

The military-administered employment camps deserve a book of their own, but our interest here is in the responsibilities the RCAMC took on as a result of their formation, and how it took care of the "twenty-centers". It seems that medical officers simply treated the new organization as they would permanent force manoeuvres or reservists' camps of instruction; they were thus inspected for proper sanitation, leading to reports such as one by Lieutenant-Colonel G.G. Corbet and Major W.H. Blake in New Brunswick. "The Sanitary condition of all parts of this Project is excellent," they stated, "the Food & Rations were excellent... The Ventilation in the sleeping quarters comply with the NB Department of Health regulations... The men were in good condition, the water supply is good... I wish to congratulate through you, all the Officers connected with the project, in the manner in which they are keeping the grounds and buildings clean and sanitary."[66] As for the illnesses and injuries associated with military operations, the employment camps seem to have been little different, K.H. Ferris, foreman for Project Number 2 in one typical report informing the headquarters for Military District Number 7 that he had ten men as sick, one with a cut finger, another with a sprained finger, yet another with a cut foot, a colleague with a sprained ankle, and six men with "La Grippe".[67]

The First World War had seen infectious disease drop in importance to the point where it was never a serious hindrance to Canadian military operations, but ensuring that remained the case required constant vigilance, which came to be applied in the employment camps as in army barracks. The same K.H. Ferris who above could relate a fairly typical casualty rate in his report had, on another occasion, to explain why "the number of men sick is in excess of the percentage noted for

66. NA, RG 24, v.5914, HQ 50-11-7, DMO 7, Med Inspection, Project No 4, 12 November 1935.
67. NA, RG 24, v.5914, HQ 50-8-7, K.H. Ferris, Foreman Project No 2, to HQ MD 7, 27 March 1936.

a Project of our strength."[68] In his defence, he wrote that "4 of these cases are Measles, the Measles were introduced into this Camp by a man returning from leave who admits that he visited an infected house while away, this man was immediately placed in isolation. 3 cases of Measles have developed during what the Project Medical Officer refers to as the incubation period these men have been isolated."

The war against epidemic disease was thus unabated, but yet another lesson of the First World War was that young men—and many not so young—often insisted on engaging in certain activities even if these put their health at risk. Venereal disease was one possible result, and the administrators of the employment camps had to prepare for it, though not always successfully. The medical officer for Project 40, for example, reported in 1933 that "he has insufficient equipment for treating these cases,"[69] relying on haphazard urethral irrigations at a time when oral medications were available—if not to him. Referring to the above and similar reports, the DGMS set about determining policy as to how such illnesses were to be dealt with. "The expense of treating Venereal Disease, especially cases of Syphilis, will be large, and it is doubtful if the staff at present employed on the different projects, is adequate, nor has the time or facilities to properly treat such cases... It would seem that the discharge from the projects, of men suffering from active Venereal Disease, both Gonorrhea and Syphilis, should be considered."[70] The Chief of the General Staff, General A.G.L. McNaughton, who had suggested forming the camps in the first place, was hesitant to simply wash the department's hands of the problem, insisting that "This is a case of very far reaching policy which will require careful consideration in consultation with the Department of Labour. Meanwhile, necessary treatments should be given..."[71]

The debate that followed was interesting in that it was the medical expert, the DGMS, who insisted that men suffering from VD, whether acquired before or after joining the camps "should be discharged from the Projects and returned to the city or town where they were taken on strength,"[72] while the Adjutant-General, responsible for discipline and personnel matters issued orders "that in the case of men who develop venereal disease while working on one of the Unemployment Relief Projects they will be retained for treatment on the Project and will not

68.   NA, RG 24, v.5914, HQ 50-8-7, K.H. Ferris, Foreman Project No 2, to HQ MD 7, 24 January 1936.

69.   NA, RG 24, v.3093, HQ 1376-11-5-3, Lt-Col C.B. Russell, Project 40, to Secy AG, 10 May 1933.

70.   NA, RG 24, v.3093, HQ 1376-11-5-3, DGMS to ORG, 11 May 1933.

71.   NA, RG 24, v.3093, HQ 1376-11-5-3, CGS to AG, 17 May 1933.

72.   NA, RG 24, v.3093, HQ 1376-11-5-3, DGMS to AG, 1 June 1933.

be handed over to the civil authorities without authority from NDHQ... Any such patients may, however, be permitted to leave if they so desire. The names and addresses of those leaving camp are to be reported to the Provincial Health Authorities concerned."[73] The perceived need to keep these men away from lives of crime or civil disobedience overrode any logistical or administrative difficulties their treatment might cause the medical establishment.

In fact, in the same way that injured soldiers often wound up in civilian hospitals, employment camps relied heavily on the same institutions for all but their least serious casualties. In the case of camp employees, however, military agreements with local institutions were made all the more important by the lack of government-administered health insurance; twenty cents a day allowed little leeway for paying hospital bills. A contract with the Chipman Memorial Hospital at St Stephen was typical, wherein "The hospital agrees to provide accommodation and nursing care for all and any cases requiring admission to the hospital from the project, together with drugs and dressings."[74] Payment would be 2.75 a day for admissions, including accommodation, nursing care, drugs, dressings, and lab investigations, but not including X-rays (to be provided at 10 per cent below regular prices), ambulance service (2.00 for the first two miles and 25 cents for each additional mile, "provided roads are passable"), or use of the operating room (5.00 per surgery).

Contracts could also be made with individual doctors, such as B.H. Dougan, though it is unknown what camp he worked for. In any case, the agreement was formulaic, requiring him to visit twice a week or whenever called by the foreman; to see all who might complain of sickness or injury and provide immediate treatment; to admit to hospital cases that could not be dealt with in the camp; to arrange for the transfer of any serious cases to the nearest civilian or military hospital; to complete and sign the necessary paperwork attending each case and any statistical work that might be required; to carry out medical exams of men requesting employment on the project; to carry out regular sanitary inspections in accordance with federal, provincial, and municipal regulations (presuming such was feasible—or even possible); to carry out any inoculations and vaccinations requested by the District Medical Officer; and to supervise the camp's hospital and first aid orderlies.[75] All-in-all, a comprehensive agreement.

73.   NA, RG 24, v.3093, HQ 1376-11-5-3, AG to Distribution, 9 June 1933.
74.   NA, RG 24, v.5914, HQ 50-11-7, Contract between Chipman Memorial Hospital, St Stephen, and His Majesty the King, 1 January 1935.
75.   NA, RG 24, v.5914, HQ 50-11-7, Contract between Doctor B.H. Dougan and His Majesty the King, 15 November 1935.

Taking care of sick and injured soldiers—as well as twenty-centers—did not distract the RCAMC and CAMC (the non-permanent force waiting until 1938 to obtain the prefix "Royal") from their responsibility of preparing for more conventional military activities, the main focus of training and indoctrination, as it had been in the years leading up to 1914, remaining the field ambulance. Its abilities were put to the test in periodic inspections and one of the latter, in 1923, can serve as a snapshot of what the military leadership expected, and can also provide some insight into the different roles of officers and other ranks. Part of the inspection was to answer questions relating to one's tasks, those for commissioned doctors centering on issues of organization. "Describe the general scheme of evacuation of the wounded from the Firing Line to the Base, naming the various medical establishments involved," was one, while "Into what 3 zones may this chain of evacuation be theoretically divided, and name the medical establishments in each' was another. Three further questions were in a similar vein: "What is the organization of a Field Ambulance, and what are its functions?"; "What main principle is to be borne in mind in the employment of Field Ambulances?"; and "What is a Bearer Relay Post?"[76] For other ranks, the questioning focussed far less on organizational and theoretical issues. "Render first aid and transport to shelter; using stretcher if required, the following casualties," was one test, the injured in question being a gunshot wound to the right thigh with fracture of the bone and haemorrhage, another to the right forearm with haemorrhage but no fracture, one to the left foot causing crushed bones and haemorrhage, and one fracturing the left lower jaw. The second question was on the normal method of carrying a stretcher, whether feet or head first, and the occasions when the technique would be altered. Finally "What are the duties of Field Ambulance Bearers?" covered organization and doctrine.[77]

Obviously, and as it had been in the First World War, first aid and evacuation were the main priorities for a field ambulance at the front, and just as obviously, officers and other ranks (or ORs) came to the task with quite different backgrounds. Doctors (and Nursing Sisters, one might add) were basically civilians—or more specifically, professionals—in uniform, who had undergone all their essential medical training before volunteering for service. Other ranks followed a different career path, not beginning their medical education until after joining up and completing a course of basic military indoctrination. Though many

---

76.   NA, RG 24, v.4625, 2-3-38, Questions, Field Ambulance—Officers, 9 December 1923.
77.   NA, RG 24, v.4625, 2-3-38, Questions, Field Ambulance CAMC—Other Ranks, 9 December 1923.

reservists had experience as orderlies in civilian hospitals, ORs were essentially soldiers first and medical practitioners second, as evidenced by R.A.L.'s experiences in the First World War.

To follow the organization and training of such units in the interwar period, the 18th Field Ambulance of Vancouver can be taken as fairly typical. In its first inspection of the era for which we have a record, the 1923 examination mentioned above, it scored only 460 out of a possible 800 points, but it should be pointed out that it lost 150 points on parade square drill, which was not as high a priority for support units as it was for the infantry. In judging the calibre of volunteers the inspecting officer gave the ambulance a 45 out of 50.[78] The CO, Lieutenant- Colonel Stanley Paulin, was judged "efficient," as well as "steady and well experienced in his duties by his services in command of a field ambulance both in Canada and afterwards in France during the War,"[79] where he had earned the Distinguished Service Order. As for the officers and other ranks, "Considering the difficulties of recruiting that have been experienced, this unit has made a good start, and should in time develop into a good and serviceable unit along the sound lines laid down by the Commanding Officer. The officers are all young, active, and with good war services to their credit. With regard to recruits special efforts have been made to select from applicants only those who appear likely with training to qualify later on as NCOs."[80] At the end of the year the District Medical Officer was still complimentary, the ambulance's only flaw being a lack of numbers. Its score at the end of 1924 was 495 out of 700, having lost 125 points on the parade square.

By early 1926 the First World War veterans seem to have moved on, and the CO was now Lieutenant-Colonel A. McP. Warner, a general practitioner, as was his second-in-command Major J.R. Atkinson; of the three other officers in the unit, two were GPs and the third a pathologist. A majority of the ORs had first aid certificates, lectures at the armouries focussing on sanitation to prevent disease, first aid to treat casualties, and organization to ensure everyone worked to a common doctrine. The unit was still not up to strength, however,[81] a problem that would persist until the end of the decade, only 30 all ranks being allowed to train. The District Medical Officer lobbied National Defence

78. NA, RG 24, v.6221, HQ 9-12-5, Annual Inspection, 1 February 1923.
79. NA, RG 24, v.6221, HQ 9-12-5, Report of the Annual Inspection of the 18th Field Ambulance Unit, 23 February 1923.
80. NA, RG 24, v.6221, HQ 9-12-5, Report of the Annual Inspection of the 18th Field Ambulance Unit, 23 February 1923.
81. NA, RG 24, v.6621, HQ 9-12-5, Report of the Annual Inspection for the Fiscal Year 1926-27 of the 18th Field Ambulance, 11 January 1926.

Headquarters in Ottawa directly to have the unit's establishment increased, his petition meeting with success, so that in October 1929 he contacted the unit's officer commanding, "writing personally to inform you of the good news. You can now go ahead and reorganize your unit on this basis, and recruit up to strength"[82] of 50 all ranks.

The peacetime militia could certainly not be accused of being spend-thrift, as exemplified by a simple item all medical personnel used either in training or in actual support of other units. In the same letter announcing the increase in 18th Field Ambulance's establishment, the District Medical Officer broached the subject of instruction materials.

> With regard to your indent for 48 Triangular Bandages for training purposes I am having the matter looked up in District Medical Stores Ledger to see how many of these articles have already been issued to you for this purpose and will let you know later. You see these articles when issued for instructional purposes are unexpendable, that is they have to be shown on the books till written off, the only way to write them off is to return them in fair condition to the Dist Med Stores or if torn and useless & etc, return the pieces representing the same with the proceed-ings of a Regimental Court of Inquiry to Dist Med Stores, when they will be condemned and replaced by new ones, otherwise deficiencies duly acknowledged are replaced.[83]

As with small items, so with large, the inspection report for 1932 complaining that "The *quarters* are so *inadequate* that this unit does *not get a chance.*"[84]

The Great Depression had as great an impact on field ambulance training as it had on almost every other feature of Canadian society, many of the unit's members being unavailable for instruction as they were out of the city to work or look for work. Of the 26 (out of 50) who showed up for the 1934 inspection, however, the standard of knowledge was high, and next year stretcher drill was even rated as "*excellent*—even recent recruits made no mistakes."[85] Personnel short-ages proved temporary, ORs being recruited in Vancouver's hospitals while officers not actually members of the field ambulance could none-theless use it as an educational facility to complete their qualifications. Training thus became more sophisticated with each passing year, so that in 1937-38 the unit not only provided demonstrations in setting splints, but carried out water supply tests and functioned as a field

82. NA, RG 24, v.4625, 2-3-38, DMO MD 11 to OC 18th Fd Amb, 7 October 1929.
83. NA, RG 24, v.4625, 2-3-38, DMO MD 11 to OC 18th Fd Amb, 7 October 1929.
84. NA, RG 24, v.6621, HQ 9-12-5, Report of the Annual Inspection for the Fiscal Year 1931-32 of the No 18 Field Ambulance, 9 February 1932.
85. NA, RG 24, v.6621, HQ 9-12-5, Report of the Annual Inspection for the Fiscal Year 1934-35 of the 18th Field Ambulance, 28 February 1935.

ambulance at summer camp, operating a small hospital. In the last full year of peace, the inspecting officer reported that "The Field work carried out may be said to be of an exceptionally high character, four days being devoted to actual field work. During this period an ADS and MDS together with sanitary requirements were constructed. On the fourth training day a detailed demonstration was given by one of the Officers in setting out an operating room with operating table, instruments, solutions, etc, at the MDS for an imaginary trephining operation,"[86] cutting a hole in the skull to relieve pressure.

The medical corps' experiences in the interwar period were thus quite complex, even after the withdrawal from Siberia brought on a period of twenty years in which Canada did not engage in war, not even a minor conflict along the lines of the Fenian Raids or the North-West expedition of 1885. It was a time to think in terms of organization, such as determining how doctors and nurses would be mobilized in time of war; a time to train a few for emergency or conflict, especially those who were members of part-time field ambulance units; a time to take care of those in the infantry, artillery, or others, who were also training for war; and, last but not least, a time to take on whatever tasks might be allocated by Parliament and its executive, such as looking after the health of young men collected in employment camps to avoid internal conflict. In short, it was a time for flexibility, which would be put to the most severe test in the war Canada joined in September 1939.

---

86. NA, RG 24, v.6621, HQ 9-12-5, Report of the Annual Inspection for the Fiscal Year 1938-39 of the 18th Field Ambulance.

Chapter Five

Preparing for War

Though for Canadian historians the Second World War began on 1
September 1939, for those of other countries hostilities opened much
sooner—1937 in China and 1935 in the Horn of Africa, to give just
two examples. For Canadian medical practitioners the conflict could be
said to have begun in Spain, where volunteers from various nations,
including surgeon Norman Bethune of Montreal, offered their services
in 1936. This narrative, however, properly begins with Colonel
Fotheringham's 1927 presentation, which we first encountered in a
previous chapter. Singing the praises of the medical profession in its
fight against disease in the First World War, he related how it had done
so through sanitation to prevent typhus, inoculation to prevent typhoid,
or rapid evacuation to prevent gangrene. Shock, however, remained a
formidable threat to the health and life of a wounded soldier, for
though medical practitioners knew of the benefits of blood transfusions
in stemming the condition, large-scale storage and transportation of the
life-giving fluid proved a continuing challenge. One of the first blood
banks was the idea of one B. Fantus of Cook County Hospital, Chicago,
in 1937,[1] and the first blood donor clinic to be established in Canada
was founded by James Potter, in Ottawa, the following year.[2]

A pioneer in the use of blood transfusions in battle at this time was,
however, the afore-mentioned Norman Bethune, a Canadian communist who made his way to Spain to work for the Loyalists in the civil
war there; though blessed with an excellent reputation as a chest

1.   NA, D187, Sise Papers, v.35, f.7, Orville F. Denstedt, The Evolution of the Clinical Use of Preserved
     Blood, Medical Meetings, Montreal Physiological Society, 90.
2.   Richard W. Kapp, "Charles H. Best, the Canadian Red Cross Society, and Canada's First National
     Blood Donation Program," *Canadian Bulletin of Medical History* (No 2, Vol 12, 1995), 38.

surgeon—he had developed new techniques and instruments for dealing with tuberculosis—Bethune decided that what was really needed was a blood transfusion service. While in London, preparing to leave for Spain, he boned up as best he could on the subject, purchasing a station wagon, complete with a kerosene-operated refrigerator.[3] Why a renowned surgeon should try his hand at something medically unfamiliar to him is of some interest; like many others, he saw the Spanish Civil War as the first stage in the campaign against fascism, and so decided to engage in activities that would be seen as uniquely Canadian—surgeons were reasonably plentiful in the Spanish army, but blood transfusion units were non-existent. According to Hazen Sise, one of Bethune's colleagues,

> I don't remember exactly what the first releases were but Bethune as I say had a brilliant sense of public relations and he also realized it was extremely important that our presence should be announced and he easily made friends with a lot of the correspondents. Herbert Matthews of the New York Times became a great friend of ours and was around at our headquarters quite a lot. And I remember Sefton Dalmer of the Daily Express, a fellow named Gallagher, I think his name was. He was a UP man. We were very palsy-walsy with them and they were very interested in this Canadian blood transfusion unit you know it caught people's imaginations.[4]

Thus, over three decades after medical practitioners had made the link between shock and the need for blood, a Canadian specialist in tuberculosis treatment could still create a niche for himself in transfusion work.

Like so much else surrounding the operations of the International Brigades in Spain, Bethune's transfusion unit had a certain amateurish quality to it. The Montrealer was the only doctor on the team, which was rounded out by Sise, an architect, and Henning Sorensen, a journalist. The first step was to gather blood, no great difficulty when it was advertised as being for soldiers at the front; universal donors (type O) made up about 75 per cent of the total, with group 2, or type A, accounting for the remainder. Working in a war zone called for some difficult choices, however. "Syphilis is endemic in Spain and so is Malaria. Normal medical procedure would be that every donor would be tested for syphilis and malaria. We didn't have the means at that point. We didn't know how to go about getting this testing done and we coldly made the decision that a man would prefer to have his life and possibly a dose of syphilis than lose his life. The syphilis might be cured later."

3. NA, D187, Sise Papers, v.10, f.9, 18-19.
4. NA, MG 30, D187, Sise Papers, v.10, f.9, 28.

Furthermore, the team was "completely innocent of any knowledge of various sub groups, Rh factors and all these things that we worry about these days,"[5] which led to serious complications later on, as we shall see.

If collection relied mainly on the health and willingness of the general populace, storage and transportation required equipment not easy to acquire or maintain in the midst of civil war. On their first night's run to deliver blood, the kerosene engine on the refrigerator gave up the ghost, and from then on the team simply plugged it in whenever they ceased operations for the day. Results could be catastrophic, as Sise admitted after describing how four French fliers were transfused after being evacuated from a plane crash: "two of them died and frankly they might have died from haemolysis [breaking down of red blood cells] because ... when I finally got this blood back to Madrid, it must have been at least a week later, I put it in a centrifuge to test it and it was very badly haemolysed and would have killed anybody who'd put it into. At any rate I remember visiting those French fliers in hospital there and I remember one of them was suffering quite a lot and he kept yelling "Ah que je souffre, ah que je souffre, ah que le diable!""[6] The architect turned transfusion practitioner also admitted that, after a while, theirs was not the only such operation in Loyalist Spain, and another was perhaps superior to their own. It was on a trip to Barcelona "that we learned of the blood transfusion work of a Dr Durand Horda who had set up a highly advanced blood bank system in Barcelona from which he distributed blood to the fronts around there, the Aragon front particularly which was rather quiescent during that period of the war. But Durand Horda I think deserves the real credit for being the first man to set up a modern, streamlined blood transfusion system."[7] Barcelona being more industrialized than Madrid allowed for better equipment, Sise suggested, but perhaps experience and training made more of a difference.

Back in Canada, Frederick Banting's old collaborator in the discovery of insulin, Doctor C.H. Best, with whom he had shared the money for his Nobel prize, was working on a different aspect of the treatment of shock—blood substitutes. After declaring war on Germany on 10 September, the country's main contribution, if it was to engage in combat, would be overseas, and no means of preserving whole blood had been developed to allow transportation across the Atlantic or to more distant theatres. Therefore, alternatives were sought, Best demonstrating how

5. NA, MG 30, D187, Sise Papers, v.10, f.9, 31.
6. NA, MG 30, D187, Sise Papers, v.10, f.9, 53.
7. NA, MG 30, D187, Sise Papers, v.10, f.9, 47.

canine serum, the liquid part of blood with red and white cells removed in a centrifuge, helped dogs recover from shock. Subsequently, according to historian Richard W. Kapp, "Under his supervision Drs John Magladery and A.L. Chute then conducted clinical trials of serum from university students on patients at the Hospital for Sick Children and Toronto General Hospital. They were able to demonstrate that serum protein increased blood volume through its ability to retain water; and that in consequence the heart had enough fluid available to restore normal circulation."[8] According to a post-war history of the Associate Committee on Medical Research, "This was the first experiment in the field of blood derivatives"[9] in Canada.

Results were sufficiently promising that in December the National Research Council's Associate Committee on Medical Research provided Best with a grant, which he used to work on concentrating the serum.[10] By March 1940 the project again made substantial progress, the doctor being asked to prepare some of his product for shipment to Great Britain, which was then still gearing up for a full-scale war. As for Canadian consumption,

> In June, 1940, the Subcommittee recommended that the Department of National Defence be asked to supply Dr Best with apparatus for drying serum on a large scale. A resolution was also passed, and sent to the Secretary of the Canadian Medical Association, the Director General of Medical Services (Army), and the Deputy Minister, Department of Pensions and National Health, asking that an organization be set up at once for laying up stores of blood or dried serum for the use of possible civilian casualties in Canada. In October, 1940, a meeting was held with representatives from the Department of Pensions and National Health and the National Research Council, at which it was recommended that financial arrangements be made for processing blood sufficient for twenty thousand shock treatments, and that the Red Cross Society be asked to arrange for donors.[11]

Work continued.

Scientists were beginning to realize, however, that wartime research differed from civilian practice—secrecy could become an issue as important as the subject under study. As Frederick Banting's most recent biographer, Michael Bliss, has pointed out, the result could be strain between those who felt that certain research, such as that into

8. Richard W. Kapp, "Charles H. Best, the Canadian Red Cross Society, and Canada's First National Blood Donation Program," *Canadian Bulletin of Medical History* (No 2, Vol 12, 1995), 33.
9. National Archives of Canada (NA), RG 24, v.312, file 8, History of the Associate Committee on Medical Research, 1938-1946.
10. Richard W. Kapp, "Charles H. Best, the Canadian Red Cross Society, and Canada's First National Blood Donation Program," *Canadian Bulletin of Medical History* (No 2, Vol 12, 1995), 32.
11. NA, RG 24, v.312, file 8, History of the Associate Committee on Medical Research, 1938-1946.

blood products, should be made readily available, and those who refused to divulge anything that might possibly be of use to the enemy. Wilder Penfield, for example, at one meeting of the Associate Committee, argued in the former vein, angering Banting, who insisted on the latter approach. Hans Selye, an immigrant scientist working in Montreal, found himself cut off from funding after publishing some of his work on shock.[12]

Such conflicts notwithstanding, research into substitutes continued, as did investigating methods of preserving the fluid complete with red cells, white cells, and platelets. Professor J.B. Collip and Doctor O.F. Densdedt of McGill University worked on the latter problem, beginning their research at about the same time as Best, their first step to study the voluminous body of knowledge on the subject before moving on to experiments of their own. Collip soon had to withdraw from the project due to pressures from his other work, but "Dr Denstedt devised a solution in which blood may be preserved satisfactorily for six to eight weeks, although twenty days is the limit for functional optimum. Blood preserved by this method was shipped to Great Britain after the invasion of Europe, as an experiment, but never in quantity for clinical use."[13] Three weeks were insufficient for a product that was to be shipped to far-flung battlefields, so the work on substitutes showed better promise—for the time being.

Though the main focus of all this research was the treatment of shock, brought on by rapid blood loss (haemorrhagic shock) or severe trauma (traumatic shock), little was known about the mechanisms, especially chemical, by which symptoms were brought on. (There was no dearth of ideas, among them a letter to Banting from Professor V.E. Henderson "suggesting that desoxycorticosterone synthesis be considered, with the prospect that that compound might be useful in treating shock.")[14] Over the years the Associate Committee on Medical Research issued grants for over a dozen projects to look into the matter, and "The results of these various investigations contributed materially to the present-day knowledge of shock. Drs Noble and Collip devised a standard method of producing shock by revolving rats in a drum. This method was adopted by other laboratories in the United States. They found that some animals resisted shock, while others did not. Resistance could be built up by repeated mild traumatism, or by an increase in the protein in the diet—a kind of commando training."[15]

---

12. Michael Bliss, *Banting, a Biography* (Toronto, 1985), 288.
13. NA, RG 24, v.312, file 8, History of the Associate Committee on Medical Research, 1938-1946.
14. NA, RG 24, v.312, file 8, History of the Associate Committee on Medical Research, 1938-1946.
15. NA, RG 24, v.312, file 8, History of the Associate Committee on Medical Research, 1938-1946.

Clinical research investigated whether the loss of essential compounds—and not just blood as a whole—might be a contributing factor, as well as such issues as the impact of shock on the kidneys and other organs, or on processes such as breathing.

The problem was one surgeons could expect to deal with every day—once operations began against the enemy—so a substantial amount of field work was done as well, much of it by the Army Blood Transfusion and Surgical Research Unit. Operating at the Southmead Hospital, in Bristol, Captain D.E. Cannell and Lieutenant F.G. Kergin, both of the Royal Canadian Army Medical Corps, reported in June 1940 that it had been decided to supply only Group O, as it had already been discovered to be a universal type for donation, and its use would greatly ease administration. As in Canada, researchers sought out alternatives to whole blood, whose storage required refrigeration facilities that might be difficult to move about a battlefield. Various possibilities were tried out, including such substances as citrated blood, haemoglobin Ringers' Solution, Ringers' Solution *tout cour*, glucose in saline, and plasma, the first two proving the most promising.[16]

In their research, the RCAMC's doctors focussed on treating haemorrhagic shock, "where it has been determined, rate of blood loss, rather than amount, is the principal factor in the production of shock. Replacement of blood or haemoglobin loss is the primary condition essential to its successful treatment"[17]—challenge enough in itself. Also, "there are at the present time investigations being pushed forward to assess the value of various preparations of serum or plasma in the treatment of traumatic shock. There is no serious question of the commonly accepted fact that blood is, and probable (sic) always will be the best substance for infusion in cases of shock associated with haemorrhage—since these cases occur in war with relative frequency we may assume at the outset that there will be a field for blood transfusion," but that still begged the question of how to get the precious substance to the soldiers who needed it. Administering blood at the front posed no technical difficulties, the apparatus provided with shipments of the life-giving fluid being more than adequate to the task, but it still had not been determined whether it was wise to hold a seriously wounded casualty at a front line Regimental Aid Post, or an Advanced Dressing Station just behind, in order to transfuse blood, or whether it was better to evacuate the patient to more complete facilities first.

16. NA, RG 24, v.12,576, 11/Blood Trans/1, A Report on the Army Blood Transfusion and Surgical Research Unit, Southmead Hospital, Bristol, 22 June 1940.

17. NA, RG 24, v.12,576, 11/Blood Trans/1, A Report on the Army Blood Transfusion and Surgical Research Unit, Southmead Hospital, Bristol, 22 June 1940.

The eventual solution was to adopt British methods, whereby Field Transfusion Units administered whole blood as far forward as possible, usually at Advanced Dressing Stations or Field Surgical Units (the latter to be discussed later). Canadian research into alternative blood products continued, however, one priority project being dried serum; meant to replace whole blood, it would obviate the need for refrigeration and was supposed to have a much longer shelf life, but even after three years results were not encouraging. At the Basingstoke Neurological and Plastic Surgery Hospital, 29 volunteers were treated with the product from 20 to 27 July, 1943. "In no case was there a really serious reaction, but there were quite a large number of annoying symptoms in the group," including high temperature and rapid pulse. The conclusion was obvious: "There is evidently present in Canadian dried serum a substance or substances which give rise to minor types of reaction," so "It is recommended that an effort be made to produce a less toxic serum than at present supplied, though it is emphasized again that none of the reactions were of a really serious character."[18] Further work was needed.

It looked, however, as if the Canadian dry serum project was headed into a dead end; not only were alternatives available, some of them being produced in Britain (closer to where the Canadians were fighting anyway), but other work pointed out the advisability and feasibility of using whole blood. The NRC's subcommittee on shock and blood substitutes, at the end of 1943, chose "to emphasize as strongly as possible the need for the use of whole blood in the treatment of traumatic shock,"[19] as well as for haemorrhagic shock. The main difficulty practitioners had faced with using the fluid was logistical, but "This has now been to a great extent overcome as it has been amply demonstrated that under optimum conditions it can be preserved up to at least seventy days and still remain physiologically active. The vicissitudes of transport by plane, ship or truck can be to a great extent circumvented by proper preservative solutions and modern refrigeration."[20]

* * *

In struggling to defeat haemorrhagic and traumatic shock, the Canadian Army faced a medical challenge that had been recognized since the First World War and earlier; in contrast, the air force, in the late 1930s and early 1940s, began to face problems rarely seen before. At the National Research Council,

18. NA, RG 24, v.12,576, 11/Blood Trans/1, Report on Canadian Dried Serum, 9 Aug 43.
19. NA, RG 24, v.12.576, 11/Blood Trans/1/2, DGMS to DMS CMHQ, 29 Dec 43.
20. *Ibid.*

During discussions arranged by Sir Frederick Banting during and immediately after the Munich Conference in September, 1938, in order to determine what part his department might take, in the war that was then obviously imminent, consideration was given to the problems of protecting fliers against blackout during tight turns of the type experienced in pulling out from a dive. This effect which manifests itself by a dimming of vision ("gray-out"), loss of vision ("black-out"), and in the most severe instances by loss of consciousness, is ascribed to a failure of the heart to pump blood to the head in opposition to centrifugal force.[21]

With the constant "G' representing the forces exerted on the body by our planet's gravity, experiments involving 540 subjects, all medically fit aircrew between the ages of 18 and 35, over 5500 runs, determined that vision dimmed between 3 and 5Gs, with the threshold for blackout between 4 and 6. Unconsciousness usually came on about 1G over that for blackout, while effects in a single individual varied by plus or minus 1G. "In fact, too frequent repetition of exposure was even found to reduce tolerance in some cases... No correlation was detected between black-out, threshold and age, weight, body measurements, resting blood pressure, pulse rate, or response of the cardio-vascular system to tilting..."[22] Much of this work was carried out at the University of Toronto, starting in the early days of the war, where "Mice which were subjected to high accelerations in the centrifuge survived if suspended in thin rubber envelopes in water, but were killed, with severe damage, if not so suspended. It was therefore decided to attempt to build a suit containing fluid, by means of which the displacement of blood and other moveable structures of the body in a direction from the head to the feet under gravitational influences would be counteracted."[23]

So, as Banting suggested in a luncheon talk in London in May, 1940, with the Battle of Britain about to begin, "We must strengthen the pilot so that he is able to withstand greater gravity." When a fighter like the Spitfire dove from high altitudes and pulled out rapidly, a man normally weighing a hundred and fifty pounds actually weighed 750, exerting that amount of weight on the seat of the plane.

That is a special problem which needs immediate attention from an investigation point of view. The first thing that happens is that he

21. NA, RG 24, v.312, file 5, History of the Associate Committee on Aviation Medical Research, 1939-1945.
22. NA, RG 24, v.312, file 5, History of the Associate Committee on Aviation Medical Research, 1939-1945.
23. NA, RG 24, v.312, file 5, History of the Associate Committee on Aviation Medical Research, 1939-1945.

becomes blind. The reason for that is that the pressure within the eye is always much higher than anywhere else in the brain, and it would seem that when the blood pressure of the brain is lowered, there isn't enough pressure to go into the eyeball, and a blindness results. It is a very temporary thing, but if the rapid descent is carried out for a longer period, or greater speed then unconsciousness results—unconsciousness simply from lack of blood to the brain. One of the reasons why there is a loss of blood from the brain is that this swinging movement on levelling off draws blood to one more dependent part of the body, the abdomen and legs, and these become a reservoir of blood, and lead blood from the heart level.[24]

Aviation technology had thus advanced beyond the human body's ability to cope.

Researchers may have been quick to arrive at basic principles, but, as many an administrator has discovered, the devil is in the details, and his presence became obvious as attempts were made to build anti-G suits. One of the pioneers in such work was Wilbur Franks, yet another of Banting's students to apply himself to wartime research, building for that purpose a centrifuge at the University of Toronto. The first problem in actually manufacturing suitable clothing was one of fit, close tailoring proving a necessity if the fluid in the suit was to apply pressure to the right areas. Also, "Certain objections were eventually raised against the suit, in particular discomfort while "at the ready", and difficulty in turning to search for enemy aircraft coming from behind." With the shift from defensive to offensive operations in 1941-42, and the near-destruction of the Luftwaffe in 1944, demand for the suit diminished as dogfights became ever rarer, so the RAF chose not to adopt it. The Royal Navy's Fleet Air Arm, however, was a different matter, its Seafire pilots having as a primary task the defence of the fleet, and Franks' suit first saw operations when the Allies invaded North Africa in November, 1942. It "was found to give valuable tactical advantages enabling the pilots to out-manoeuvre the enemy. The anti-G suit received considerable operational use in the Fleet Air Arm and the objections found in the RAF do not appear to have outweighed the advantages of its use. The existence of greater operational need probably accounts for this difference."[25]

G-forces were mainly a phenomenon of lower altitudes, where aircraft did much of their manoeuvring, but higher up pilots faced problems that at the beginning of the war were only vaguely understood, though at least one researcher had no doubts as to their impact.

24. University of Toronto, Fisher Rare Books, Banting Papers, Box 20, file 8.
25. NA, RG 24, v.312, file 5, History of the Associate Committee on Aviation Medical Research, 1939-1945.

"It was a firm conviction of Sir Frederick Banting that flight at high altitude would have great tactical importance in the war that had just begun," which was confirmed by an extended visit by Dr Harry G. Armstrong of the United States Army Air Corps to the Department of Medical Research, University of Toronto, in 1940-41. It brought to the attention of researchers there certain medical hazards of high flight quite separate from those dependent on a lack of oxygen, including "aeroembolism', the formation of gas bubbles in the blood, as well as a high altitude fatigue of an obscure and chronic type. Experimental ascents to simulated high altitudes were carried out by Banting and others in the department's decompression chamber in 1940, and consideration was also given to the general physiological aspects of the subject by various researchers, Banting referring to high altitude flying as "The greatest problem that faces Aviation Medical Research Today."[26]

The University of Toronto had Canada's only decompression chamber at that time, and as Banting explained,

> We had constructed it for purposes of carrying out research, but we found it also important for examination purposes and for training purposes of pilots that have just come to us from the initial air training. Procedure is this—16 come to the laboratory, 8 in the morning and 8 in the afternoon. We run from 8:00 to 6:30 sometimes. Four at a time these young pilots are taken and an oxygen mask fitted to them. They are fully instructed in the use of these masks. They are then taken into the chamber, which is soundproof and has telephonic communication, altimeters and full equipment. The chamber is evacuated, and we set the pressure within the chamber to correspond with about 2,000 feet per minute altitude. When we get them to 5,000 feet altitude, we level off. They are then given a simple code to decipher. When they have finished (they are stopped at the end of three minutes) they are asked to write their name and address, and the regimental number, and the name "Canadian National Exhibition." There is also a medical graduate in the chamber with them, or a person who is perfectly familiar with the whole procedure, for safety measures. In some cases our medical graduates have had too strenuous a time, and we have had to put in our own technicians, but there is a medical graduate always present—sometimes outside the chamber, observing, because it is a dangerous procedure. The observer within the chamber is breathing oxygen, so that his faculties are perfectly normal. The ascent is then made to 17,000 feet, at which level we again levelled off. There is a daylight bulb in the chamber, and they are asked to observe their finger nails. They see them and compare them with the observers in the chamber, and they see them turning blue, and finally almost purplish, then their lips get blue at 17,000 feet altitude. It is explained to these pilots also that what they see in their fingernails is

26.   U of T, Fisher Rare Books, Banting Papers, Box 20, file 6.

occurring in each tissue in their bodies, including the brain cells—in other words, they have a visible demonstration of lack of oxygen. Then they are asked to take cognizance of their feelings. Some of them say "I feel fine—I don't need oxygen". Others say "I feel sleepy". Others say "I don't feel well". Others "I don't feel anything". After making the 17,000 feet they are again presented with the de-coding decipher, and then one by one the oxygen masks are again adjusted to their faces.

Observing that their fingernails were returning to normal pink colours,

> They are then taken up to a level corresponding to 30,000 feet. As they go up they often find the top of their trousers are tight, or they require to break wind, because as the gas escapes the intestines spread and give that sensation, and it is explained that it is not against good society to break wind at high altitudes. At 30,000 feet, breathing oxygen, it is explained to them that without oxygen they would be dead in about one to three minutes. They are then asked to do the code test the third time, and then they descend at the rate of 2,000 feet a minute for the first 10,000.[27]

Since Germany had 80 decompression chambers to Canada's one, Banting and his staff had a lot of catching up to do.

Similar studies, from December 1940 to December 1941, showed a worrisome frequency of incapacitation at the 30 to 40,000 foot mark, and "It was therefore clear that it might become a serious hazard in military aviation if operations of several hours' duration were carried out within that range of altitude." The Flying Personnel Medical Section, established at Halifax in August, 1941, greatly augmented the available data, but by 1943 it was determined that, contrary to previous predictions, bombing would not be carried out at altitudes where aircrew would face serious medical risks, so the section was closed down. By then, however, much had been learned, some 7000 subjects making 20,000 ascents in decompression chambers, and "Pain in a limb was the most common symptom, and this was usually described as occurring in or about a joint. In severe cases there was a general muscular stiffening and signs of impending collapse. In a smaller number of cases a burning sensation was felt in the respiratory tract. Sometimes coughing occurred. In severe cases of this kind there was a rapid onset of collapse. Other symptoms included headache and skin rash or itching."[28] The lowest altitude at which symptoms became manifest was 25,000 feet, though this was only in a single case; 35 per cent ran into difficulties at 35,000 feet over two hours, though "the rate of incidence at a given altitude decreased during successive intervals of continuous

---

27. U of T, Fisher Rare Books, Banting Papers, Box 20, file 8.
28. NA, RG 24, v.312, file 5, History of the Associate Committee on Aviation Medical Research, 1939-1945.

exposure." As to the cause, the general assumption was that gas was being released either in the bloodstream or in tissues, leading to experiments to try to counteract it. Breathing oxygen at ground level for an hour before ascent seemed to flush nitrogen out of the pilot's system and "gave a considerable degree of protection to all but the most susceptible cases." The problem's main cure, however, was to use the decompression chamber as a testing device to weed out those who could not handle high altitudes for extended periods of time.

Concentrating on the problem of providing sufficient oxygen at higher altitudes, Colonel A. James, whom Banting called the grandfather of aviation medical research, explained that "For anyone who has not been familiar with flying, perhaps you do not realize what that involves—it is an entirely new field. In the last war, of course, they simply flew—if birds went up in the air, then humans could go up there—there was no question of oxygen." Though researchers knew that there was not much of the life determining gas at higher altitudes,

> nevertheless they struggled and flew to almost 20,000 feet. How many individuals were brought down through lack of oxygen ... we do not know. To give you an example of the effect of lack of oxygen on a person—there was one case recited to me recently by one of the officers who had been with one of the early RAF medical services. A highly trained and experienced photographer went up to 16,000 feet—he was instructed to take photographs of the battle area. He opened the back of the camera, urinated into same, and took the pilot's photograph, and came down. He was absolutely incompetent—didn't know what he had done—suffering from anoxaemia.[29]

The challenge was easy enough to meet, and by 1941 at least three different oxygen systems had been devised.

Another difficulty, related to oxygen deficiency, proved trickier to correct, however.

> The total atmospheric pressure at an altitude of about 37,000 feet above sea level is equal to the pressure of oxygen alone at sea level. Thus at altitudes above 37,000 feet a man using the conventional type of oxygen mask in which equalization of pressure with the outside atmosphere is permitted cannot obtain at his mouth the pressure of oxygen to which he is normally accustomed. It was shown at Wright Field in 1942 that a man's physiological ceiling could be raised by the use of "pressurized breathing", which is a system by which the pressure of gas at the mouth is raised in excess of that in the surrounding atmosphere.[30]

29. U of T, Fisher Rare Books, Banting Papers, Vox 20, file 8.
30. NA, RG 24, v.312, file 5, History of the Associate Committee on Aviation Medical Research, 1939-1945.

Research was carried out at the University of Toronto, and then within the RCAF's own facilities, the results of which were made available to the British testing establishment at Farnborough from 1943 to 1945. "It was found that the modified equipment was particularly suitable to meet an operational need of unarmed photographic reconnaissance pilots who depended on their speed and altitude for their security," and the necessary operational equipment was subsequently produced.

Research went much deeper than aviation technology, also investigating those who would have to use it, and in that regard the RCAF was not only interested in an individual's physical characteristics, but in the workings of his mind as well. "In the spring of 1939 a program of the possible uses of psychology in aviation selection was formulated by the Department of psychology, University of Toronto. Work was begun in September of that year on devising and validating tests for use in selecting pilot candidates," eventually focussing on intelligence, steadiness, distance perception, and form relations. Whether such testing was valid was itself evaluated by following candidates through their training to see how well their initial scores had predicted their subsequent performance. The results pointed to the need for two major types of tests: mental ability and sensory-motor coordination, for which procedures were prepared in early 1940.[31]

*   *   *

While the RCAF attempted to deal with challenges that had been unheard of a few decades before, the Royal Canadian Navy operated in an environment that had been familiar for millennia, which perhaps explains why naval medical research took longer to get started. Whereas Sir Frederick Banting ensured aviation matters were looked into as early as 1938, it was not until the middle of 1941 that naval issues came to the fore, and even then it was not the RCN that took the initiative. In a 14 June letter to Colonel Maclachlan, Acting Deputy Minister of National Defence, acting president of the NRC C.J. Mackenzie pointed out that the issue of doing naval work had recently come up at a meeting of the Associate Committee on Medical Research, and suggested a subcommittee be established under Doctor C.H. Best. The naval staff assenting, a first meeting was held on 10 July in which two reports were presented: one on illumination inside ships and night vision, the other

---

31.   NA, RG 24, v.312, file 5, History of the Associate Committee on Aviation Medical Research, 1939-1945.

on auditory frequency discrimination in naval personnel (the latter no doubt to help choose effective asdic—later called sonar—operators).[32]

Other projects followed in quick succession, many of them supervised by Doctor D.Y. Solandt, a future *doyen* of Canadian research; they were certainly not going to break the bank, work on engine room noise receiving $570, with $550 for a process called slit lamp examination of eyes and 200 for designing a lantern to test colour vision. Interestingly, the engine room noise investigations having been designated a war project, in the interests of secrecy it was assigned a code, subsequently being referred to as Project Number NM6 to dissimulate it from the enemy's gaze. Other work was as varied as the number of researchers interested in navy matters, and at the second meeting of the Associate Committee on Naval Medical Research, reports included "Some Observations on Local Fluid Loss in Relation to Death from Tourniquet Shock in Rats," "A Method for Evaluating Blood Substitutes," "Study of Peripheral Vascular Phenomena Associated with Shock," protective clothing, special goggles for "Following Tracer Bullets into the Sun," "The Effect of Training on Pitch Discrimination in ASDIC Operators and Fatigue of Hearing in ASDIC Operators," "Suggestions for Rendering ASDIC Trace Visible Under Red Illumination," and many more.[33]

One obvious project for naval medical research was an investigation of seasickness, especially in a navy where well over 90 per cent of the sailors were unseasoned newcomers. Jim Galloway, for example, described his first experiences aboard *Agassiz* after it left St John's in early July, 1942.

> The ship began to rise and fall with the long, rolling waves. The sardines I had for lunch started to swim around. I laid down on top of the foot lockers. My first watch was on the bridge as lookout on the port side. The first lieutenant was on the same watch. Each time I would remove the binoculars from my eyes, he would growl at me, saying I had to make continuous sweeps from dead ahead to 90 degrees on the port side... The motion of the ship climbing up and down each rolling swell got my stomach heaving. The next thing I knew I was throwing up all over that corner of the bridge.
>
> The first lieutenant called me a few choice names and ordered me below to get a bucket and rags to scrub the bridge clean... I went below and

32. NA, RG 77, Acc 88-89/049, Box 5, 4-M-6-7, Mackenzie to Col Maclachlan, 14 Jun 41; Acc 88-89/046, Box 35, 4-M6-5, Agenda for Subcommittee on Naval Medical Research, First Meeting, 10 Jul 41.
33. NA, RG 77, Acc 88-89/046, Box 35, 4-M6-6, NRC, Proceedings of the Second Meeting of the Associate Committee on Naval Medical Research, 7 Oct 43.

got two buckets and cleaning equipment. I spent the rest of the dog watch scrubbing with one bucket and throwing up in the other bucket.[34]

In one extreme case, an unnamed officer in HMCS *Louisbourg* was recommended for transfer to a larger ship because of "continued seasickness," the "only fault of which his commanding officer complains."[35]

Researchers looked into the issue in great depth, and a report by B.P. Babkin, whose main area of expertise was physiology, gives a good indication of the sophistication and breadth of such work. "The problem of seasickness is extremely complicated because one of its manifestations is vomiting, of which the physiological mechanism is not well understood. The symptoms are very widespread; besides nausea and vomiting one sees vertigo, skin anaemia, cold sweat, and changes in heart-rate and blood pressure (the last two often decreased)."[36] One possible avenue towards a better understanding of the process might be a study of acetylcholine, which transmits nerve impulses and might be responsible for certain automatic bodily reactions. Thus

> a first approach to the problem could be made by studying the concentration of acetylcholine in the blood. A tentative approach to this aspect could be made by examining sea-sick persons whose blood would be drawn on ship and stored until brought to the laboratory. Preliminary tests would have to be made to determine how long blood could be stored until brought to the laboratory. Or the whole problem could be studied in the laboratory, which would require, first, the building of an apparatus in which one could subject animals (dogs or cats) or human subjects to various swinging movements and stimulate the different parts of the labyrinth,

part of the inner ear that controls balance. Studies already done had shown that "all signs of sea- sickness can be induced experimentally by continued labyrinth stimulation. Blood would be taken before and after the production of the symptoms of sea-sickness and tested for acetylcholine..." Narcotics were already known to alleviate the symptoms of motion sickness, but were not considered appropriate to administer to sailors on duty.

Experiments may have caused volunteers, including many sailors, regrets for having offered their bodies to science. One swing, developed by Doctor André Cipriani, consisted of an electrically driven seesaw; requiring a room 20 by 35 feet to house it, "a poor sailor' was placed in a cage at one end. He was provided with a "tin cup clasped to his chest, so that he would not be without solace if and when the machine produced what is scientifically termed "motion sickness". The rating,

---

34.   Mac Johnston, *Corvettes Canada* (Toronto and Montreal, 1994), 120.
35.   *Ibid*, 129.

by means of electrical controls, could be thrown up and down through a distance of 12 feet, while independently controlled rockers tossed him from side to side, either in rhythm with the seesaw, or in sudden unrelated movements. Altogether it was a most unpleasant experience."[37] It seems that Doctor Cipriani had been inspired by devices at Belmont Park, in Cartierville, such as the ferris wheel, but also by "rides' with such names as "Shoot the Chute," "Flip-Over," and "Loop the Loop," in a rare instance of the entertainment industry making a direct contribution to scientific research.[38]

The ailment was not only of interest to clinicians, however, and policy makers, researchers, and staff officers also awaited results, though they were not of one mind on the issue. While J.B. Collip, chair of the Associate Committee on Medical Research, could report that one of his American counterparts was "very enthusiastic about the necessity for a further serious study of this age-old affliction,"[39] Wilder Penfield related an opposing view, that of the Royal Navy's Medical Director General. "Admiral Dudley states that *sea sickness* is no problem in the Navy. It is never of importance except when they have soldiers and parachute troops. He states they have had an excellent opportunity to study sea sickness among soldiers being transported to and from Iceland!"[40] The good admiral seems to have been an exception, however, as there was a general interest in dealing with the problem, Penfield himself, of the Montreal neurological institute, chairing a committee of sixteen, of whom ten were affiliated with universities or research institutes, two were medical practitioners, and four were uniformed doctors.[41]

In fact, popular interest reached such levels as to raise no little amount of contempt in the NRC's C.J. Mackenzie. "Friday afternoon Dr Collip and Captain King in re the Navy seasick pills. I have never seen anything like the fuss that is being kicked up all over the world, requests for the formula, etc. It is a first class hoax because all they are is German pills with a little additional vitamins in them and also only slightly better than the British have had for a couple of years without making any fuss about it. Captain King wants to get the thing patented and there is a great todo [sic] from all quarters. I would not want to be in Charlie Best's place."[42] How the co-discoverer of insulin felt about

36. NA, RG 77, Acc 88-80/046, Box 35, 4-M6-14, B.P. Babkin, Physiology, to J.B. Collip, Biochemistry, 1 May 41.
37. R.C. Fetherstonaugh, *McGill University at War* (Montreal, 1947), 205.
38. *Ibid*, 206.
39. NA, RG 77, Acc 88-80/046, Box 35, 4-M6-14, J.B. Collip, Chair—Ass Cttee on Med Res, to Morris Fishbein, Journal of the AMA, 8 May 41.
40. NA, RG 24, v.5383, S.47-6-3, Wilder Penfield, Report to the Chairman of the Associate Committee on Medical Research et al, Nov 41.
41. NA, RG 77, Acc 88-80/046, Box 35, 4-M6-14, Wilder Penfield to Cook, 9 Dec 42.

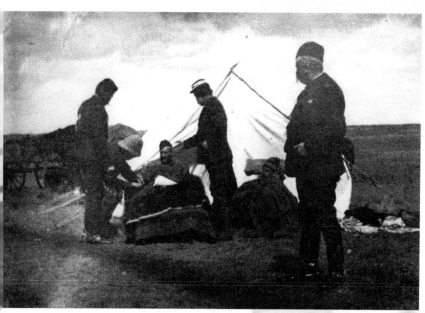

Medical facilities at Batoche, ANC C 3453

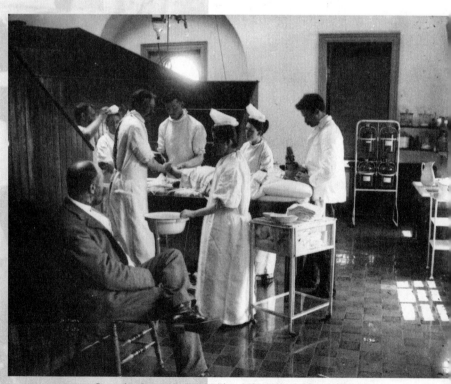

Operating Room No 2 at Halifax, 1898-1907, ANC PA 028421

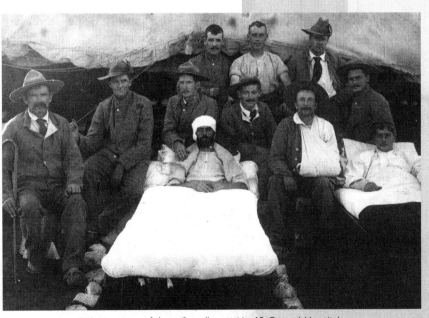

Patients, some of them Canadian, at No 13 General Hospital,
Johannesburg, April 1902, ANC PA 113 049

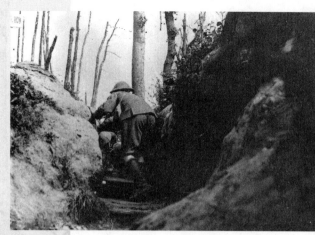

A member of the 5th Battalion is evacuated from the trenches by stretcher bearers, August 1916, ANC PA 000545

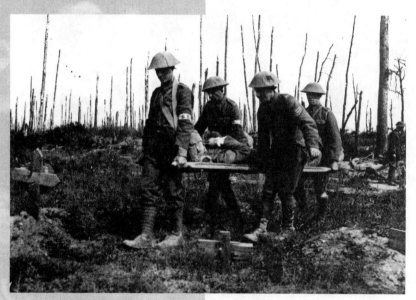

They then carry him to a light railway terminal, ANC PA 000549

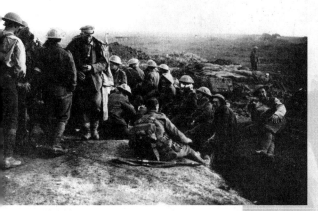

He awaits treament at an Advanced Dressing Station, ANC PA 000618

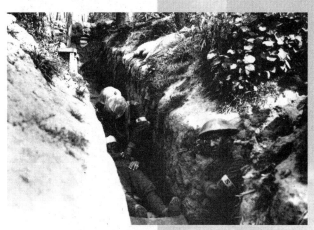

He receives treatment. Note the trench to provide
shelter from shell fire, ANC PA 000794

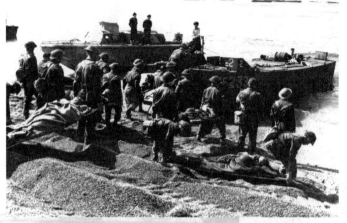

Members of the Royal Canadian Army Medical Corps treat "exercise"
casualties during a rehearsal for the Dieppe Raid, 1942
ANC PA 113242

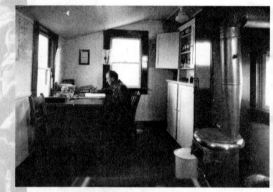

A Medical Officer's office, RCAF station Vancouver,
October 1937, ANC PA 133582,

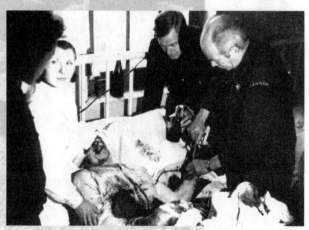

Norman Bethune, assisted by Henning Sorensen, performing
a transfusion during the Spanish Civil War, ANC C 6745 1

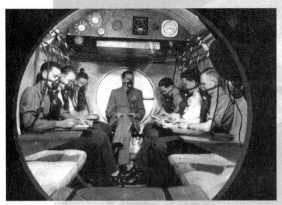

RCAF medical research, with six airmen and an instructor
in a pressure chamber, June 1942, ANC PA 140655

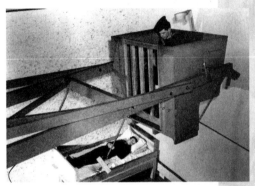

A seasickness machine at the Montreal Neurological
Institute, November 1943, ANC PA 136886

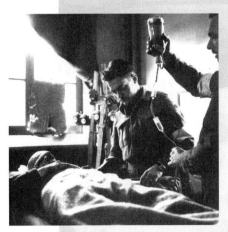

Sgt T.F. McFeat and Pte J. Viner
of 23 Field Ambulance admininister plasma
in France, June 1944, ANC PA 132723

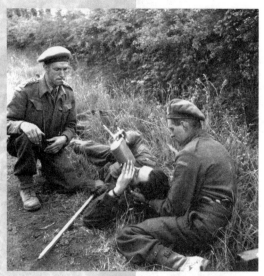

Sgt W.G. Grant is given first aid near Bayeux, France,
June 1944, ANC PA 152089

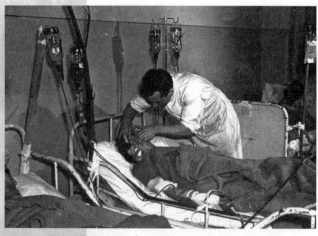

Pte McCauley attends a patient at 5 Field Dressing
Station and Surgical Unit, Germany, March 1945, ANC PA 153192

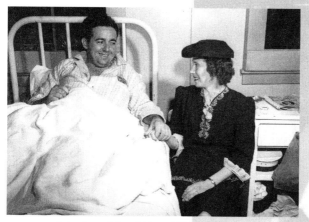

A survivor of the sinking of HMCS Esquimalt
at the RCN hospital in Halifax, April 1945, ANC PA 157022

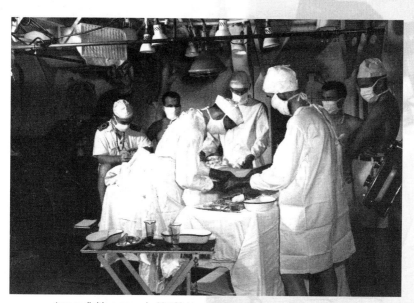

Appendicitis surgery in HMCS Uganda, August 1945, ANC PA 151507

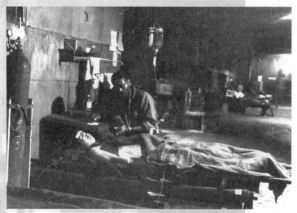

The post-op ward of the 43rd MASH, Korea,
March 1953, ANC PA 128834

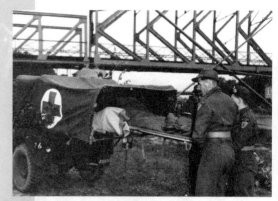

Canadian Infantry Brigade Group jeep ambulance
during Exercise Spearhead II, in Germany,
August 1952, ANC PA 140127

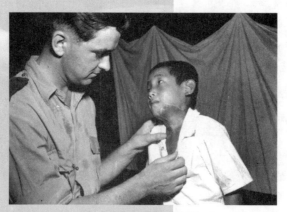

Maj. Louis Lavallée, RCAMC,
examines a Korean boy, August 1953, ANC PA 140411

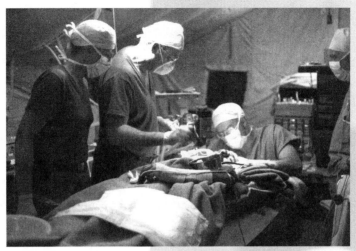

Surgery in the Gulf War, Canadian Forces Photo Unit ISC 91-60 60-1

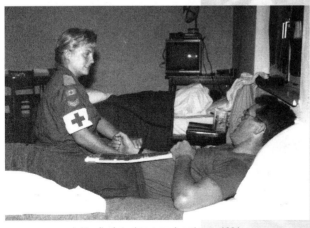

A Medical Assistant and patients, 1991,
Canadian Forces Photo Unit ILC 91-019-138

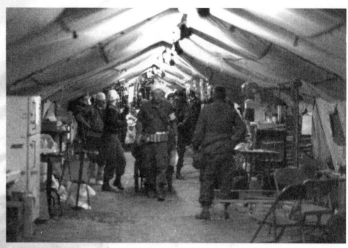

A Field Hospital in the Gulf War, Canadian Forces Photo Unit ISC 91-60-72-2

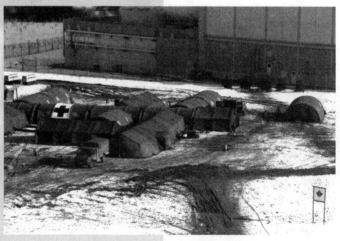

A Field Hospital set up outside NDMC, 1995,
Canadian Forces Photo Unit MPC 95-014-44

the whole issue has unfortunately been lost to the historical record, but the pills in question, though they may have helped mitigate symptoms somewhat, were no cure.

By the end of 1943 one could say that there were two main schools of thought on how to treat the problem, the navy's method consisting in "making men carry on at their normal duties as if seasickness had not occurred (except for having to clean up the mess). One hears of Naval personnel who have been consistently sick for years,"[43] according to one major report. The other approach suggested sufferers keep to their beds and take sedatives, and "Both methods have the same objective—to keep the patient going until his natural immunity has been established." That might work for people who would be on board ship for an extended period, but

> The problem of seasickness in assault troops is entirely different from either of these methods. It is that of a large number of fit but unsalted men having to be tidied over a brief but possibly stormy period in a landing craft and brought ashore capable of fighting strenuously and for a long time.
>
> Obviously strong sedatives, hypnotics and the bed find no place in their treatment, neither does the expectant treatment of the Navy.
>
> It is well known that recovery from the prostrating effects of violent seasickness is rapid on reaching land, but it has been shown that it is not rapid enough for the first few minutes ashore after an assault landing which may prove vital in an operation.[44]

One remedy, tested in trials in late 1943, consisted of a combination of hyoscine hydrobromide, hyoscyamine hydrobromide, and niacin (whatever they are), and showed much promise. Further tests, involving 1500 members of the 3rd Canadian Infantry Division, slotted to go ashore on D-Day, were scheduled for January 1944.[45]

From the common soldier's point of view, research into motion sickness does not seem to have alleviated his lot much—the landings in Normandy were carried out by some very ill troops. Reginald Roy, in his description of the battle, related how in the final run-in to the beach "Many were seasick and thought only of getting on shore, even if it was enemy-held territory,"[46] while a history of the 1st Hussars refers to men getting into amphibious tanks as "The sea-sick crews."[47] C.P. Stacey's

42. NA, MG , C.J. Mackenzie Papers, v.1, 1-15, 10 Dec 43.
43. NA, RG 24, v.12,641, 11/Seasickness/1, Report on Seasickness Alleviation Trials, Sep-Nov 43.
44. NA, RG 24, v.12,641, 11/Seasickness/1, Report on Seasickness Alleviation Trials, Sep-Nov 43.
45. NA, RG 24, v.12,641, 11/Seasickness/1, Report on Seasickness Alleviation Trials, Sep-Nov 43, Brig J.A. Meakins for DGMS to DMS CMHQ, 4 Dec 43; M.H. Brown AMD 5 to DMS CMHQ, 21 Jan 44.
46. Reginald H. Roy, *1944: The Canadians in Normandy* (Ottawa, 1984), 10.

account, part of the official history of the Canadian Army, was no different, relating how "The landing ships and craft tossed and pitched; many soldiers and some sailors were miserably sick."[48] The problem was one that remained unsolved to the end of the war, and even today holds many mysteries to those who study it.

From the navy's point of view, however, research was a very small part of the medical establishment's support of the war effort; there were also recruits to examine, training establishments to keep free of epidemic disease—and casualties to prepare for. Of the three services, it was perhaps the RCN which faced the biggest challenge in that regard, as it would see a fifty-fold expansion of its personnel, but had only a tiny nucleus of a medical service to take on these responsibilities at the outbreak of war. As Surgeon-Captain A. McCallum explained, in a somewhat Dickensian vein, after the First World War,

> whilst the Medical Branch of the permanent Navy was dead, a flicker of life remained in the medical activities of some half dozen of the twenty Divisions of the Royal Canadian Naval Volunteer Reserve which functioned in twenty cities throughout Canada. In these six Divisions a practicing physician took an interest in Naval activities through the examination of recruits; by the occasional attendance at midweek training periods; by turning out to ceremonial parades or inspections; by taking part in the ships' companies' social functions; and by infrequent visits to the Naval Base at either coast for a week or fortnight's training, or possibly short cruise.[49]

When war broke out, these few doctors were allocated in equal numbers to the major naval bases at Halifax and Esquimalt where "they took up the work of final appraisal of fitness for service of the thousands who poured into these establishments; and they supplied the subsequent medical care."[50]

Meanwhile, the Reserve Divisions acted as recruiting centres, but with the doctors that had served with them now working in the two larger establishments, new arrivals were examined by medical personnel who were themselves recent entries into the navy. In the course of the conflict they would put 105,000 volunteers through their paces, rejecting just a little more than 10 per cent of them, while of those accepted 3.5 per cent would later be eliminated for medical reasons. According to McCallum, "Since the wear and tear of service life in six years of warfare would give cause for more than half of these discharges,

47. Bill McAndrew et al, *Normandy 1944: The Canadian Summer* (Montreal, 1994), 33.
48. C.P. Stacey, *The Victory Campaign* (Ottawa, 1966), 91.
49. NA, RG 24, v.8138, NS 1440-11, The Medical Branch of the Royal Canadian Navy in World War II, by Surgeon-Captain A. McCallum.
50. *Ibid.*

it is seen that the error of the recruiting medical officer would be little more than one per cent, and this figure would include the recruit who wouldn't admit to epilepsy, ulcer, or other conditions not readily discernible in the type of physical examination it is possible to conduct at recruiting centres."[51]

Such results may have been due in large part to simple good fortune, but regardless of how effective—or lucky—selection procedures might be, there was still a need to hospitalize those who might fall prey to sickness or injury while on active service. For this purpose the RCN, which had no hospitals when war broke out, formed nine such institutions in the course of the conflict, with a total bed capacity of over 2000. Not all of them were organized in Canada, one being formed at HMCS *Niobe*, the naval service's base in the British Isles, and according to McCallum the facility "was of great comfort to those employed on the convoy routes who became ill or injured in this strenuous service. It was literally a haven for the nautical human flotsam and jetsam who were always turning up in odd ways from strange places."[52] As a small hospital far from home its staff maintained a close liaison with the Royal Canadian Army Medical Corps, which could provide training, courses, and even personnel on occasion.

In keeping with civilian practice, the actual care of patients in these nine institutions was the responsibility of nursing staff, and in the autumn of 1941 a Nursing Service Branch was formed, its members recruited not only among qualified graduates of accredited schools but within the Royal Canadian Army Medical Corps as well. It eventually grew to a strength of 343 by the end of the war, under the command of a Matron-in-Chief, Nursing Sister Marjorie Russell, after September 1943. Training was limited to naval matters, their civilian education being deemed appropriate for their medical duties, and they were then commissioned as sub-lieutenants, though they were specifically barred from serving in ships, the navy of the 1940s not yet prepared for dual-gendered combat units. In post-war interviews, many regretted not having had that opportunity, but in that regard, as in the recruiting of nurses in the first place, the navy was reflecting the general and medical values of Canadian society as a whole.[53] On the other hand, women serving in these hospitals were allowed greater autonomy than in their previous careers, only their male comrades at sea able to exercise greater independence. As Marguerite McGrattan related, "I am amazed when I

51. NA, RG 24, v.8138, NS 1440-11, The Medical Branch of the Royal Canadian Navy in World War II, by Surgeon-Captain A. McCallum.
52. NA, RG 24, v.8138, NS 1440-11, The Medical Branch of the Royal Canadian Navy in World War II, by Surgeon-Captain A. McCallum.
53. G.W.L. Nicholson, *Canada's Nursing Sisters* (Toronto, 1975), 182-183.

think of all the procedures we were trained to do, and did, in contrast to all the things RNs are not permitted to do without a doctor's written order nowadays!' including giving injections.[54]

The Royal Canadian Air Force did not establish its own medical branch until September of 1940, with 202 medical officers as a nucleus. Even the Canadian Army Service Force, that portion of the land element allotted to go overseas, expected to rely on the British for any care required further back than field ambulances, though that policy changed late in November 1939, with such units as Number 1 Neurological Hospital and Number 4 Casualty Clearing Station being mobilized.[55] As for recruiting doctors, following discussions that had begun in 1930, if not before, the Medical Council of Canada informed the Minister of National Defence that "we deem it inadvisable to disturb medical students in their studies; and that staffs of hospitals and faculties be given consideration in mobilization."[56]

The need to avoid denuding communities and institutions of their health-care professionals was, as we have seen, a lesson of the First World War; so was the careful screening of volunteers. As Lieutenant-Colonel R.S. Pentecost, an ear, nose, and throat specialist, informed his superiors, in the previous conflict he had recategorized hundreds of soldiers from "'A' to 'B' and even 'C'" as a result of "chronic conditions which had undoubtedly existed for a number of years," many of them applying for pensions after the war.[57] To avoid such waste, the Canadian Medical Association offered to help in the selection process,[58] and it quickly grew in sophistication. As Lieutenant-Colonel F.S. Park explained later in the war,

> It is only by appreciation of the long-time point of view that certain apparent absurdities are justified. To reject "Butch Riley', the boss of a lumber camp, because he has had a discharging ear since childhood, and to accept little Billy Smith, a stripling just out of school whom the lumber-jack could break across his knee, would be poor judgement if the Germans were marching through our cities tomorrow. But after a year's training in half a dozen camps, exposed to many infections from all parts of the country, the probabilities are (and experience seems to prove it) that Riley would be a casualty in hospital because of his ear—to be

54. S.T. Richards, *Operation Sick Bay* (West Vancouver, 1994), 49, 52, 60.
55. G.W.L. Nicholson, *Canada's Nursing Sisters* (Toronto, 1975), 182, 189, 116.
56. NA, RG 24, v.6519, HQ 393-8-103, Med Council of Cda to Ian Mackenzie, 11 September 1939.
57. NA, RG 24, v.6001, v.6519, HQ 1982-1-109, v.4, Pentecost to DMO MD 2, 26 September 1939.
58. NA, RG 24, v.6519, HQ 393-8-167, Secy CMA to C.G. Power, Min Pensions and Nat Health, 1 September 1939.

discharged with a pension—while Smith, filled out and developed, proceeds overseas to fight.[59]

The battle to keep an army healthy in the field thus began long before its soldiers donned uniforms.

The 1st Canadian Infantry Division moved to Great Britain in December 1939, to be followed by four other similar formations in subsequent years. Though their first major operation, the disaster at Dieppe, would not come until August 1942, and their next, the landings in Sicily, until July 1943, training and the daily life of an army were sufficient to keep medical practitioners busy. When Number 15 General Hospital moved to England in the early summer of 1940,

> Their arrival from Canada had not been a moment too soon. Road accidents were taking a heavy toll as army motor-cyclists were learning to negotiate the narrow English lanes, often in the blackout; and twenty-four major operations a day were not uncommon when the hospital became fully operational. Soon there were wards full of fractured femurs. "Give the Canadians enough motor-cycles," the Germans are reputed to have said, "and we don't need to worry about them."[60]

Many of these accidents produced injuries analogous with those of combat, such as compound fractures, providing experience that would be useful later, especially in deciding whether or not to amputate. According to a Medical Research Council memorandum, "the main indication for amputation is irreparable interference with the blood supply," regardless of the severity of skin destruction, damage to bone, or contamination of tissues.

> If the main blood vessels are not destroyed, the limb can usually be saved. Severe infection may be controlled by adequate drainage, immobilisation, and chemotherapy; skin destruction even over the whole circumference of a limb may be treated successfully by skin grafting; non-union of fractures can be prevented by continuous and prolonged fixation in plaster or splints; stiffness of joints and disuse atrophy are avoided by early active exercise of uninjured joints; excellent function may often be regained even when first inspection suggests that the limb is injured beyond repair. A surgeon who amputates because of the severity of the local injury assumes a grave responsibility—particularly in the case of the upper extremity—and *a second expert opinion should always be sought before proceeding to this drastic step.*[61]

---

59. NA, MG 30, B85, Harris Papers, v.5, Lt-Col F.S. Park, Causes of Rejection from the Army and Incidence of Defects in Recruits, 30 April 1943.
60 . G.W.L. Nicholson, *Canada's Nursing Sisters* (Toronto, 1975), 121.
61. NA, MG 30, B85, Harris Papers, v.5, Medical Research Council Memorandum No 5, Emergency Amputations, May 1941.

Though at least one doctor, Gordon Dale, could write that experience following the First World War "leads one to feel that amputations are among the most satisfactory of surgical procedures,"[62] his seems to have been a minority view.

For techniques developed in the 1914-1918 conflict proved that in a large number of cases amputation could be avoided as a means of treating infection. In mid-1942 J.A. MacFarlane was a consulting surgeon to the Canadian Army Overseas (meaning England at this time), and he advocated keeping serious wounds open, as in the previous conflict, for it is in the closed wound that certain bacteria, which cannot reproduce in the presence of oxygen, find a most hospitable climate. Canadian surgeons were again discovering that there was an important difference between operating in a civilian hospital and taking care of wounded on or near a battlefield. As Doctor F.W. Bancroft explained, "The ideal conditions of a healthy patient, a clean skin, a wound made by a relatively sharp and clean instrument, repair of the wound within six hours after it was inflicted, and opportunity for the surgeon to use meticulous care in the treatment of the wound and to watch it during the time it is healing, are hardly likely to be found in war surgery."[63] He also advocated delaying suture until the patient was further to the rear.

One had to watch, however, for various sources of infection along the line of evacuation, especially a bacterium called haemolytic streptococcus. As MacFarlane reported in late 1940, "Dr Ronald Hare sent me before I went overseas the manuscript of a very interesting paper on streptococcal infection. He has been able to show very clearly that during the previous war this infection became progressively more common as the soldier journeyed down the long line of communication to the base."[64] Another source suggested that

> this organism finds its way into wounds, not from the skin of the patient, but from the ministrations of the attendants and dressers, from the air of the dressing stations and hospitals, where other infected wounds are being continually tended and in the soiled dressings which, even with the greatest care, distribute organisms throughout the air; from the blankets which cover such patients, from the dust which, in spite of precautions, is stirred by the inevitable movement in a busy ward.
>
> Efforts are being made in England to combat this dust-born [sic] infection. Greater care is encouraged in dressing technique. In some hospitals

---

62. NA, MG 30, B85, Harris Papers, v.5, Gordon Dale, Amputations, November 1943.
63. F.W. Bancroft, "Delay Sewing Up War Wounds," *Science News Letter*, reprinted in the *Canadian Medical Association Journal* (January, 1941), 79.
64. J.A. McFarlane, "The Trends in Military Surgery in the First Year of the War," *Canadian Medical Association Journal* (December, 1940), 543.

the floors are treated with spindle oil in an effort to trap the dust. A method of treating blankets with minimal amounts of oil have been recommended, with the idea of lessening the danger of airborn [sic] infection.[65]

Anti-bacterial work was not to be limited to English hospitals, and in March 1943 the NRC's Associate Committee on Medical Research advised the DGMS to create a special unit, formed as Number 1 Research Laboratory, to study the problem of infection in a battle area.[66] (It will reenter our story in the next chapter.)

Meanwhile, a competing mode of treatment for wounded soldiers came to the fore in the work of a Doctor Trueta of Oxford; originally developed in Barcelona during the Spanish Civil War, the technique was a complete departure from accepted methods. As an article in the *Canadian Medical Association Journal* explained,

> In the great majority of serious war wounds they are left open and the cavity filled with plain sterile gauze or a lightly coated vaseline pack. The whole limb is then included in a plaster cast, including the joints above and below the area, thus ensuring perfect immobilization. The wound is not inspected for at least ten days and sometimes 30 days. The removal of the plaster, which in the meantime has developed an offensive odour, shows a non-oedematous granulating surface. The whole area is cleansed and the plaster is renewed. The initial operative procedure is followed as a rule by three or four days of fever, but the patients are comfortable and can be transported from the area of immediate danger within a very short time. In a limited number of cases we have had an opportunity to use this method and the results were gratifying.[67]

Based on the theory that nature works best if the limb is completely at rest, of 1200 cases Trueta treated during the Spanish Civil War, by his account less than 1 per cent died.

The Barcelonan doctor explained that the inspiration for his approach came from the 1853 work of an English surgeon named Joseph Gamgee, so that it predated the aseptic and antiseptic work of Joseph Lister. As Edward W. Archibald suggested in the *Canadian Medical Association Journal*, "The immediate question in minds trained for more than a generation in Listerian principles, demanding daily dressings and the washing away of pus with antiseptic lotions, was, how can such a procedure avoid disaster from retained infection?"[68] He

65. NA, MG 30, B85, Harris Papers, v.5, J.A. MacFarlane, Consulting Surgeon to Cdn Army OS, Wounds in Modern War, June 1942.
66. NA, RG 24, v.312, file 8, History of the Associate Committee on Medical Research, 1938-1946.
67. J.A. McFarlane, "The Trends in Military Surgery in the First Year of the War," *Canadian Medical Association Journal* (December, 1940), 542-543.
68. Edward W. Archibald, "New and Old in War Surgery," *Canadian Medical Association Journal* (August, 1942), 97.

answered his own question in pointing out that there was no real antagonism between the two techniques, as Listerians also insisted on rest while the Barcelonan, like his First World War predecessors, carried out careful debridement. His technique did in fact allow drainage, the plaster absorbing pus and hence accounting for the foul odour, but Canadian practitioners continued to use the open-wound method, no doubt because it was simpler than Trueta's approach and achieved the same results.

In addition to such alternatives, medical practitioners could make use of a greater chemical arsenal against infection than their predecessors, though the research of the latter half of the 1930s has since been relegated to the footnotes of historical studies by the later development of penicillin and other antibiotics. The compound in question was a brick-red sulfonamide dye called prontosil rubrum, whose existence and properties were announced to the world in a German medical journal by Gerhard Domagk, who would later earn the Nobel prize. Before his 1935 article, according to a physician of the time, the only drugs known to treat specific diseases were quinine for malaria, salvarsan for syphilis, insulin for diabetes, and liver extract.[69] As early as the First World War, however, it was discovered that certain dyestuffs, such as one called flavine, could be fairly efficient antiseptics and were relatively free of side effects. Fifteen years later Domagk found that a derivative of a dye called chrysoidin cured mice infected with streptococci. Soon after, French researchers discovered that the active agent in the dye was sulfanilamide, and though it was not a true antiseptic, it performed well as a bacteriostatic, keeping the organism in a state of enfeebled existence until the body's own immune system could destroy it.[70]

As J.A. MacFarlane explained in an October 1940 article of the *Canadian Medical Association Journal,* "It has been the practice in the British army to administer a prophylactic dose of sulfanilamide by mouth to all wounded. In certain hospitals the powdered drug has been used locally in wounds, particularly in those cases where it has been impossible to give it by mouth. I have not seen any critical analysis of results of such treatment. From experimental work, however, it would seem that the administration of sulfanilamide either by mouth or into the wound is a justifiable prophylactic measure."[71] As if to provide an example where war hindered rather than promoted medical research, MacFarlane

---

69. S.E.D. Shortt, ""Before the Age of Miracles": The Rise, Fall and Rebirth of General Practice in Canada, 1890-1940," Charles G. Roland, ed, *Health, Disease and Medicine: Essays in Canadian History* (Hamilton, 1982), 130.
70. Frederick F. Cartwright, *A Social History of Medicine* (London and New York, 1977), 147.
71. J.A. McFarlane, "The Trends in Military Surgery in the First Year of the War," *Canadian Medical Association Journal* (December, 1940), 541.

added that "It is unfortunate that many of the seriously wounded in the BEF had to be abandoned in France," during the evacuation of Dunkirk and similar operations, "and it will only be at the termination of the war that we can get the records of results in that group."[72]

Such setbacks aside, by the end of 1940 the British were sufficiently confident to prescribe three tablets totalling 1.5 grams of sulfanilamide as an initial dose, with a tablet two hours later and another every four hours over four days, or a total of 13.5 grams. When used locally they suggested rubbing 5 to 15 grams of powdered sulfa into the wound.[73] Even gas gangrene might prove less lethal with the proper application of sulfa drugs, though the War Office warned in May 1941 that "The most fatal complication of war wounds is gas gangrene. Recent statistical evidence shows that of 107 reported cases, 37 ended fatally."[74] The first line of defence was proper debridement, as in the First World War, but as well "Chemotherapy should be instituted at the earliest opportunity, and it is to be emphasized that local application by packing the wound, after excision, with one of these agents should be carried out." With the war a year-and-a-half old, and British troops having been involved in campaigns in France and Belgium, the Mediterranean, and North Africa, among others, there had been plenty of opportunity to test such approaches, though "Scrutiny of the returns made indicates that the dosage given in such cases is inadequate and frequently too long delayed... Particular attention should be paid to giving a detailed and accurate record of the sulfonamide derivative employed, the route of administration, the date, time and the dose of the drug administered. In many instances sufficient detail has not been given in the returns already made. The evaluation of this line of treatment has therefore been rendered difficult or impossible."[75]

As promising as they might be in treating infection and as safe as they may have seemed, sulfonamide derivatives, like all such chemicals, produced side effects, though these do not seem to have been severe. Two of them, sulpha pyridine and sulphathiozole, when used in the large doses necessary to help fight off infection, could crystallize out in the upper urinary tract, including the kidneys, sometimes to the point of causing blockage. The solution was a simple matter of good nursing, intake and output being monitored to ensure a soldier's system was working as it should. In a 1942 bulletin, Britain's Army Medical

72. J.A. McFarlane, "The Trends in Military Surgery in the First Year of the War," *Canadian Medical Association Journal* (December, 1940), 541.
73. J.A. McFarlane, "The Trends in Military Surgery in the First Year of the War," *Canadian Medical Association Journal* (December, 1940), 541.
74. DHist, FN 46, *Army Medical Directorate Bulletin No 2* (1 May 1941), 2.
75. *Ibid.*

Directorate recommended that, for a dose of 6 grams of sulpha pyridine in 24 hours, "it is essential that *at least 4 pints of fluid* be administered. If this quantity cannot be taken by the mouth it must be given by the rectal or intravenous route."[76]

Unclear at the time was the possible impact of antibiotics such as penicillin, though their potential had been known for some time. As Wilder Penfield informed the Associate Committee on Medical Research in August 1941, Alexander Fleming had described the effects of penicillin over ten years before, having discovered that it inhibited staphylococci and streptococci bacteria. At Oxford, however, which Penfield had recently visited, "The chemical analysis of the substance has not yet succeeded. It is rapidly absorbed but the dose is so large and the material so difficult to produce that it has no practical application at the moment. It does not work very well by mouth, being destroyed by acid in the stomach. Intravenous administration is probably best."[77] Potentially more effective that the sulfonamides and their derivatives, more work was needed before the true worth of antibiotics could be determined.

One problem was the nature of the product. Penicillin is itself a life-form, and waiting for it to reproduce naturally so as to provide sufficient quantities of drug for research—let alone for use in the field—was simply out of the question. Though it was in fact work in the United States that would solve the problem, much was done in Canada as well, and in January 1943 the Associate Committee on Medical Research recommended the erection of a pilot plant to explore large-scale production. Within a few months it was producing up to two million units, or 1.2 grams, a day for the treatment of some infections (those of staphylococcal origin which can cause boils or abscesses) as well as for further research.[78] At about the same time, in March 1943, British work in the Middle East provided further information for Canadian medical practitioners, tests performed on seven soldiers in a Cairo hospital leading to the conclusion that "Penicillin is obviously a remarkably interesting substance, with well-defined bacteriostatic powers in vitro [petri dishes] and in vivo [live animals] against staphylococci and streptococci,"[79] the latter capable of causing pneumonia, intestinal

76. DHist, FN 46, *Army Medical Directorate Bulletin No 6* (June, 1943, Canadian reprint), 2; *Army Medical Directorate Bulletin No 10* (April, 1942), 3.
77. NA, RG 24, v.5383, S.47-6-3, Wilder Penfield, Report to the Chairman of the Associate Committee on Medical Research et al, Nov 41.
78. NA, RG 24, v.312, file 8, History of the Associate Committee on Medical Research, 1938-1946, 16.
79. NA, RG 24, v.12,628, 11/Penicillin/1, Report from the Middle East Forces to the War Office on the action of Penicillin (Florey) on War Wounds, March 1943.

disease, and a host of other ailments. Researchers warned, however, that these patients had received special care, and that sulfa medications were sometimes equally effective.

Treating the wounded was thus far more than a matter of surgical technique, which is not to deny the latter's critical importance, but to understand developments in that field it is necessary to return to the career of Norman Bethune. Having set up a blood transfusion service in Spain, he returned to Canada, where he learned that Mao Zedong's army was in critical need of surgeons in its campaign against the Japanese invasion of China. As he made his way to the scene of battle, however, Bethune could not have gone further in time and space; for he did not travel to the China of Shanghai, or Peiping, or even Nanjing, but to the north-west, where little had changed in hundreds or even thousands of years. There, almost invisible to Europe and North America, pitched battles were being fought between armies numbering in the hundreds of thousands as the communist Chinese and the Japanese Empire made war against each other. Bethune had already gained fame and his ideological credentials were certainly in order, but the medical challenge that faced him as he made his way across China to join the 8th Route Army was immense. A formation of 200,000 troops, with 2500 in hospital at any given time, it had available only five doctors and 50 apprentices;[80] the Canadian had his work cut out for him.

Coming to grips with the role of the surgeon in modern war, in the last two months of 1938 the Marxist doctor from Montreal carried out work which would have been familiar to his Huguenot and Scottish forebears. Referring to the prevalence of bone infection in certain wounds, he wrote:

> All osteomyelitis cases, involving the thigh, should have amputation as the quickest and most humane method of getting them out of hospital. It should be kept in mind, that, irrespective of whether or not these cases are treated conservatively or radically, that they will never be able to return to the front and their usefulness, as soldiers, is finished. We dislike as much as they, to be forced to amputate, but it is the most merciful procedure. At least we have saved their lives, even though they have only one leg, and in addition, have saved them months and possibly years of suffering—which, even though they endure, will leave them with a leg which is not capable of bearing weight. In addition, to leave them in their present condition, with uncontrolled infection of the bone, is merely to await a slow death from chronic sepsis. So, all would point to amputation or nothing done.[81]

---

80. NA, MG 30, D187, Sise Papers, v.35, f.2, Bethune to General Nieh, 7 Dec 38.
81. NA, MG 30, D187, Sise Papers, v.35, f.2, Bethune to Hu Chia Ch'aun, 17 Nov 38.

A surgeon of the War of 1812 would have agreed, not only with the need for the technique, but in the humane motives that underlined it.

In another sphere, however, the Canadian attempted to bring about change, and went about it in his usual bull-in-the-china-shop style. On 22 November he and his staff began operating on 35 wounded soldiers who had spent three gruesome days in transit, and Bethune reported that he subsequently berated the brigade commander for the delay. The officer "promised that on the next occasion of a planned action, that our Mobile Unit should be placed immediately behind the regiments in action, to render operative First Aid."[82] A week later the situation had already improved, the Canadian gleefully noting that "We received our first patient at 5:15 p.m.—seven hours and 15 minutes after he had been wounded,"[83] he and his team operating on 71 cases, of whom only one, suffering from near-hopeless wounds to the abdomen, succumbed. After further work of this nature, Bethune was much encouraged. "We have demonstrated to our own satisfaction and I hope to the satisfaction of the Army commanders the value of this type of treatment of wounds. It is expected that it will revolutionize our present concepts of the duties of the Sanitary Service. The time is past and gone in which doctors will wait for patients to come to them. Doctors must go to the wounded and the earlier the better. Every Brigade should have at its disposal such a Mobile Operating Unit such as ours."[84]

Making a similar report to supporting committees in New York, Hong Kong, and London, the surgeon punctuated his argument with a compelling anecdote.

> I will mention the two cases of perforation of the intestine by rifle bullets operated on. The first case was operated on 18 hours after wounded and the second 8 hours after being wounded. Both cases had almost identical wounds—the bullet entering the abdomen at the level of the umbilicus. Both had ten perforations and tears of the small and large intestine with escape of intestinal contents into the abdominal cavity (including round worms!) Also there was in both cases a big haemorrhage from tear of the mesenteric artery with the abdomen full of blood. Both were operated on at night in a dirty Buddhist temple by the light of candles and flash lights. The first case died the following day but the second made an uneventful recovery, in spite of being transported 60 li [roughly 30 kilometres] every night for the following week on a rough stretcher. The difference between life and death was the difference between 8 hours and 18 hours.[85]

It could not have been clearer.

82. NA, MG 30, D187, Sise Papers, v.35, f.2, Bethune to General Nieh, 7 Dec 38.
83. *Ibid.*
84. *Ibid.*
85. NA, MG 30, D187, Sise Papers, v.35, f.2, Bethune Report to Committees in New York, Hong Kong, and London, 1 Jul 39.

It was, however, the recommendation of a lone Canadian working in the hinterland of the largest continent on earth, and when Bethune died on 12 November 1939 his ideas had not percolated beyond the Chinese army he worked with. However, they re-emerged independently two years later in a report by Lieutenant-Colonel J.A. MacFarlane, who noted that "For some time the whole question of operating facilities in the forward area with motorised units has been under consideration."[86] Sweeping battles in Syria and East Africa had shown that Casualty Clearing Stations (somewhat rearwards in the casualty evacuation organization, behind stretcher-bearers, Regimental Aid Posts, Advanced Dressing Stations, and Main Dressing Stations) were incapable of sufficient mobility to operate on a flowing battlefield, while Field Ambulance units, though well-mounted on a variety of vehicles and operating close to the front, lacked the necessary equipment for anything but the most rudimentary surgery. The solution was obvious, to form a mobile operating unit, perhaps with sufficient dressings and supplies for 30 to 50 surgeries, capable of being carried in a few trucks. Thus, in a rapid campaign, patients could be transported by ambulance to some form of forward operating post before being evacuated further to the rear.

A colleague of MacFarlane's, a divisional Director of Medical Services, R.M. Luton, agreed with the need for such a unit in "a campaign of rapid movement," suggesting the army acquire specially constructed vehicles on 3-ton chassis. Other equipment would include a generator for keeping lights burning, a 60-gallon water tank, sufficient linen for 30 to 40 operations, and a 15-hundredweight truck for carrying baggage, rations, and personnel. The surgeon and nursing sisters would travel in a station wagon. As for staff, he suggested a surgeon "who must have sound training and experience in all branches of traumatic surgery, preferably young, and must be of good physical condition."[87] Completing the team would be another surgeon with hospital experience in traumatic surgery, an anaesthetist, two nursing orderlies, and two nursing sisters, though the latter would only join a given unit at the discretion of the Corps' Deputy Director of Medical Services. (The military hierarchy was still uncomfortable with the prospect of women working close to the front.)

In the first days of 1942, therefore, it seemed that the creation of forward surgical units had been worked out in every detail, but the very concept of such an organization was still a subject for debate, and the proper location for a surgeon was not, in the eyes of some, near the

86.   NA, RG 24, v.11,621, 11/Mob Oper/1, MacFarlane to DMS, 22 Nov 41.
87.   NA, RG 24, v.12,621, 11/Mob Oper/1, DMS to DAG CMHQ, 19 Jan 42.

fighting. One divisional Deputy Adjutant General, Beament by name, insisted that

> In clearing a battle field, the first consideration is, as far as possible, to evacuate surgical cases to as far back a fixed hospital installation as possible. The theoretical ideal, therefore, would be if one could evacuate directly from collecting posts in the battle area to a general hospital... This desirable feature of making long evacuations to rear areas is in many surgical cases considerably aided by the development in medical science. I am now informed that in many cases of gunshot wounds it is now possible to pack the wounds with a sulfanilamide dressing and the wounded man will keep without operative treatment and without danger of gangrene for about 48 hours.[88]

Beament thus concluded that surgeons would be needed in the rear, not in the battle zone, though there were still arguments for some form of forward surgery, if on a small scale. For "cases will undoubtedly occur, where early operative treatment would result in the eventual recovery of the soldier... Further, it seems to me that it would be unfortunate, from the point of view of morale, if the idea were to become prevalent that surgical cases, who could not wait to reach a rearward installation, were abandoned to die." He therefore supported the creation of one surgery team per division.

Thus by June 1942 the function and organization of such a unit was ready to move from theory to practice, MacFarlane describing its role as follows: "Mobile warfare has presented a new problem to the surgeon, he must put himself, his assistants and the essentials of equipment into vehicles which can move [as] quickly as the armoured division which he now serves. He must be prepared to set up his theatre in whatever shelter he can find, and do it quickly. He must be able to disband it rapidly and move forward to another area on short notice, and unfortunately sometimes he must be ready to move it rearwards out of enemy hands when the battle sways against his comrades."[89] The consulting surgeon to the Canadian Army concluded that "I am convinced that something of this sort is the answer to the problem of bringing early surgery to the wounded in this war," the result being the Field Surgical Unit, or FSU, though it would be more than a year before Canadian surgeons followed troops into battle. (Dieppe being designed as a raid, all casualties—that did not fall into enemy hands—were dealt with in hospitals in Britain, as we shall see.)

While surgeons, at least on paper, were getting closer to the front, so were the blood products they would need to treat shock—and the

---

88. NA, RG 24, v.12,621, 11/Mob Oper/1, Beament to BGS, 16 Feb 41.
89. NA, MG 30, B85, Harris Papers, v.5, MacFarlane to Cdn Army OS, 15 Jun 42.

technicians to administer them. After the Fall of France in June 1940, Canadian land forces in Great Britain concentrated on defending England against invasion, Dieppe being the main exception. Even aside from that disastrous raid, as we have seen Canadians suffered casualties to illness and accident, and if transfusions were necessary they were able to rely on British supplies, but they also had to prepare for operations in other theatres.

> It is likely that any Canadian force will be part of a larger British force. In such an event, British plans are to establish a forward transfusion base in the new area, and from this base supplies will be forwarded to the various formations and distributed through the forward transfusion unit...
>
> This unit consists of one officer, a driver and two other ranks. They are provided with a refrigerated truck, capable of carrying large quantities of plasma, blood serum—as well as the crystalloid solutions, together with giving sets. Such a unit would be based on the CCS, but would be free to travel anywhere in the forward area where large numbers of cases are concentrated and are in need of resuscitation measures...
>
> It would seem, therefore, that the question of providing four such units in the Canadian Army should have early consideration. I am satisfied that the provision of such supplies should tie in closely to the British scheme, which seems to me to be excellent, and is working out satisfactorily in the campaigns in the Middle East.[90]

Able to learn from British experience, the Canadians thus formed Field Transfusion Units, or FTUs.

Their organization thus closed a circle as Canada prepared to go into battle, the FTUs bearing a striking similarity to Bethune's transfusion team of the Spanish Civil War. In some ways it might have been preferable to wait longer before joining the British, Americans, and other United Nations allies in combat operations, especially with research into such issues as blood substitutes and motion sickness still ongoing, but in war there is never sufficient time to perfect technology and technique before both are put to the test. At least the Canadian medical corps had had the opportunity to learn from others in the years leading up to 1943, and was thus able to organize specialist units to help mitigate some of the horrors of war. They would be put to their first major, large-scale test in Operation Husky, the landings in Sicily, on 10 July 1943, though only after a catastrophic dress rehearsal at Dieppe on 19 August 1942.

---

90. NA, RG 24, v.12,576, 11/Blood Trans/1, Consulting Surgeon for DMS CMHQ to DMS, 10 Apr 42.

Chapter Six

In the Face of the Enemy

Unlike the First World War, when the Canadian Army's first engagement at Ypres led to the loss of a third of its contingent, its first two forays of the Second World War were, thankfully, accompanied by minimal casualties. The first, in June 1940, was a brief expedition to France, just as the country was falling, and ended when Canada's 1st Infantry Brigade was evacuated back to England without encountering the enemy; the second had a similar outcome when 500 Canadian troops went to Spitsbergen, an island north of Scandinavia, to destroy coal facilities there so they could not be used by the Germans in Norway. It was thus the navy and not the army that would first have to deal with the casualties of war in large numbers, and in doing so RCN doctors would, in the main, rely on the baggage of knowledge they had accumulated before joining the armed forces. This was especially the case with those 40 or so Canadians who served in Royal Navy establishments on two year loan,[1] many of them accompanying British forces when they suffered their worst disasters of the European war, at Dunkirk, Greece, and Crete. The first was the result of the British Expeditionary Force and the French Army being unable to stem *Blitzkrieg* in north-west Europe, leaving German forces in command of France, Belgium, Luxemburg, and the Netherlands by June 1940; the others were more Churchillian, Britain coming to the aid of Greece in early 1941 to retain some kind of foothold on the European continent, while the Germans cleared their southern flank in preparation for their main campaign against the Soviet Union. The result was defeat and retreat for British armies and severe losses among the ships that attempted to evacuate them.

---

1. "Canadian Medical War Services," *Canadian Medical Association Journal* (April, 1943), 367.

Surgeon-Lieutenant W.M. Tait was witness and participant in the retreat from Greece, reporting how his ship began to suffer casualties from dive bombing before even reaching the rendez-vous area where it was supposed to begin taking on survivors. Thankfully, "Casualties from this show were few; three men partially suffocated with smoke, one fractured femur and four badly lacerated scalps and faces from flying splinters. These were promptly dealt with."[2] Arriving at its destination, Tait's ship remained some two miles offshore while troops were ferried from the beaches. As the naval surgeon related, "We in the medical department found ourselves almost snowed under with wounded, walking and stretcher cases. It was a sight difficult to describe by word of mouth or pen to anyone who has not actually witnessed it." The ship, with an intended capacity of 3000, took on about 5000, 200 of whom were seriously wounded. "I remember saying to myself: How will we ever get them sorted out and dealt with?"[3] Every man requiring treatment was ministered to, however, with only two fatalities; no doubt those too seriously wounded to stand the trip had been left behind or died, a pattern we will see repeated when discussing the withdrawal from Crete. Off Greece, Tait's ship returned for a second load of troops, though the doctor noted that the bulk of medical supplies had been exhausted on the first trip. Struck by a bomb, the vessel was, however, put out of action, and Tait's third trip to the beaches was on board a destroyer, which picked up about fifty survivors from previous sinkings, who were stripped, cleaned, and treated as the ship made its way to Alexandria.

Surgeon Lieutenant M. McRitchie's experiences were similar as the British withdrew from Crete, the Germans' next target after Greece, and which they invaded with paratroops in one of the largest such operations of the war. Having left his practice in Fernie, British Columbia, in the fall of 1940, by 1 December McRitchie had been appointed to the Royal Navy's tented hospital. Arriving at Suda Bretein, Crete, on 8 May, he and his comrades set up a 60-bed facility with a staff of nine officers, six non-commissioned officers, and 32 sick berth attendants (or SBAs, a trade to be discussed later in this study). German paratroopers and gliders assaulted the island on the 20th, and within a week the small hospital was attempting to accommodate 450 cases. "We had them sleeping under the Olive trees and in stretchers and in the semi-protection of a nearby monastery... In the hospital we were working far

---

2. Surg-Lt W.M. Tait, "The Evacuation from Greece," *Canadian Medical Association Journal* (October, 1943), 315.
3. Surg-Lt W.M. Tait, "The Evacuation from Greece," *Canadian Medical Association Journal* (October, 1943), 315.

past the point of exhaustion. We worked in relays of threes. One would operate and one would administer the anaesthetic," there being little room for specialization. "Out of that inferno everything passed for all of us like a dream. You never quite knew or realized whether it was day or night or night or day. The planes were over all the time. The bombs were falling and the machine-gunning was almost continuous."[4]

McRitchie recalled one incident which "remains over all else... We were operating at the time. The patient was under the anaesthetic. All was going quite well until a trench mortar landed close by and put the whole lighting system on the blink. Fortunately it was daytime. While everything was heaving and swaying about like mad we picked up our unconscious patient and laid him on the floor and then continued with the operation. It was a nightmare."[5] As the month of May neared its end the military situation worsened, lots were drawn to determine who would remain with the most seriously wounded, with capture the inevitable consequence, and who would evacuate the hospital with those injured who could travel. McRitchie was one of the latter, but even though he would, for the time being, avoid the uncertainties of becoming a prisoner of war, he could still remember how "I was never so tired or frightened in my life." Carrying stretchers until they could find vehicles to transport them, the now-nomadic band of staff and patients made its way to an army hospital, where they discovered that the military situation was deemed hopeless and it had been decided to leave the island. The evacuation, however, was to take place from beaches in the south, some 40 miles away. As the Canadian related, "It was a nightmare," a word he used with understandable frequency. "We could only travel by night, as by day it was death to be on the roads. During the day we hid in the rocks or lay beneath the Olive trees. All through the journey we were picking up casualties along the road. Everywhere was death and desolation."[6] Leaving their vehicles to be destroyed by enemy aircraft, McRitchie, his comrades, and their charges boarded the second-to-last ship to leave the island on the 30th.

Such experiences, whether in ship or ashore, seemed to indicate that medical practitioners joining the navy would further their education more in its tactical than its technical aspects. Unlike Tait and McRitchie, however, most doctors who joined the RCN served in the Atlantic, where their shipmates took on ever greater responsibilities, shepherding

4. DHist 4430, vol 1, Medical Branch, Experiences of Surgeon Lieutenants M. McRitchie and Wm Tait in Evacuations at Benghazi, Greece and Crete.".

5. DHist 4430, vol 1, Medical Branch, Experiences of Surgeon Lieutenants M. McRitchie and Wm Tait in Evacuations at Benghazi, Greece and Crete.".

6. DHist 4430, vol 1, Medical Branch, Experiences of Surgeon Lieutenants M. McRitchie and Wm Tait in Evacuations at Benghazi, Greece and Crete.".

merchant vessels through U-boat patrolled waters—the voyage often
ending in tragedy with scores of casualties. By mid-1942 the service
could count a surgeon-captain, three surgeon-commanders, 18 surgeon-
lieutenant-commanders (including one a prisoner of the Germans), and
173 surgeon-lieutenants (though one was posted as missing) among its
medical personnel.[7] It should be noted, however, that the wartime
Royal Canadian Navy was made up mostly of hundreds of small ships
used as escorts for merchant convoys—and medical officers were not
numerous enough to assign to all of them. Thus a corvette or mine-
sweeper would most likely rely not on a licensed doctor, but on a sick
berth attendant (or SBA), whose medical responsibilities nonetheless
differed little from his university-trained counterpart. At the outbreak
of war there were just 20 such sailors in the RCN, but that number
expanded to 1200 as the conflict wore on. Similarly to the rest of the
navy, training had to be somewhat truncated, the one or two-year course
of the interwar period being replaced by a much shorter indoctrination.
Surgeon-Captain Archibald McCallum related that "A large part of the
male Sick Berth rating's duties was performed in fighting ships on the
convoy routes. Since many of these ships carried no medical officer, the
Sick Berth rating was given responsibility for the health of the ship's
company and had to rely upon the training he had received and his own
judgment."[8]

Though the RCN actively sought out "recruits with related civilian
training and experience," and though from the early days of the war it
managed to attract a number of registered and graduate male nurses (and
at least one apprentice embalmer), newcomers still required some further
education to ensure they worked from the same knowledge base. Additional indoctrination thus included lectures in anatomy and physiology,
bacteriology, communicable diseases, and first aid along with
demonstrations of basic nursing procedures in sick bay wards; since the
instructors, who were often medical officers or nursing sisters, had
themselves been civilians shortly before, these were effectively civilian
techniques taught in traditional manner. Most graduates then went on
to work in corvettes, small escort vessels originally built for coastal
work but which found themselves serving as anti-submarine workhorses
throughout the North Atlantic theatre.[9] One example of the relation-
ship between an SBA, a ship's complement, and the practice of medicine is provided by Stanley B. Mosher, who in a post-war interview

7. "Nominal Roll of Medical Officers Royal Canadian Naval Service as on June 1, 1942," *Canadian Medical Association Journal* (August, 1942), 175.
8. NA, RG 24, v.8138, NS 1440-11, The Medical Branch of the Royal Canadian Navy in World War II, by Surgeon-Captain A. McCallum.
9. S.T. Richards, *Operation Sick Bay* (West Vancouver, 1994), 42-44, 86.

complained how some sailors waited too long before coming to see him with their problems. "One such case involved a man who cut his finger while on watch but it had stopped bleeding by the time he came off so he didn't think it worth bothering me about. About a week later he came to me with a badly infected finger and a sore arm. First, he got a "blast" from me for not reporting sooner, then told he had "blood poisoning". His finger was badly swollen, red streaks ran up his arm. The lymph glands in his armpit were tender, swollen and hard. After several days of epsom salts and glycerine poultices along with sulpha drugs he started to improve."[10]

The tasks of MOs and SBAs (the latter as assistants or working on their own) were thus made up mostly of routine, which is not to say that life aboard ship was easy for them, as Archie McCallum explained. "When a Naval doctor sets sail in wartime he doesn't know if the next few months will see him dealing with the common colds and pneumonias of the northern climates, or with the Malarias and sunstrokes of the Tropics. Nor are his facilities for dealing with the sick always to his liking. Truly in some of the larger men-o'war the sick quarters and operating rooms are surprisingly spacious and well equipped; but in hundreds of the smaller craft which carry a Medical Officer, the "Sick Bay" is crowded when he and the patient and one assistant are all in it at the same time."[11] One whose career was more eventful than most was Surgeon-Lieutenant T. Blair McLean of Edmonton, who survived the sinking of HMCS *Fraser*, after a collision, then later survived again when HMCS *Margaree* went down.

In some ways daily routine was similar to that of a general practitioner ashore, starting with sick parade, when sailors presented themselves with various illnesses and injuries. Some symptoms might be serious and require emergency surgery, while others were no more than the vague aches and pains of men seeking a little extra time to rest. As a despatch to the *Star Weekly* put it, "When a rating shows up on sick parade and says: "I have a pain—just here... it may call for anything from the traditional Number Nine to an immediate operation, or it might be the first signs of an epidemic liable to sweep through the entire ship."[12] Included in daily routine were visits to those who had been excused duty, essentially a round of hammocks, followed by the paperwork that accompanied any modern medical activity. Where the process differed from similar operations ashore was in the realm of logistics, a ship's medical officer or SBA having to work with whatever

---

10. S.T. Richards, *Operation Sick Bay* (West Vancouver, 1994), 123.
11. DHist 4430, Medical Branch, vol 1, The Naval Doctor, by Surgeon-Commander Archie McCallum.
12. DHist 4430, Medical Branch, vol 2, Despatch to *Star Weekly*.

had been made available before sailing, with further supplies probably a thousand miles distant.

For the most part, this does not seem to have been a problem, if Surgeon-Lieutenant J.R. Bingham can be taken as fairly typical. During his nine months' service in a destroyer in the North Atlantic, he treated a total of 242 cases worth mentioning (minor complaints such as headaches and mild indigestion were not reported), 54 of them all at once when an influenza epidemic broke out; fortunately, the vessel was in port at the time and simply delayed sailing. Other cases included 41 assorted eye, ear, nose, and throat complaints, 26 digestion problems, and two of appendicitis. Injuries required the setting of 11 fractures, the treatment of four burns covering more than 25 per cent of the body, and dealing with an assortment of hernias and bullet wounds (the destroyer had obviously seen action).[13] Surgeon Lieutenant-Commander W.C. Mackenzie, writing in the *Canadian Medical Association Journal*, reported in like manner, noting that a practitioner's "assignment may entail long periods with a small body of normally healthy men, and one may feel that his professional knowledge is not being adequately utilized." But, "Suddenly, without warning, disaster is upon them and the medical officer has every opportunity to test his ability and ingenuity. He is on his own, without the service of a consultant. A medical officer at sea, may, in addition, be called upon to minister to a patient in another ship of the convoy. The hazardous trip in a small boat from ship to ship in a heavy sea is long to be remembered."[14]

How difficult his task might be differed from one vessel to another; for example, while a meeting of the Subcommittee on Naval Medical Research could discuss how "On the *St Laurent* there was no evidence that the healing of wounds was appreciably delayed," as "The inspections of the superficial wounds, which were incurred, was prompt and the treatment effective," the same could not be said of HMCS *Snowberry*. According to one of the ship's officers, Sub-Lieutenant Cowan, who spent two weeks in the corvette, "the conditions were far less satisfactory."

> From his own observations and those of Lieutenant Kelly, Captain of the Snowberry, it appeared that a large number of ratings suffered from boils, infected cuts, sores, ear infections, inflamed eyes, sore throats and ulcerated mouths. In Sub-Lieutenant Campbell's own experience, every minor cut or scratch appeared to become infected and took a long time to heal. This may have been due in part to the very concentrated solutions of iodine ... but more probably was related to the dietary conditions

13. DHist, 4430, Medical Branch, vol 2, Report to Star Weekly.
14. Surg Lt-Cdr W.C. Mackenzie, "Surgical Problems in the Royal Canadian Navy," *Canadian Medical Association Journal* (November, 1942).

or perhaps to the exposure and wetting with salt water to which the men had to be subjected.[15]

Delayed healing was also observed at hospitals in Halifax and Newfoundland, so it was not a phenomenon limited to life on board ship. Researchers hypothesized that nutritional (underlined in red in the minutes of the above meeting) factors might have played an important role in such circumstances, but also suggested that "this subject needs further study."[16]

Even avoiding minor injury did not mean avoiding infection, as endemic in these vessels was a condition which was eventually called "sailor's skin," a rash brought about by lack of water for washing, the prevalence of oil and dirt in even the best-maintained ship, the use of harsh soap (originally designed to remove oil and grease), uniforms made of wool which encouraged perspiration, and close personal contact between individuals whenever they ate or slept. About all that could be done was to urge men to keep as clean as possible, but, nonetheless, "A large percentage of cases reporting to our sick bays have to do with "skins"."[17] Higher powers were not overly concerned by rashes, however, and after investigation Admiralty Fleet Order No 3154 could proclaim that "Modern research has shown that scabies," an ailment more serious than sailor's skin, "is rarely transmitted by clothing or bedding," so that "The routine disinfection of clothing and bedding may therefore be discontinued. Treatment of clothing should, however, be carried out if, in the opinion of the Medical Officer, the nature of the case demands it, as in very heavy infestations or where there is a superimposed infection." However, "Disinfestation of clothing is necessary in the treatment of body louse infestation, and is always to be carried out,"[18] an order with which no one would argue. Nevertheless, dermatology was a specialty that seemed to be more mystery than science, leading to such ship-to-ship messages as "Please can you let me have some sort of medicine for some sort of rash."[19]

Complicated surgery on board ship, a domain limited to MOs, was rare, appendicitis cases and similar problems usually being dealt with conservatively, the patient made comfortable (if such was possible in a pitching, rolling ship), while the medical practitioner focussed on alleviating symptoms. There were occasions, however, when it might be hazard-

15. RG 24, v.8130, NS 1287-7, Proceedings of the Second Meeting of the Subcommittee on Naval Medical Research, 28 Jan 42.
16. Ibid.
17. Surgeon-Lieutenant Roy Forsey, "The Problem of the Sailor's Skin," *Canadian Medical Association Journal* (March, 1943), 213.
18. NA, RG 24, v.11,706, NB 1854-1, PMO, Admiralty Fleet Order No 3154, 15 Jul 43.
19. James B. Lamb, *On the Triangle Run* (Toronto, 1986), 53.

ous to wait until the vessel made port, leading to experiences such as that of Surgeon-Lieutenant B.A. Cambpell in conducting the war's third appendectomy aboard a Canadian destroyer, in this case HMCS *Haida*. The patient first felt ill while the ship was in Murmansk, having escorted a convoy to the USSR, but unwilling to place his fate in the hands of Soviet medicine he did not report to sick bay until the destroyer was well on its way back to the UK, by which time his situation was critical. The doctor had to transfer from another ship, a process made easier by fair weather, and set up in the captain's day-cabin, the dining table serving for the operation, while sterilizers were positioned on a writing desk and light was provided by one of the ship's Torpedo Gunners. Oxygen equipment was run by a quickly-trained paymaster. The operation had to be postponed for a while as the ship manoeuvred to avoid a U-boat reported nearby, but "The destroyer then abandoned her zig-zag, reduced speed, and settled on a course designed to cut down the ship's motion to a minimum. Incidentally, this made her a slightly better target for any U-boat which could get close enough to launch a "fish"." The intervention was a success and the patient, Able Seaman A.H. King, recovered completely.[20]

Other cases were far more difficult, especially when injuries to limbs were so severe that a doctor deemed amputation was called for. Arriving at such a conclusion must have been accompanied by no little trepidation, given that the surroundings for such surgery were extremely primitive when compared with the average operating room in a Canadian hospital (though in rural areas such work was often still done in family kitchens). One typical case was Telegraphist Charles Kent, seriously wounded in an attack by a radio-guided bomb in August 1943, who had both legs removed below the knee on an improvised operating table in the captain's cabin. "Dr Wallace gave great praise to Able Seaman Ike Mengoni for not only volunteering to keep the anaesthesia progressing but also for his cheerful chatter which helped to relieve a lot of the pressure at that time."[21] Another example was described by Leading SBA William Oneschuck, an engine room artificer who survived, though barely, the sinking of HMCS *Regina* off the coast of Cornwall in August 1944. "The ERA was in a badly shocked condition with a severely mangled left leg below the knee. Both the tibia and fibula were fractured and protruding through a large gaping wound. The main arteries were severed. He was treated for shock and given morphine, it being recognized that an amputation would be required

20. DHist 4430, Medical Branch, vol 2, Press Release; S.T. Richards, *Operation Sick Bay* (West Vancouver, 1994), 114.
21. S.T. Richards, *Operation Sick Bay* (West Vancouver, 1994), 147.

after the morphine had taken effect." Surgeon Lieutenant G.A. Gould had also been rescued, and though suffering from broken ribs, "on the rolling deck, proceeded with a complete amputation of the leg. A large shot of brandy and a padded stick for the patient to clench his teeth on, served in the absence of an anaesthetic," which was often unavailable, as it was in many remote parts of Canada at the time. As for the patient, "The stump was dusted with sulfanilamide, shell dressings were applied and tightly held in place with bandages."[22]

Though such incidents were challenging enough, it was perhaps in dealing with large numbers of survivors that navy medical practitioners' knowledge and training were truly put to the test. Relating the experiences of Surgeon-Lieutenant George Maughan while serving in a destroyer, Surgeon Lieutenant-Commander W.C. Mackenzie recalled that the doctor once had to deal with 22 men rescued from a tanker, one of them dying in spite of a barrage of morphia, coramine (to stimulate the heart), hot coffee, general heat, and "several plasma transfusions administered at sea."[23] In another case a torpedoed tanker left 44 men requiring treatment, and as was usual the convoy escort was made up of corvettes and minesweepers, none of which carried medical officers as part of their normal complements. It was thus left to sick berth attendants to begin the process by which these men's lives would be saved as they provided relief for frost bite, gave their charges hot food and liquids, and attempted to put their minds at rest after a horrific ordeal. Oil was a two-fold problem: caking a crewman's skin, it could only be stripped and scraped away with difficulty—and much tenderness if the attendant was to avoid adding injury in the process; swallowed, it could release toxins into the body, an attack that proved fatal in many cases. Treatment had to be immediate and comprehensive, as such patients might not see a doctor until the ship that had rescued them made its way into port, which could be days away.[24]

A common and limb-threatening condition, especially in a convoy that might see several sinkings and hence dozens of survivors, was immersion foot, and unlike the Canadian Corps of the First World War, which focussed on prevention, the Royal Canadian Navy of the 1939-45 conflict had no choice but to deal with it post hoc. What eventually emerged was a mode of treatment encapsulated in a report to a Subcommittee on Surgery (part of the NRC's structure for medical research) in early 1942.

22. S.T. Richards, *Operation Sick Bay* (West Vancouver, 1994), 107.
23. Ibid.
24. DHist 4430, Medical Services, Medical Treatment of Survivors.

When survivors, who have had their feet frozen or immersed in icy water, are picked up, the cold extremities should be kept cool and only allowed to thaw or warm up extremely slowly, while heat is applied to the rest of the body. It should be remembered that bad results have followed heating extremities before a galley stove. In the case of one frozen foot, the unaffected limb should be immersed in hot water to produce reflex dilatation in the affected limb; if both feet are frozen, the arms should be placed in hot water...

Extreme care should be exercised in handling such a limb while it is still numb so that local injury may be avoided. Friction should not be employed at any time. The skin should be kept clean and, in severe cases, sterile. It is recommended that the limb may be placed in dry cotton wool and pressure points carefully avoided.[25]

Within a month or so, reports from the hospital in Halifax confirmed the validity of such an approach, survivors of a sinking being monitored by researchers from Canada and the US, including Doctor Omond Solandt from the former. They determined that, aboard the rescue ship, feet should be left open to the air and kept cool, without friction or massage, while the rest of the body and other extremities were warmed up.[26] Immersion foot was thus another example of civilian research applied to a navy medical problem, though with a far more successful outcome than in the case of seasickness.

Dealing with burns, tragically common when fuel from sinking ships ignited on the water's surface, was more controversial. Such injuries are among the most painful and damaging, and to this day treatment procedures are not always satisfactory; the Subcommittee on Surgery noted as late as March 1943 that the RCN, RCAF, and the Department of Pensions and National Health were all "interested in a recommendation for standard treatment of burns."[27] The reason a common mode for dealing with such problems had not yet been developed was because the challenge faced by medical practitioners, be they doctors, nurses, or sick berth attendants, was multi-layered. First it was necessary to allay the initial pain while also fighting infection, burn injuries providing an excellent medium for the multiplication of bacteria. Similarly, the patient had to be kept in as aseptic an environment as possible, doctors, nurses, and orderlies wearing masks and gowns much as they would in an operating room, while dust had to be swept in accordance with special precautions (i.e. no dry brooms). Debridement, or cutting away dead

25. NA, RG 24, v.8129, NS 1287-3-1, Proceedings of the First Meeting of the Subcommittee on Surgery, 16 Feb 42.
26. NA, RG 24, v.8129, NS 1287-3-1, Proceedings of the Second Meeting of the Subcommittee on Surgery, 27 Mar 42.
27. RG 24, v.8129, NS 1287-3-1, Proceedings of the Second Meeting of the Subcommittee on Surgery, 27 Mar 42.

tissue, was an effective means of reducing the immediate medium of infection, but it was often impossible to remove all affected areas, especially if they covered the face or large portions of the body. Finally, it was necessary to replace the patient's skin through grafting, a process that in the Second World War still incorporated many experimental elements.[28]

One medication that had been in use since 1925 was tannic acid, but by early 1943 or thereabouts research was beginning to put its usefulness into doubt. After evidence began to emerge that the compound caused liver necrosis (in effect, the death of the organ, which would be inevitably fatal), rats were exposed to it for periods up to 28 days, though without causing any harm. Other shortcomings were soon apparent, however, one report to the Subcommittee on Surgery suggesting that it could actually cause damage by destroying capillaries below the burn layer, while hindering drainage and thus increasing the chances of infection.[29] The compound had to be eliminated from the pharmacopoeia, though no effective substitutes were immediately available and the search for effective treatment continued until the end of the war, as it does to this day.

More straightforward to deal with were the various injuries suffered by survivors either as a direct result of enemy weapons or in abandoning a sinking ship; often, rescued surgeons found themselves their first patients, patching themselves up as best they could so they could tend to their comrades. On other occasions SBAs had to perform the necessary first aid, as happened when *Weyburn* struck a mine in February 1942 while sailing from Gibraltar to the UK. Most of the ship's complement survived to be picked up by HMS *Wivern*, but the Surgeon-Lieutenant from the first ship was incapacitated with two broken ankles, so the SBAs from both vessels treated the injured, including five in dangerous condition and one who died of blast injuries (a problem to be described below). Having done the best they could with the others, they then operated on the MO's leg without anaesthetic, a common enough procedure, as we have seen.[30] In another incident, the sinking of HMCS *Chebogue* in late 1944, "The injured were mostly suffering from shock, badly cut and lacerated faces, broken limbs and blast damage." According to Leading SBA Hugh Lees, "As soon as aboard, there being no Medical Officer, the SBAs working together, commenced treatment. As part of this activity they hurriedly applied a total of 126

28. NA, RG 24, v.8129, NS 1287-3-1, Proceedings of the Sixth Meeting of the Subcommittee on Surgery, 16 Oct 42.
29. NA, RG 24, v.8129, NS 1287-3-1, Proceedings of the Seventh Meeting of the Subcommittee on Surgery, 9 Jan 43.
30. S.T. Richards, *Operation Sick Bay* (West Vancouver, 1994), 99.

temporary sutures to close wounds and dust with sulfanilamide. Morphine was given as necessary for patient comfort."[31]

The great bulk of Canada's war at sea was carried out against the U-boat, and the weapon most used in that conflict was the depth charge, a simple device consisting in its essentials of explosives, a casing, and a detonator designed to go off at a chosen water pressure. The weapon was fitted with a safety device so that if an escort was sunk survivors would not be killed or seriously injured by underwater blasts, but there were occasions when destroyers, corvettes, or minesweepers (which were equipped more and more with depth charges so they could play an anti-submarine role) were struck by torpedoes with their weapons fully armed. The result was casualties among those who managed to survive the U-boat's original attack, and Surgeon-Commander D.R. Webster, in the *Canadian Medical Association Journal*, noted that there had been three such cases during the evacuation from Dunkirk, with various doctors reporting 10, 35, and similar clusters as the anti-submarine war gained in intensity.[32]

In one incident, the sinking of HMCS *Charlottetown* in Canadian waters, 15 men sustained abdominal injuries from an exploding depth charge, and "The survivors all gave a fairly uniform history of feeling that they had been struck a tremendous blow in the abdomen, 4 stating that they were paralyzed or knocked unconscious for a short period," one officer having a cigarette lighter flattened in his pocket. All were rescued, but at least one regretted it, as "his pain was so agonizing that he begged to be shot or thrown overboard." His comrades also suffered from severe abdominal pain, which continued after they were admitted to hospital ashore; they also vomited repeatedly, several bringing up blood and bile, while nine suffered from bloody diarrhoea; fever averaged 102 degrees. One man died the first day, another on the second, a third five days after rescue, and a fourth after six weeks. Five months after the incident four men still suffered from symptoms, and an investigation concluded that some of the fatalities might have been saved by early surgical intervention.[33]

The tragedy demonstrated both how devastating depth charges could be and how insidious the injuries they inflicted. Torpedoed in the Gulf of St Lawrence, most of the ship's complement managed to abandon ship, but "The fearful detonation of her own charges killed more of *Charlottetown*'s sailors than either of the two German torpedoes," includ-

31. S.T. Richards, *Operation Sick Bay* (West Vancouver, 1994), 104.
32. Surg-Cdr D.W. Webster et al, "Immersion Blast Injuries of the Abdomen," *Canadian Medical Association Journal* (July, 1943), 1.
33. Surg-Cdr D.R. Webster et al, "Immersion Blast Injuries of the Abdomen," *Canadian Medical Association Journal* (July, 1943), 1.

ing the captain, William Bonner, whose "distorted face showed how he had died." Survivors were put ashore at Gaspé pier but "men who seemed quite fit could suddenly develop the dreaded symptoms—retching, bringing up blood—of internal injuries due to the detonation of the ship's depth charges. Telegraphist Edmund Robinson insisted on his fitness, only to collapse as he walked up the pier. Five days later he died in hospital, leaving fifty-four survivors from a ship's company of sixty-four."[34] The threat of one's own anti-submarine weapons loomed sufficiently large whenever an escort was torpedoed that it was considered a selfless act to put the weapons to safe as the ship went down. Such was the case when *Valleyfield* was torpedoed in May 1944, three ratings making their way aft, "clutching at every handhold, and climbing upwards as the sinking hull tilted ever more sharply,"[35] to do just that. They were never seen again.

Injury due to blast was very unusual in peacetime, and thus presented a rare example of a purely naval (or military) medical challenge. Surgeon-Commander D.R. Webster was instructed to look into the matter, making detailed recommendations in the summer of 1943. The first, that naval personnel should be warned of the danger so they could swim out of the area as quickly as possible, was somewhat redundant, sailors being all too aware of the hazards posed by depth charges in sinking ships. Further, the suggestion that life preservers cover the abdomen and chest was not accompanied by any kind of explanation as to how this would help—a few inches of kapok would certainly make little difference against a shock wave that could flatten cigarette lighters. In the area of treatment the doctor was on firmer ground, recommending that shock and blood loss be dealt with quickly, through transfusions if necessary; that physicians in coastal areas be taught to appreciate the urgency of early treatment; that naval base hospitals either fly the necessary equipment to the scene of a sinking or transport patients ashore promptly; and that doubtful cases have laparotomies, surgical incisions through the abdominal wall, presumably to relieve pain and pressure.[36]

Another area in which navy medical treatment differed from that of civilian practice was in dealing with psychological damage; for though psychoanalysis was well-established in Canada, it was available only to higher-income families and focussed on subconscious phenomena rather than psychic trauma. For the RCN, the issue was especially of

34. James B. Lamb, *On the Triangle Run* (Toronto, 1986), 120-122.
35. James B. Lamb, *On the Triangle Run* (Toronto, 1986), 164.
36. Surg-Cdr D.R. Webster et al, "Immersion Blast Injuries of the Abdomen," *Canadian Medical Association Journal* (July, 1943), 1.

interest in cases such as the above-described loss of HMCS *Valleyfield*. Torpedoed by U-548, its survivors had to watch as a nearby ship, HMCS *Giffard*, first tried to pull some of them on board—though without stopping because of the risk of torpedo attack—sucking one or more of them into its propellers before continuing on and seemingly abandoning them to their fate. *Giffard* returned after searching, unsuccessfully, for the enemy, and took those still alive to the RCN hospital in St John's. Of the frigate's complement of 163, only 38 made it back to port alive, and psychological evaluations began immediately. Reflecting the RCN as a whole, the majority were under the age of 25, none had been torpedoed before, and a little less than half had a year's experience or more. Very few had previously seen action, and for the first hours after the explosion had been subjected to severe physical and mental stress. According to an article in the *Canadian Medical Association Journal*, "While in the water they thought of being rescued, their folks at home and their mess mates... On the rescue ship the majority of the survivors felt nervous, thankful or felt cold. They were thinking about their mess mates, their personal safety and their folks at home... A day after arrival in hospital about one-third were already anxious to return to sea," demonstrating remarkable resilience.[37] In spite of this, survivors generally did not want to discuss their ordeal until the third day or so after the torpedoing, and according to the article's authors "It is our opinion that immediate rest is the most important therapy for patients subjected to this type of experience. Adequate sedation is indicated and, if the condition progresses, psychotherapy may be necessary."[38]

If blast injuries and psychological trauma were relatively unknown or mainly untreated in peacetime Canada, the hospitals where sailors received medical attention, such as the already- mentioned RCN facility at St John's, were effectively civilian organizations, even after over four years of war. When *Valleyfield*'s survivors were brought ashore, it was to an institution which was "in the forefront of the Battle of the Atlantic,"[39] according to James Lamb. "Nowhere on this side of the Atlantic was there a medical facility with more experience of survivors, those shivering, sodden, oil-soaked wretches, half drowned, fearfully burned or mangled, plucked from torpedoed merchantmen, burning tankers, rammed escorts, or crashed aircraft, and brought, often more dead than alive, to the huddle of wartime emergency buildings that comprised the RCN hospital in St John's." Nevertheless, the hospital

---

37. Surg-Lt J.F. Simpson and A/Surg-Cdr Marvin Wellman, "Emotional Reactions in Survivors of HMCS Valleyfield," *Canadian Medical Association Journal* (October, 1944), 321.
38. Ibid.
39. James B. Lamb, *On the Triangle Run* (Toronto, 1986), 203.

staff was made up of personnel who had been civilians a few years—or months—before, and according to *Operation Sick Bay*, a history of sick berth attendants, "Their work would no longer be confined only to sick bays concerned with sick parades, recruit examinations, immunizations and the treatment of minor diseases and injuries. Large numbers would now work in hospitals where patients could receive high levels of medical and surgical care. Moreover, they would be working with and trained by a wide range of professional personnel in wards, clinics and special departments." Since many brought with them skills they had learned before joining the navy, though working relationships with officers were generally professional the "problems which did arise can be traced to either perceived or actual failure to grant ratings appropriate recognition for pre-entry civilian training and experience."[40]

Thus by the time the army first came to grips with Axis forces the navy had been doing so for over two years, but the land service's casualty rates would soon dwarf those of the RCN. Its first units to see combat were the Royal Rifles of Canada and the Winnipeg Grenadiers, at Hong Kong, and the result was catastrophic, encompassing the loss of the entire force. Attacking the garrison in the days after Pearl Harbor, the Japanese accepted the colony's surrender on Christmas Day, 1941, and among the prisoners were 1700 Canadians whose ordeal in captivity led to the most difficult medical problems faced by Canadian medical practitioners in that war, as will be discussed in the next chapter. The attack against Dieppe, in northern France on 19 August 1942, was even worse; it was the largest raid organized by Britain's Combined Operations, the largest operation to date for the Canadian Army, and an unmitigated disaster. Involving the 4th and 6th Brigades of 2nd Canadian Infantry Division, as well as attached troops, the entire formation was nearly destroyed, leaving over 900 Canadians dead and almost 2000 in enemy hands.

As for the wounded, G.W.L. Nicholson describes how the day of the raid "found Canadian medical units in Britain hurriedly preparing to receive casualties from across the Channel—hurriedly, for due to the necessary security enshrouding the operation their commanding officers had been told about the raid only that morning,"[41] after the initial landings. Patients already resident in British-based hospitals who could be moved were rapidly discharged to other facilities so designated institutions could focus on the surgical and other work the Dieppe wounded would need; almost 600 of the latter had been evacuated from the beaches, with an equal number left behind to be treated by the enemy.

40. S.T. Richards, *Operation Sick Bay* (West Vancouver, 1994), 49, 52, 60.
41. G.W.L. Nicholson, *Canada's Nursing Sisters* (Toronto, 1975), 129.

Since they were placed on board landing craft as soon as possible and taken immediately across the Channel there was little processing, and hospitals were thus effectively operating as front-line units. "Many casualties arrived with their complete battle equipment, and with live hand grenades in their pouches,"[42] Nicholson relates, while according to one anonymous nurse, it was "the first time we *really* worked." Similarly, Assistant Matron Kennedy-Reid of Number 1 General Hospital reported how "I never thought that our staff of fifty-eight nurses could handle so many bad cases" as 95 operations were performed in 19 1/2 hours.

The sheer scale was something unheard of in city hospital work, one area where military medical operations differed markedly from their civilian equivalent. There had been problems, of course, and according to the Committee on Medical Research, which looked into the lessons of Dieppe as they applied to treating the wounded, "Two general complaints of the Canadians were the lack of liaison—not knowing when the raid was planned and hence not being able to prepare adequately for casualty reception—and the necessity of changing all their arrangements in the middle of the show. (Incidentally, also in the middle of a very wet night)."[43] The committee had to point out, however, that such difficulties would always exist to some degree, rigid security always preceding operations while, ironically, flexibility and confusion accompanied their execution. "One thing that became very clear," the Committee reported, "was that the chief duty of the surgical CO of a base hospital was the rapid inspection of the wounded, application of resuscitation measures, determination of the order for operation, etc, instead of doing any actual operating himself."[44] From wounding to first dressing had required 1 1/2 hours, with 15 hours needed to reach England; seven hours to get men into hospital, and another 11 before being operated on. "One serious break in liaison came when it was found that the stretchers on which the wounded had been brought back would not fit the ambulances (from another service) drawn up near the dock to receive them. The obvious lesson is the urgent need for standardization of equipment in all branches of the fighting forces."[45]

With such a long chain of evacuation, only the hardiest survived, accounting for a fatality rate after arrival at hospital of only 2.5 per cent,

42. G.W.L. Nicholson, *Canada's Nursing Sisters* (Toronto, 1975), 129.
43. NA, MG 30, B85, Harris Papers, v.5, Office of Scientific Research and Development, Committee on Medical Research, News Letter No 20, 26 September 1942.
44. NA, MG 30, B85, Harris Papers, v.5, Office of Scientific Research and Development, Committee on Medical Research, News Letter No 20, 26 September 1942.
45. NA, MG 30, B85, Harris Papers, v.5, Office of Scientific Research and Development, Committee on Medical Research, News Letter No 20, 26 September 1942.

or 15 men overall. Of 16 soldiers with wounds to the lower torso, three died before they could be operated on and another three in the post-operative ward, an abdominal death rate that would haunt surgeons and nurses for the rest of the war; similarly, of 11 men with head wounds, four died, three without being operated on. The busiest hospital in the immediate aftermath of the raid was Number 15 General, with 221 casualties arriving in a three-hour period, 112 of whom required major surgery. They were taken care of in a 28-hour "blitz", with three teams working the first half of the period and five teams the remaining half, for an average of one victim per hour per team.

> They found it worthwhile to have one team exclusively for the handling of minor wounds. This team needed less equipment and actually set up in the dental clinic of the hospital for its work. There was a great deal of discussion as to the proper relationship of the medical men in the pre-operative or shock wards and the surgical teams; also as to the best organization of wards and operating rooms as to selection of cases, placing in the wards, and post-operative care. One fact that was emphasized was that when outside assistance is obtained, as was the case here in the later hours, one of the local surgeons should be on each team. The mistake was made in this instance of having visiting surgeons on separate teams of their own and thus post-operatively none of the local group knew about a considerable number of patients. Another practical point is the necessity of having all the chest cases in one ward with a medical man permanently assigned to their care.[46]

The main medical lesson to be derived from the catastrophe at Dieppe was that, regardless of one's credentials, much would have to be learn-ed through experience, and we shall see that this was especially the case in the realm of combat surgery.

There would be plenty of opportunity for on-the-job training in the Canadians' next major operation, the landings in Sicily alongside American and British allies on 10 July, 1943. Thankfully, 1st Canadian Infantry Division, at least for the first few days of the campaign, found itself fighting Italian coastal troops with little interest in dying for fascism, so one of the first enemies the medical corps had to contend with were not the wounds of shrapnel, shell, or bullet, but the minute bite of the anopheles mosquito, carrier of malaria. Occupying the island took almost until the end of August, by which time 756 Canadians had come down with the disease, with a further 1184 suspected cases, compared to 562 killed in action and 1664 wounded (the latter including 15 staff members of No 5 Canadian General Hospital). The mosquito having accounted

---

46. NA, MG 30, B85, Harris Papers, v.5, Office of Scientific Research and Development, Committee on Medical Research, News Letter No 20, 26 September 1942.

for the equivalent of an infantry battalion (of which there were nine in 1st Canadian Division), it comes as no surprise that a draft history of the Mediterranean campaign referred to malaria as "a medical disaster."[47]

The malariologist for the formation had a somewhat different view, insisting that "The operation recently completed proves that it is possible to train and embark troops in a non-malarious area and land them in a highly malarious area with less than 1% of casualties from malaria in the first 31 days of active operations, in the malaria peak season,"[48] in effect pointing out that the loss rate could have been much higher. But, as yet another report related,

> planning for protection against Malaria offered many problems, mostly caused by lack of clear information on conditions to be met, and inexperience with the disease in general... Information trickled in slowly and seemed incomplete. Time for planning was brief, and there was no time for extensive training of special personnel. Equipment was provided so late that no one had time to see it, let alone become familiar with it. [Headquarters] Middle East was most helpful, but not knowing the general state of indecision and ignorance of the subject, could, at first, help only with suggestions,[49]

hence the appointment of the divisional malariologist to provide advice, assist in microscope work, and help in diagnosis and treatment.[50]

He was not alone, anti-malaria squads of an NCO and three ORs each carrying the war to their tiny enemy, their arsenal including such weapons as mosquito nets and insect repellent, though the latter was not too popular with the troops: "This cream was so sticky, greasy and objectionable that it was not used to any appreciable extent."[51] Mepacrine, taken in pill form, had proven effective in other armies, but after arriving in Sicily the division found supplies were strained, so only 40 to 50 per cent of Canadian troops had the medication available to them. Simple devices such as helmet veils and gloves do not seem to have been plentiful, or at least worn often enough to have an impact on sick rates. The result was what we have seen above, so that

> September and October were busy months for the nursing staff of No 5 General. The majority of cases resulted from the attention of anopheles mosquitoes which had taken full advantage of a laxity in anti-malaria

47. G.W.L. Nicholson, *Seventy Years of Service* (Ottawa, 1977), 165.
48. RG 24, v.12,642, 11/Sicily/1, Report on Malaria in 1 Cdn Div from D to D 31, 10 August 1943.
49. RG 24, v.12,621, 11/Sicily/1, Report on Employment of Medical Units in Sicilian Campaign, 25 August 1943.
50. RG 24, v.12,617, 11/Malaria/1/2, Malarial Summary, First Canadian Division, 10 November 1943.
51. RG 24, v.12,617, 11/Malaria/1/2, Malarial Summary, First Canadian Division, 10 November 1943.

precautions by Canadian units and individuals during and after the recent campaign. Because of restrictions on sending malarial patients from Sicily, there were times when the hospital's normal bed capacity was greatly exceeded, and nurses had patients on the balconies, in the corridors, and even on the roof.[52]

In the end, cooler weather did far more to protect Canadian troops from malaria than their own efforts or those of their supporting medical practitioners.

In evacuating battle casualties the latter were in far more familiar territory, such having been part of their training since before the war; as soldiers fell, stretcher-bearers removed them to Regimental Aid Posts, from which they were evacuated towards dressing stations, and hence to casualty clearing stations and into hospitals. The workhorse of this organization was the field ambulance, which we have seen develop from before the First World War, and which would continue to evolve in the Second. One issue of interest in studying the Sicilian campaign was the use of a light field ambulance to support armoured formations, in this case the 1st Canadian Army Tank Brigade, later renamed the 1st Canadian Armoured Brigade. With the 2nd Canadian Light Field Ambulance under command, it operated independently of the infantry division, taking its orders from General Bernard Law Montgomery's Eighth British Army, which had made its name famous fighting against Rommel. Describing its operations in Sicily (and in the early campaigning in Italy), the medical unit could not help but emphasize "tropical heat, hyperendemic malaria, the most primitive standards of hygiene and sanitation, and a march of 800 miles over the worst possible roads and country..."[53]

The Tank Brigade was made up of three armoured regiments, and whenever one of these was detached to support an infantry attack, or for other duties, personnel from the light field ambulance accompanied it to clear any casualties in its sector, whether British, Canadian, or enemy. Admissions to dressing stations totalled 1466 in July and August, of which 356 were quickly discharged back to their units. Sick parades averaged about 3000 a month, the ambulance insisting that "It is most important that it be realized that sickness, no matter what climate or country is being considered, will always be a greater factor of wastage than battle casualties. *Consequently experiences have shown that a Lt Fd Amb is absolutely essential for an independent armoured*

---

52. G.W.L. Nicholson, *Canada's Nursing Sisters* (Toronto, 1975), 137.
53. NA, RG 24, v.12,617, 11/2 Lt Fd Amb/1, Report re 2 Cdn Lt Fd Amb, in Sicilian and Italian Campaign 12 Jul 43-15 Oct 43.

brigade. This is particularly the case with regards a Cdn force operating as part of a British or Allied force and having the natural attendant difficulties with regards re-enforcement problems."[54]

The reader should not be confused by the statement that the sick were more numerous than battle casualties, as previous references to the effectiveness of hygienic and other measures in the prevention of disease focussed on fatality rates. Epidemics having been brought under some form of control in the opening months of the First World War did not mean that men did not continue to come down with all manner of illnesses, but it did ensure the great majority of these would survive, recover, and return to their units. The reinforcement problem is also worthy of further explanation; in its report 2nd Light Field Ambulance was referring to the difficulties of getting replacement troops to a brigade operating outside the administrative control of the parent for-mation. Later in the Italian campaign, however, and again in north-west Europe, Canadian forces would find themselves severely short of trained infantry, making it even more important for medical units to be able to treat the sick and wounded so they could return to the fighting.

Part of that process involved the transfusion units that had been formed in England before the Sicilian campaign started, and which quickly integrated themselves into the larger medical system. As one member of Number 1 Canadian Field Transfusion Unit wrote, he and his colleagues were joined up with two Field Surgical Units (or FSUs) to support a Field Dressing Station (abbreviated as FDS). Triage, which in this case meant separating the wounded into those who did not require surgery, those who did, and those who would not survive an operation, was done by an admitting officer; if he determined that a case required resuscitation, the soldier was sent to a special ward where warmth and blood products were used to fight shock. Deciding on the timing of surgery was a joint decision by the transfusion officer and—of course—the surgeon who was to carry out the procedure.[55]

As one might expect, performing such operations in close proximity to the front meant working in less-than ideal conditions, as a certain Doctor Roche reported to Colonel MacFarlane. "John R. and I started operating about 24 hrs after landing—i.e. a filthy stable—using the equip-ment that an English FSU had brought ashore in packs on their backs—we next worked in a wine cellar, then a house, a tent, a school, a cathedral and finally a school." Cases arrived in batches, so that "our

---

54. NA, RG 24, v.12,617, 11/2 Lt Fd Amb/1, Report re 2 Cdn Lt Fd Amb, in Sicilian and Italian Campaign 12 Jul 43-15 Oct 43.
55. NA, RG 24, OC Army Blood Supply Depot Bristol to Dir Pathology; Extract from letter from 1 Cdn FTU.

work is anything but steady—periods of rush alternating with longer periods of idleness." Working with Number 2 Field Surgical Unit, he and his partner performed about a hundred procedures, but "We have not had an opportunity of following any of them after their discharge from the FDS so cannot tell whether our work is good or bad."[56] In some ways the lessons of Dieppe were relearned, six of 11 abdominal wounds succumbing, while a horror of the First World War, gas gangrene, made a reappearance, killing one man admitted with a compound fracture of the femur.

Numbers 1 and 2 Field Surgical Units carried out 229 operations in the two months of the Sicilian campaign, with an overall mortality of 17 per cent. "The fatal cases were for the most part abdominal cases, sucking chest wounds, severe burns and cases of clinical gas gangrene. 24 Abdominal cases were operated on at an average of 7.7 hrs after being wounded. The mortality rate was 54%,"[57] a horrific toll that would change little in the course of the war. Doctor Bruce Tovee, with his partner Frank Mills, reported losing about 40 per cent of their abdominal cases, but also pointed out another characteristic of military injuries; of their 100 or so patients, many "were major problems, almost every one being not only *one* bad wound but several."[58] At a professional level, Tovee actually found cause for satisfaction, as "I really feel after this campaign that I now am much better able to handle my hands, and I have seen and done much of what might be called emergency surgery. It certainly peps up ones [sic] heretofore questionable opinion of how one would act with these emergent [sic] cases, and I would not have missed this opportunity."[59] Part of the satisfaction was no doubt derived from carrying out surgery in the field which, back home, would have been limited to the most sophisticated hospital operating room.

What happened to these patients after surgery—or treatment for illness—was something of an issue, the army wanting the survivors to get back to the business of defeating fascism and Nazism as soon as possible. "Early in the Sicilian campaign it became evident that a large number of Casualties including the slightly wounded and the mildly ill were being evacuated from the island and lost to their units for an indefinite period. Where as [sic] convalescence in a suitable place would have assured prompt return to action. Furthermore, the evacuation of such casualties and their return to the island involved the use of ship-

---

56. NA, RG 24, v.12,621, 11/Sicily/1, Roche to MacFarlane, 16 August 1943.
57. NA, RG 24, v.12,642, 11/Sicily/1, Report on Activities of 1 & 2 Cdn FSUs during the Sicilian Campaign, 18 August 1943.
58. NA, RG 24, v.12,621, 11/Sicily/1, Bruce Tovee to Col MacFarlane, 14 August 1943.
59. NA, RG 24, v.12,621, 11/Sicily/1, Bruce Tovee to Col MacFarlane, 14 August 1943.

ping facilities already heavily taxed."[60] The solution was the formation of a new unit on 3 August, the Canadian Medical Rest Station, though whether it was inspired by the rest stations (its name implied it might have been) of the First World War is not known.

For those who needed long-term care or treatment not available in theatre, hospitals waited for them in North Africa and, if necessary, Great Britain. Getting them there could be much quicker than in previous conflicts, as theoretical discussions around the use of aircraft to transport sick and wounded had turned into reality by the time the Allies invaded Sicily. In some ways, however, theory was not reflected in practice, such as the 1941 suggestion by Canada's Wilder Penfield to the NRC's Associate Committee on Medical Research that "The lives of men could be saved who are fighting over widely scattered districts. Abdominal wounds, chest wounds, and head wounds are apt to be fatal unless the injured man can reach a properly equipped hospital within 12 to 24 hours after the injury. Wounds of the extremities may be cared for at dressing stations but months of convalescence, as well as frequently fatal complications, can be prevented by early arrival at base hospitals."[61] As we have seen, however, certain wounds needed immediate treatment, not quick evacuation, and even then severe injuries to the abdomen proved highly fatal. In the course of the Sicilian campaign and afterwards, rather, aircraft were used to move soldiers, totalling about 15,000, who had already been sufficiently treated to be medically stable. Under control of the Royal Air Force, they were transported by planes which had brought in supplies or reinforcements, some of them having conversion equipment aboard so they could take ordinary field stretchers. There were, in fact, few air ambulances per se, ordinary cargo aircraft proving sufficient to the task.[62]

In the medical world of 1943, it was not enough to prevent disease through hygiene and sanitation and treat the sick and wounded, practitioners also sought to apply the discoveries of modern science. Thus, in June, a special unit was formed within Canada's medical corps, as "The need for a Medical Research Laboratory had been felt for some time." Though originally suggested in 1942, it was felt by higher authority that Canadian specialists could simply work with the British Army or the Medical Research Council of Great Britain. A month before the landings in Sicily were scheduled to go ashore, however, the ubiquitous Colonel MacFarlane tried again to form a purely Canadian unit, and a

60. NA, RG 24, v.12,642, 11/Sicily/1, Canadian Medical Rest Station, 25 August 1943.
61. NA, RG 24, v.5383, S.45-6-3, Wilder Penfield, Report to the Chairman of the Associate Committee on Medical Research et al, November 1941.
62. NA, RG 24, v.5393, HQS 60-1-46, Canmilitry to AG, 1 September 1943.

more nationalistic (and as we shall see, pragmatic) approach prevailed. Number 1 Research Laboratory was thus authorized to form on 26 August, a few days after the campaign in Sicily wound down.[63] According to its instructions from Ottawa, "the first studies will be those dealing with the physiological, Biochemical and bacteriological aspects of wounds. Provision is made for a mobile laboratory and staff to proceed to the forward areas in the field to see and study the cases as early as possible after wounding. There is also to be a static laboratory and staff at the base to receive cultures, specimens etc for further study and identification of the material collected at the front, besides following the further progress of the cases on arrival at the base."[64] Staff was small, consisting of three officers and three laboratory technicians, consistent with a research as opposed to a diagnostic unit.

At the time the germ theory of disease only went so far, and in dealing with other ailments—those of the mind—medical practitioners saw a clear distinction between the physical and the psychological. Injuries to both could, however, be dealt with in similar fashion; as Lieutenant-Colonel A.M. Doyle explained in a post-war article. "Experiences of the last war, and those of our British and American colleagues in this one, has indicated that Psychiatric services were required in the field and should be available as far forward as possible."[65] The result for 1st Canadian Infantry Division was the appointment of a formation psychiatrist. "For six months prior to invasion, he had handled the Neuropsychiatric work of the Division and had participated in the training, schemes, and practise landings on the beaches of the Clyde, that were later to be reduplicated upon the Sicilian beaches." Number 15 General Hospital in North Africa contained a Base Neuropsychiatric Centre, and "Any soldier whom it was felt would be fit for duty in the theatre within 9 days, was considered suitable for treatment,"[66] which consisted of psychotherapy, "prolonged narcosis," essentially stupefying the patient with drugs, and the use of electro-shock. "Valuable assistance to the unit in the way of occupational therapy was provided by the Red Cross, and full use of opportunities for employment within the General Hospital were made," meaningful work being considered an important part of psychiatric treatment. Closer to the front, the divisional psychiatrist himself dealt with 45 cases in the course of the campaign, of whom 29 were returned to duty and 16 evacuated. Of the latter, "14 gave a

---

63. NA, RG 24, v.15,598, No 1 Research Laboratory, September 1943.
64. NA, RG 24, v.15,598, War Diary, No 1 Research Lab, September 1943, Introduction.
65. Lt-Col A.M. Doyle, "Psychiatry with the Canadian Army in Action in the CMF," *The Journal of the Canadian Medical Services* (January, 1946), 93.
66. Lt-Col A.M. Doyle, "Psychiatry with the Canadian Army in Action in the CMF," *The Journal of the Canadian Medical Services* (January, 1946), 95.

bad history of neuropsychiatric disorder in civilian life and in the other 2 a satisfactory history of previous health could not be obtained. Six of the 14 gave a history of hospital treatment for nervous or mental disorder. It is felt that all of these cases could have been recognised as unfit for combatant duty had they been surveyed by a Neuropsychiatrist prior to the campaign. All the cases returned to duty were under treatment less than 7 days."[67]

Blaming difficult cases on the recruiting system may seem something of a cop-out, but in spite of Captain H.P. Wright's work in the First World War, in 1943 neither the army nor the psychiatric profession had yet admitted that every soldier had a limited reserve of courage or fortitude which, when used up, led to what could be termed psychological injury. This would not be recognized until later, though in the realm of treatment the divisional psychiatrist was on very solid ground. "In view of the high percentage that can be returned to duty in a period of a week, it is felt that neuropsychiatric service should be maintained as far forward as possible. By and large all that a recoverable patient requires is rest and reassurance and security from enemy action and some sedation. In a few cases special treatment such as hypnosis was employed with success but no special equipment is required for such treatment."[68] Thus, like surgeons, psychiatrists sought to operate as close to the front as feasible.

As for those who did the fighting, Terry Copp and Bill McAndrew have pointed out in their seminal work, *Battle Exhaustion: Soldiers and Psychiatrists in the Canadian Army, 1939-1945*, that infantry commanders were generally supportive of the efforts of Lieutenant-Colonel Doyle and his colleagues. It seems that "their main concern was to rid themselves of unstable, jittery soldiers who lost control of themselves in action. Not only were they a danger to themselves, they were also an operational hindrance, because good soldiers had to be diverted to look after them. According to Doyle, combat commanders judged that there were few malingerers among the exhaustion cases."[69] As the psychiatrist reported, "Though they frequently use such uncomplimentary terms as yellow they usually recognize that the soldier with an anxiety neurosis just can't help it."[70] It was one of the most dramatic medical lessons of the campaign.

Unknown to Canadian soldiers fighting in Sicily, there would be plenty of time to absorb the lessons learnt there, as the campaign in the

---

67. NA, RG 24, v.12,642, 11/Sicily/1, Report of Neuropsychiatrist 1 Cdn Division, 25 August 1943.
68. NA, RG 24, v.12,642, 11/Sicily/1, Report of Neuropsychiatrist 1 Cdn Division, 25 August 1943.
69. Terry Copp and Bill McAndrew, *Battle Exhaustion* (Montreal and Kingston, 1990).
70. Ibid.

Mediterranean had another 16 months to go before German forces finally surrendered (Italy agreed to an armistice in September 1943). The next step after securing the island was to assault the Italian boot on 3 September, in operation Baytown, landings that went so smoothly one medical report boasted that "No lessons in combined operations were learned because everything went according to plan."[71] By the end of the month casualty evacuation was over 250 miles on a single road, though the same report insisted that "the normal high standard of treatment was maintained," and there is no evidence to the contrary. As for dealing with illness, contagious and otherwise, "It is worthy to note that in spite of the strain imposed by long drives, lack of sleep, malarious and unhygienic state of the country traversed in general, the percentage of sick remained at .28%, as compared with a conceded normal of .3% per day."

In the course of the campaign the field ambulance proved to be something of a jack-of-all trades, its focus shifting with the intensity of battle, its role changing as the front stabilized and turned fluid again. Number 24 Field Ambulance, for example, landed at Naples on 8 November and moved to Altamura, where it remained until the following January; while there it "was occupied in caring for local sick, equipping itself, and general training."[72] Taking over a local Italian military hospital, it ran an 80-bed establishment "caring for all types of minor sick," as well as victims of gonorrhea. "Serious medical and surgical cases were evacuated by motor ambulance" to 54 British Hospital and later to Number 1 Canadian General Hospital. In all it deal with 518 casualties while at Altamura, most due to fighting but including 89 accidents and 6 self-inflicted wounds, while also treating 422 sick, including VD, hepatitis, a case of diphtheria, a few dozen of flu, many respiratory, a similar number of gastric, some twenty nervous, over forty dermatological, and a large group of miscellaneous cases. A little over 60 per cent were evacuated further back down the line, the remainder being returned to their units.[73]

December 1943 proved one of the busiest months for RCAMC personnel, the Canadians attempting to capture the fortified town of Ortona, leading to fighting so heavy some soldiers referred to it as "little Stalingrad." The cost, 692 killed and 1738 wounded, was added to by about 500 cases of battle exhaustion.[74] Fighting continued into January, Number 24 Field Ambulance reporting that "On the 16 Jan

71. NA, RG 24, v.12,642, 11/Sicily/1, Lessons from Operation "Baytown", 27 September 1943.
72. NA, RG 24, v.12,596, 11/7 FSU/1, Quarterly Report, 24 Cdn Fd Amb, 1 Dec 43 to 31 Mar 44.
73. NA, RG 24, v.12,596, 11/7 FSU/1, Quarterly Report, 24 Cdn Fd Amb, 1 Dec 43 to 31 Mar 44.
74. G.W.L. Nicholson, *Seventy Years of Service* (Ottawa, 1977), 170.

44 preparations were made for the handling of the large number of casualties that were expected in the next few days."[75] Part of the unit moved well forward and set itself up as a Casualty Clearing Post (or CCP), with accommodation for 50 casualties if necessary. Forward evacuation was by ambulances able to carry four stretchers each as well as 3-ton lorries, and after treatment at the CCP wounded were removed by a detachment of a British MAC (Motorized Ambulance Column); serious casualties went to Number 2 Canadian Field Dressing Station, others to Number 4 Casualty Clearing Station, with exhaustion cases, which formed about 9 per cent of the total, being sent to Number 4 Canadian Field Ambulance. Of 192 victims, only five were returned to their units.

In the months that followed, the Allies continued to grind away at a series of defensive lines the Germans constructed across the peninsula in an attempt to keep American and British armies away from Austria and the Balkans. Ironically, it was when Canadian troops were most successful that evacuation procedures faced the severest tests, wounded having to travel ever farther as the front made its way towards Rome. In the campaigning of February and March, for example, a survey of a hundred wounded who moved through Number 4 Casualty Clearing Station found that the average elapsed time from injury to admission was 12 $\frac{3}{4}$ hours. Over three hours were then required for resuscitation, pre-operative procedures, X-rays, and other exams, making a total from wounding to surgery of just under 16 hours. The fastest was six, the longest a near-fatal 40. Later, however, in the Liri Valley fighting that helped clear the way to Rome in May and June, the CCS was closer to the front, allowing a reduction in average evacuation and preparation times from 16 hours to 12 $\frac{1}{2}$.[76]

The Eternal City fell to American forces on 4 June, and by then the lessons of the first part of the Italian campaign had been reported and discussed for some months. One issue which would remain near the fore for some time to come was the proper employment of nursing sisters, whose training in civilian life made them near-perfect for certain tasks such as monitoring patients in the critical days following major surgery. Number 3 Field Surgical Unit, for one, thought they should work closer to the front, as FSUs often operated alongside Main Dressing Stations, well-forward of the Casualty Clearing Stations where nursing sisters normally performed their tasks. According to one surgeon,

---

75. NA, RG 24, v.12,596, 11/7 FSU/1, Quarterly Report, 24 Cdn Fd Amb, 1 Dec 43 to 31 Mar 44.
76. G.W.L. Nicholson, *Seventy Years of Service* (Ottawa, 1977), 183.

There is no comparison of the ease of working at the CCS, where there are well organized Post-Op wards, with Sisters, and well trained nursing orderlies, as compared with the MDS where there are no sisters and the quality of nursing is not as good. At the MDS we did the supervision of the Post Op wards and had to watch such details of nursing as the care of a patient's back, had to be sure that the NOs [nursing orderlies] turned an unconscious patient, and sometimes to show them how to do it, etc, and we could not go to bed with the same ease of mind that one would like. Possibly I am not taking into full account the fact that the patients were all more serious cases, but the very presence of Sisters in a ward is of greater benefit than one would think.[77]

As for the women who might carry out their work further forward, according to their semi-official historian "To be a nursing sister serving in a field surgical unit, close enough to the forward troops to be within range of the enemy's guns, was an envied role to which few nurses did not aspire."[78]

If the competence of personnel was a known quality, the same could not be said of new medicines, even those that later came to be accepted as wonder drugs, such as penicillin. As late as October, 1943, reports on administering the antibiotic could still name patients as individuals, there having been so few Canadians treated with it, and in early 1944 Number 1 Research Laboratory advocated special cards be attached to those receiving the compound so their progress or decline could be traced in detail.[79] Though its ability to hinder the reproduction of certain bacteria had been demonstrated long before, practitioners were still unsure of how to take advantage of that characteristic, a typhus research team in North Africa, for example, finding no improvement after administering the drug.[80] The treatment of gas gangrene seemed more encouraging, though the fatality rate in Italy was still high, 33 of 48 dying between 1 September and 30 November 1943, though only nine of 30 victims died in December. According to the Eighth Army's Major J.D. MacLennan, "Despite the stress rightly laid in recent years upon the value of serotherapy and chemotherapy, it must not be forgotten that, as matters now stand, these measures are still ancillary to adequate operative treatment."[81]

---

77. NA, RG 24, v.12,596, 11/3 FSU/1, Monthly Report, 29 January 1944.
78. G.W.L. Nicholson, *Canada's Nursing Sisters* (Toronto, 1975), 145.
79. NA, RG 24, v.12,628, 11/Penicillin/1, MacFarlane to Cairns, 5 October 1943; RG 24, v.12,628, 11/Penicillin/1, Maj A.L. Chute, CO No 1 Res Lab RCAMC to DMS CMHQ, 3 February 1944.
80. NA, RG 24, v.12,628, 11/Penicillin/1/2, Typhus Research Team, British North African Force, 6 April 1944.
81. NA, RG 24, v.12,628, 11/Penicillin/1/2, Report on Gas Gangrene in the Eighth Army, April 1944.

Perhaps the best example of the experimental nature of penicillin was described by G.W.L. Nicholson as he related how two members of Princess Patricia's Canadian Light Infantry suffered loss of limb from a German shell, with gangrene soon threatening their lives.

> The efforts of the Corps DDMS Brigadier McCusker, promptly secured two million units of penicillin, brought by special courier from Canadian sources in Naples, and half of this was turned over to the advanced surgical centre. The brief instructions accompanying the shipment failed to give scale of dosage, and it was mistakenly assumed that the entire batch was to be used on the two casualties. "It was consequently decided, in true quartermaster fashion, to husband some of it by giving each patient 600,000 at the rate of 100,000 units per day. Recovery was not only prompt but truly remarkable. When the package had been emptied, the manufacturer's bill was found lying at the bottom. The price tag?—just under $500,000.00 Canadian."[82]

By May 1944 penicillin was administered in a more rational fashion, the patient receiving a first dose at a Casualty Clearing Station or Advanced Surgical Centre, with subsequent treatments on ambulance trains, ships, or at any other convenient time. "Doses spaced as above are necessary to maintain the concentration of the Penicillin in the blood at an effective level, until definitive surgery has been completed,"[83] according to wisdom current at the time.

As for the physical, so for the psychological, procedures to deal with injured minds evolving—at least a little—in the months leading to the fall of Rome. The 1st Canadian Division's psychiatrist became the Corps psychiatrist after the arrival of 5th Canadian Armoured Division at the end of 1943, and the new, larger, formation that resulted had a Corps Exhaustion Centre, usually attached to a Casualty Clearing Station, a Field Dressing Station, or any medium-sized (that is with about 200 beds) hospital. Treatment began with the forward psychiatrist, and consisted simply of rest with sedation, bath facilities, clean clothing, new equipment, and psychotherapy in the form of explanation and reassurance. In the course of the Mediterranean campaign about one in four such patients returned to duty; for the others, there were Special Employment Companies.

> They did all the loading of ammunition and petrol for Corps, and many other duties at workshops, medical units, stores, dumps, etc and became a highly successful and valued part of the military organization. Neuro-psychiatric casualties were sent to the Special Employment Companies directly without passing through a Medical Board. Very often the

---

82. G.W.L. Nicholson, *Seventy Years of Service* (Ottawa, 1977), 186.
83. NA, RG 24,v.12,628, 11/Penicillin/1/2, Instructions for the Use of Penicillin in Severe War Wounds as a Prophylactic against Gas Gangrene and Sepsis, 30 May 1944.

casualty was posted to the SEC within 2-3 days of having been evacuated from his unit and the therapeutic value inherent in the policy of putting the casualty to work as soon as possible was very evident. This was particularly true while the Corps was still in action where the casualty, having failed to stand up to battle stress, still was able to carry on a job that was important to the immediate battle. During rest periods, a Medical Board at Corps level was set up to deal with those soldiers who had been posted to the SECs.[84]

The special companies took much of the burden of treating exhaustion cases off the hospitals and other medical units, who could thus focus on those with more "traditional" wounds or illnesses.

Total exhaustion cases among Canadian formations in the Mediterranean numbered about 5000, of whom a little more than a fifth returned to duty. Attitudes towards these men and their condition demonstrated both conservatism and change, and as late as 1946 a practitioner publishing in *The Journal of the Canadian Medical Services* could state that 85 per cent of these cases were chronic. "By "chronic" is meant that they suffered from some form of Neuropsychiatric disorder prior to enlistment. These were mainly—Chronic Neuroses, Inadequate Personalities (Psychopathic Personality—Inadequate Type) and Mental Defectives. It was felt that a large number (perhaps 50%) of these could have been recognized as unsuited to combat duties prior to going overseas."[85] If this may seem rather harsh in light of the view that each soldier has a limited reserve of fortitude which runs out sooner or later, at least practitioners did not blame the patient for his illness. The same psychiatrist quoted above also related how "It was the policy in the forward area that all Neuropsychiatric casualties evacuated from a combatant unit would be labelled "Exhaustion". This is a procedure that has long been used by both our American and British colleagues and the reasons for its adoption were as follows: (1) The term "Exhaustion" suggests a mild and recoverable condition to the soldier. (2) The stigma of a psychiatric diagnosis was not attached. (3) It was a simple, administrative diagnosis for the busy MO."[86] The writer had to admit, however, that only the latter reason was valid, as stigma attached to the diagnosis anyway.

The fall of Rome to the Americans on 4 June was one of those events historians subsequently used as a milestone in the Mediterranean campaign, though to most of the participants, such as the Canadians fighting

---

84. Lt-Col A.M. Doyle, "Psychiatry with the Canadian Army in Action in the CMF," *The Journal of the Canadian Medical Services* (January, 1946), 97.

85. Lt-Col A.M. Doyle, "Psychiatry with the Canadian Army in Action in the CMF," *The Journal of the Canadian Medical Services* (January, 1946), 98.

86. *Ibid*, 100.

in another part of the peninsula, it was far less important than the patch of ground they were currently trying to wrest from the enemy. In any case, the city's liberation was eclipsed by events to the north and west, as two days later one of the largest amphibious operations in history placed allied divisions on the coast of Normandy, preparatory to a campaign aimed at ending the war. In the battles that followed medical practitioners would rely on some of the lessons of the Mediterranean campaign while facing problems of their own, including what were perhaps the most intense three months in the history of Canada's armed services.

The doctors, nurses, and medical staff of the 2nd and 3rd Infantry as well as the 4th Armoured Divisions had been training for the northwest European campaign since their arrival in England, some of them as early as 1940. As the FSU surgeon John Burwell Hillsman related in a later autobiography, indoctrination sometimes focussed on skills, critically important as they were, that the lay-person would not think of when considering combat medicine. For example,

> We began training attached to a Casualty Clearing Station in January 1944. Our first consideration was to teach the men to erect the tent under varying conditions. We spent three weeks literally living in mud, putting up the tent and taking it down. The canvas was wet and heavy but we soon got to the point where we could set up in blackout conditions in twenty minutes and take down in fifteen...
>
> At nights we practised night driving. Each man was given map references and required to find his way to various locations in the blackout by directing the driver what roads to take and what turns to make... I considered the men sufficiently trained in map reading when I noticed they invariably managed to get lost within a few hundred feet of a pub.[87]

Having mastered the basics, the FSU could practise its role along with other units. Thus, "On the first of March, 1944, things began to look up. the invasion was obviously approaching. Headquarters ordered all seven of the Field Surgical Units along with two Field Transfusion Units into the field to be attached to a Field Dressing Station at Cranleigh. The next month was spent practising combined set ups with this Unit and in combination with other Field Dressing Stations."[88]

The invasion of 6 June was more difficult than the landings in Sicily and Italy, as it was carried out against troops who, if not exactly first-rate, were thicker on the ground and with more armoured support than previous adversaries; over 1000 Canadian soldiers became casualties the first day, and losses mounted in the three months that followed. German mortar crews were well- trained and motivated, so evacuating the

---

87. John Burwell Hillsman, *Eleven Men and a Scalpel* (Winnipeg, 1948), 12-13.
88. Ibid.

wounded was often under fire, forcing the units responsible to adapt; thus 11 Field Ambulance found it was better to use its own vehicles as well as those of the infantry it was supporting to by-pass the Regiment-al Aid Post and the field ambulance's forward section to transport injured soldiers directly to a Casualty Clearing Post.[89] The unit further reported that, "As a result of this abnormal situation, the first place the wounded received skilled first aid was in the CCP. This was in a thick-walled building, which withstood several hits by shells, and aerial and mortar bombs. It could be well blacked out, and was reinforced with sand bags. Necessary plasma was administered here, and splints and bandages applied."[90] Thus even the CCP was under fire, as was the entire line of evacuation leading back to it, so that additional casualties were inevitable. "During these few days the unit had two men killed, and one badly wounded. One jeep was totally demolished, and several other vehicles were badly holed, but repairable. We learned to dig deep slit trenches, and protect the patients by digging and sand-bagging. At no time was the rush of patients greater than could be handled com-fortably, and we were able to study the problem of giving the best care possible to each case."[91]

Combat is a different universe from the classroom, drill square, and training area, so it comes as no surprise that medical personnel spent the first part of the campaign learning on the job. One lesson relating to casualty evacuation, made clear by the experiences of 11 Field Ambulance related above, was the limited role of the Regimental Aid Post during intense operations. Set up in haste to deal with the wounded as quickly as possible, it was almost always within range of enemy mortars and vulnerable to their bombs. As the unit explained, "In the forward areas the section and RMOs were only able to dig narrow slit trenches. These could not be blacked out at night, and were most unsatisfactory for treating patients. The necessary labour could not be found to make deep dugouts, and any undue digging attracted a great deal of enemy fire."[92] It was thus a site for quick treatment and even quicker evacuation by jeep or car, so that "ambulance personnel at the RAP over and above those necessary for loading and unloading these cars, and very occasionally to assist in the active treatment of casualties in the RAP, are unnecessary and in most cases merely a nuisance and an embarrassment to the RMO."[93]

89. NA, RG 24, v.12,593, 11/11 Fd Amb/1, 11 Fd Amb, Quarterly Report, 12 Jul 44.
90. NA, RG 24, v.12,593, 11/11 Fd Amb/1, 11 Fd Amb, Quarterly Report, 12 Jul 44.
91. Ibid.
92. NA, RG 24, v.12,593, 11/11 Fd Amb/1, 11 Fd Amb, Quarterly Report, 12 Jul 44.
93. NA, RG 24, v.12,593, 11/10 Fd Amb/1, 10 Fd Amb, Quarterly Report, 30 Sep 44.

The nature of soldiers' wounds in some ways reflects the nature of the battle they are fighting as well as the treatment required, so it may be of interest that, according to 15 Field Ambulance, only a little over 10 per cent were caused by rifles, 17.5 by machine guns, 14.5 by mortars, and almost 43 by artillery. Of those who survived their injuries long enough to be evacuated to this particular unit, which totalled 1688 for the Normandy campaign, almost 15 per cent had wounds to the head, 8 $^{1/2}$ to the chest, 5 to the abdomen, 31 to the upper extremities, 28 to the lower extremities, and 2.7 to the back, in many ways reflecting the immediate chances of succumbing to such trauma. Almost 27 per cent of patients brought in had multiple wounds, another reflection of the severity of modern warfare. Easing the medical unit's burden somewhat was that over half the soldiers it treated had slight injuries, with over a third considered severe and only a little over 10 per cent categorized as dangerous.[94]

For those suffering from shock, the first order of business was resuscitation, often the responsibility of Field Dressing Stations; Number 5 FDS, for example, focussed on dangerous cases, which often required its staff to go to some lengths to deliver the blood products the wounded needed. "As no whole blood was available, the Unit Nursing Orderlies donated 14 pints to these casualties. All personnel of the Unit had been previously typed. It was discovered that although the majority of these severe casualties could be resuscitated, they suffered a relapse by the time they had travelled the 8 miles to the CCS,"[95] a lesson from the Italian campaign being relearned in north-west Europe. According to the Assistant Director Medical Services, a nearby ADS was also used as a resuscitation centre, but "This was found to be impracticable, as it involved an extra transfer of the casualty, and meant delay in essential treatment."[96] Fighting shock was thus not a matter just for specialists, but over time became the responsibility of all medical units serving near the front line.

Number 12 Light Field Ambulance would have agreed, reporting that "No separate section of the ADS was reserved for resuscitating shocked casualties. When required plasma was administered on the treatment table while the patient's wounds were being dressed. In this way, the average time of delay in evacuation of the patient caused by giving plasma was only about fifteen minutes."[97] The unit also noted that resuscitation was an ongoing process, as "Usually two pints were

94. NA, RG 24, v.12,593, 11/15 Fd Amb/1, 15 Fd Amb, Quarterly Report, 30 Sep 44.
95. NA, RG 24, v.12,592, 11/5 FDS/1, Quarterly Report, 18 Jul 44.
96. NA, RG 24, v.12,593, 11/11 Fd Amb/1, 11 Fd Amb, Quarterly Report, 12 J ul 44.
97. NA, RG 24, v.12,617, 11/12 Lt Fd Amb/1, Quarterly Report, 30 Sep 44.

given while the casualty was at the ADS and a third pint during his journey back... All our ambulance orderlies were capable of changing plasma bottles en route and discontinuing the transfusion if necessary,"[98] in what by the end of the campaign had become an established routine. At one FDS, for example, wet clothing was removed, including boots, the patient being wrapped in blankets and hot water bottles. If necessary, a pillow was provided to make him comfortable, as was a cigarette, hot sweet tea (unless he had an abdominal wound), food (often in the form of stew), and reassurance. Always on the alert for fresh haemorrhage, staff splinted all fractures, closed sucking chest wounds, treated burns, and provided morphia for pain. "Blood plasma transfusion was given if indicated by Blood Pressure, which was taken on all severe wounds, or general condition of patient or as routine in wounds with extensive tissue damage."[99]

As for its effectiveness, according to 21 Field Dressing Station,

> The use of plasma and whole blood for resuscitation has given phenomenal results when used in forward areas. On many occasions patients have been admitted in the most severe shock, both from severe wounds and from minor wounds in individuals who have lain out for long periods after being hit. There is often no palpable pulse at the wrist, no recordable blood pressure and Cheyne-Stokes [laboured] respiration has started. After two, three or four pints of plasma, and proper posturing the whole picture may change, breathing improves, pulse becomes palpable and BP starts rising, and within one to two hours the patient can be evacuated. It has been noted that if there is no response within one hour, there is not likely to be any at all... Unfortunately it has not been possible to follow cases after evacuation, but what reports are available indicate that once BP has reached about 100 systolic and the patients' general condition seems good, they travel fairly well provided plasma is continued during the journey. Condition may deteriorate somewhat, but further resuscitation at CCSs or ASCs is effective.[100] [The ASC was the Advanced Surgical Centre, to be discussed below]

As part of an ongoing discussion on the relative merits of plasma and whole blood, 21 FDS opted for the latter, "particularly in exsanguinated patients ... The proportion of one pint blood to each three pints plasma has been found to be a good working rule though of course conditions vary considerably in different cases."

In this evolving organization field transfusion units had an important role to play, though at least one complained that it was "grossly under staffed," its responsibilities running to more than the administering of

98. NA, RG 24, v.12,617, 11/12 Lt Fd Amb/1, Quarterly Report, 30 Sep 44.
99. NA, RG 24, v.12,592, 11/4 FDS/1, Reports by Officers Commanding Medical Units, 4 Cdn Field Dressing Station, 1 Jul—30 Sep 44.
100. NA, RG 24, v.12,593, 11/21 Fd Dressing Stn/1, 21 FDS, Quarterly Report, 30 Sep 44.

blood and including injecting narcotics, medications, penicillin, and carrying out a variety of other pre-operative procedures.[101] Overworked they may have been, along with everyone else fighting in Normandy, but FTUs could still observe the effectiveness—or lack thereof—of their procedures in hopes of improving them. In a section headed "Time lag between wounding and resuscitation," 4 Field Transfusion Unit maintained that

> Both FSU and FTU officers agree that this factor is all-important. When we started in at Caen, the time lag was 2-3 hours, nearly all cases under 6 hours. These cases were, on the whole, easy to resuscitate and did well before, at, and after operation. When the front opened out and our cases started arriving 12-16-24 hours after wounding, they were difficult to resuscitate... There is, of course, the exception to this—the cases that are so seriously injured that would die before arriving at an ASC if it were placed a long distance away, and which do die at an ASC when it is close. These cases increase the mortality rates of an ASC when it is close to the fighting front.[102]

Another unit, 7 FTU, had a different perspective, complaining of having been matched up with a relatively inactive Casualty Clearing Station when, some 5 to 10 miles away, other CCSs were operating to capacity "with overworked Resuscitation personnel." Its main lesson of the campaign was that "On the whole it was felt that in general not enough use was made of the high mobility of the FTU," to send it where it was most needed.[103]

That some units would be strained to their limits while others were under-used was an expected consequence of the confusion of battle. Generally, it would seem that those wounded who required resuscitation received the necessary treatment, many or most of them then moving on to surgery. This was mainly the responsibility of Field Surgical Units, often linked with Field Dressing Stations to form Advanced Surgical Centres (or ASCs). For the FDS, whose repertoire could include such tasks as holding convalescents from an epidemic of gastroenteritis, such surgical work was more satisfactory, "as the personnel and equipment of the FDS were fully used, yet not overtaxed. Medical Officers worked according to roster and on no occasion was there evidence of undertreatment. When a rush of casualties occurred, Medical Officers off duty assisted until the situation was eased."[104]

At least one Casualty Clearing Station, 6 CCS, reported in like manner, suggesting that "The most useful role of a CCS during battle appears

101. NA, RG 24 v.12,596, 11/6 FTU/1, Quarterly Report, 30 Sep 44.
102. NA, RG 24 v.12,596, 11/4 FTU/1, Quarterly Report, 30 Sep 44.
103. NA, RG 24 v.12,596, 11/7 FTU/1, Quarterly Report, 30 Sep 44.
104. NA, RG 24, v.12,592, 11/5 FDS/1, Quarterly Report, 18 Jul 44.

to be as a forward Surgical Centre," or Advanced Surgical Centre, but to fulfil this role it needed to be supplemented by an FTU and two FSUs.[105] Number 10 Field Surgical Unit advised that "we believe that the FSU, FDS, combination is more satisfactory than the FSU CCS arrangement. This [is] probably primarily due to the fact that the personnel of a CCS are numerically not sufficient to handle the patients of four operating teams and not from a lack of co-operative spirit, while the entire resources of an FDS are available for its function as a parent Unit to its two FSUs."[106] Number 9 FSU agreed, relating that "During this period certain observations were made. An FDS with two Field Surgical Units are mutually complimentary [sic]. They are flexible, readily adaptible [sic] and are able to move with great facility... Good cooperation between FDSs and FSUs has been universally [sic]... FSUs and CCSs are incompatable [sic]."[107]

Even 6 CCS, which preferred operating as a surgical centre to its other, perhaps more mundane roles (such as treating convalescents), had to admit: "It became apparent that, during a busy period, a CCS acting as a Forward Surgical Centre really needs one extra Medical Officer,"[108] while also reporting that, later in the campaign, it needed an FDS to take care of triage. Though the resulting "CCS-FDS combination worked exceedingly well," that was because the FDS half of the organization was responsible for "freeing CCS personnel from the arduous task of admission..." The main role played by the Casualty Clearing Station in such an operation was immediate post-operative care, but that kind of work could be carried out by a few nursing sisters, which as we have seen some FSUs and FDSs were demanding. With FTUs, FSUs, and FDSs handling casualties close to the front and hospitals treating convalescents further back, it would thus seem that the CCS had an ever shrinking role to play on the Second World War battlefield.

Field Surgical Units were a different matter, and for many of their members Normandy was a baptism of fire, few surgeons and supporting practitioners in the Canadian Army ever facing a more difficult initiation. John Burwell Hillsman, for one, related how he tried to ease his staff into the performance of combat medicine.

> The time came for us to perform our first operation. The boys were standing by scrubbed and grinning but it was obvious that they were a little nervous. I went into the Resuscitation Tent and had a talk with the

105. NA, RG 24, v.12,578, 6 CCS, Quarterly Report, 1 Jul to 30 Sep 44.
106. NA, RG 24, v.12,596, 11/10 FSU/1, Quarterly Report, 30 Sep 44.
107. NA, RG 24, v.12,596, 11/9 FSU/1, Quarterly Report, 30 Sep 44.
108. NA, RG 24, v.12,578, 6 CCS, Quarterly Report, 1 Jul 44 to 30 Sep 44.

Transfusion Officer. The tent was full of wounded but I chose a trivial wound of the arm for our first case. I didn't want to take on a big case until the men's nervousness had cleared a bit. The case was brought in. The arm was painted and the operation began. Soon we were through. As I put on the bandage I noticed the men were laughing and joking among themselves, proud as peacocks. I slipped into the Resuscitation Tent and chose an abdominal case. It went smoothly. From then on we took the cases as they came. By morning we were a weary, happy Unit—and I knew I had a team that could work with the best.

We operated in Secqueville for ten days and covered the attack that took the City of Caen. During those ten days we changed from mere soldiers to war-wise veterans. We saw the tragic sights from which we were never to be free for ten long months. Men with heads shattered and grey, dirty brains oozing out from the jagged margins of skull bones. Youngsters with holes in their chests fighting for air and breathing with a ghastly sucking noise. Soldiers with intestines draining feces into their belly walls and with their guts churned into a bloody mess by high explosives. Legs that were dead and stinking—but still wore a muddy shoe. Operating floors that had to be scrubbed with lysol to rid the Theatre of the stench of dead flesh. Red blood that flowed and spilled over while life held on by the slender thread of time. Boys who came to you with a smile and died on the operating table. Boys who lived long enough for you to learn their name and then were carried away in trucks piled high with the dead. We learned to work with heavy guns rocking and blasting the thin walls of our tent. We learned to keep our tent ropes slack so that anti-aircraft fragments would rain down harmlessly and bounce off the canvas. We became the possessors of bitter knowledge that no man has ever been able to describe. Only by going through it do you possess it.[109]

An infantryman or armoured trooper would not have said different.

Professionally, surgeons at FSUs faced a grim task as the fatality rates among their patients were without doubt the highest of any medical unit. While field ambulances could claim that well over 90 per cent of the wounded they picked up were still alive when they were dropped off at an advanced surgical centre or advanced dressing station or similar institution, and while hospitals experienced a death rate in the low single digits, FSUs saw the darker side of medical operations. Number 6, for example, which arrived in France in July, reported working on 41 victims that month, another 61 in August, and a further 35 in September, of whom 10 died in July, 14 in August, and 1 in September, for a total death rate of 25 out of 137, or just over 18 per cent, almost all of them from chest and abdominal wounds. Surgeons and staff obviously expected such a catastrophe, however, 6 FSU

109. John Burwell Hillsman, *Eleven Men and a Scalpel* (Winnipeg, 1948), 34-35.

reporting that "the unit as a whole has had a fairly happy three months."[110]

Since soldiers with abdominal wounds had by far the lowest survival rate, it is not surprising that they were much studied, one of the most detailed reports on the subject coming from Italy. According to A.L. Chute, who had carried out an analysis of such injuries from 23 August to 30 September, the most striking point about the problem was that half of these unfortunates died within 24 hours of having surgery. Though "It has now become a firmly established principle that all preoperative cases must have careful *minute* by *minute* supervision by a competent resuscitation officer," the same could not be said of postoperative care.

> Most officers on post operative wards find their hands full juggling with gastric suctions, aspirating chests and in attending to the general needs of their patients. During the night except in cases of real emergency no medical officer is on the wards. Even during the day time patients just returned from the OR are left to themselves to come out of the anaesthetic. Blood pressures are rarely taken and unless the patient is in extremis no particular attention is paid to him. It may be that if the same careful observation of pulse, blood pressure etc were made in the post operative ward and the same energetic type of resuscitation were carried out that a considerable number of serious or potentially serious cases might be saved from a rapid decline and death. This raises the question when does resuscitation cease? When the patient goes to OR? at the end of operation?—or when the patient is safely past any danger of post operative collapse?

> Patients who have had to undergo major operative procedures—no matter how skilful or careful the surgeon may be—have in many cases suffered as great an insult to their constitution as from their original injury. It would seem reasonable therefore that they would require the same care post operatively as in the preoperative ward...

> Careful observation combined with active methods of resuscitation during the 6-12 hours immediately following operation would seem to be the means by which these high mortality figures can most readily be reduced.[111]

As for the severely wounded generally, 10 FSU in Normandy reported that "Nursing Sisters have been of the greatest value in the post operative treatment of the high priority cases on which we have operated. It is impossible to overstate their marked effect on morale, Ward Routine, and recovery of seriously ill patients. It is also significant that they

---

110. NA, RG 24, v.12,596, 11/6 FSU/1, Quarterly Report, 1 Nov 44.
111. NA, MG 30, B85, Harris Papers, v.5, A.L. Chute, Analysis of Abdominal Casualties in Advanced Surgical Units, AAI.

are both able and willing to live under primitive difficult and dangerous conditions."[112]

Their main role in the Normandy Campaign, however, was to take charge of post-operative and other wards in various hospitals and hospital-like institutions dotted about the French countryside, where not only the wounded but the sick were treated and kept for convalescence. One should note, however, that in a campaign as combat-intensive as Normandy, illness caused far fewer serious casualties than the enemy, 10 Field Ambulance, for example, reporting at the end of the campaign that it had dealt with 1832 battle casualties (including the dead), 587 ill (excepting VD cases), 17 cases of venereal disease, and 168 accidents.[113] The sick are worthy of mention nonetheless, and among the many possible roles of a field dressing station was to set up as a hospital to treat illness, as did 11 FDS in the latter part of August. "Approximately 50 of our 70 beds were occupied most of the time, principally with cases of Gastro-enteritis," its commander reported, his attitude towards such work reflected in the statement that "Although we were very busy we still did not feel we were doing much since as yet we had not treated any battle casualties."[114] Number 6 FDS made no such comment, but one must wonder how its staff reacted to becoming a VD clinic when some of its sister units were acting as advanced surgical centres. It also handled exhaustion cases, minor wounds, and illnesses, and it is perhaps yet another indication of the severity of the fighting that, though it was responsible for all venereal cases in First Canadian Army, it only treated 182, as compared with 1184 wounded and 1670 men with battle exhaustion.[115]

The latter were dealt with in part according to lessons learned from the fighting in Italy, though it should be noted that there was a greater emphasis on discipline in north-west Europe. As Copp and McAndrew relate in *Battle Exhaustion*, "The Senior Officers of the [IInd] Corps and the 2nd Canadian Division had decided that psychiatric casualties were largely the creation of psychiatrists and had refused to integrate such services into the corps or divisional medical system."[116] The Canadian Army that went to Normandy nevertheless had procedures in place to triage and treat psychological injuries. Number 4 FDS operated as a divisional recovery centre for such casualties from 24 July to 10 August, responsible for screening them, then retaining the mild and moderately

---

112. NA, RG 24, v.12,596, 11/10 FSU/1, Quarterly Report, 30 Sep 44.
113. NA, RG 24, v.12,593, 11/10 Fd Amb/1, 10 Fd Amb, Quarterly Report, 30 Sep 44.
114. NA, RG 24, v.12,593, 11/11 Fd Amb/1, 11 Fd Amb, Quarterly Report, 8 Dec 44.
115. NA, RG 24, v.12,592, 11/6 FDS/1, Quarterly Report, 30 Sep 44.
116. Terry Copp and Bill McAndrew, *Battle Exhaustion* (Toronto and Montreal, 1990), 121.

severe for 48 to 72 hours in the hope they would recover while still with the division. In the 17-day period mentioned above, its staff looked at 182 soldiers suffering from symptoms of severe stress, retained 143, of whom 113 were discharged to the divisional advanced reinforcement company for reassignment to front-line duty. Immediate treatment consisted of a bath, pyjamas, a bed, and clean blankets, patients required to parade for meals and wash their own utensils to remind them that they were still in the army. Tranquillizers were used, the unit commenting that the "dosage seemed ample sedation as patients slept through bombing raids."[117]

Not all who complained of psychological symptoms were, in fact, treated for exhaustion, the army and its medical personnel being on a constant look-out for malingerers of all kinds. For example, Lieutenant-Colonel C.U. Letourneau, No 18 Field Ambulance's CO, thought that, of those admitted, more than half had been misdiagnosed, dividing potential cases into two main groups parallelling Captain H.P. Wright's First World War classification (hysterical versus neurasthenic). The first was made up of "Men who were inaction [sic] for the first time, or who were under fire for the first time. These cases generally exhibited symptoms of sheer fright and, in my opinion, should have been treated in the battalion by stern disciplinary measures." The second group comprised "Men who had been in action for some time, subjected to severe enemy fire while in static positions, fatigued by lack of sleep, suffering from cold and exposure. These were true exhaustions and did not reach a very high number." There was another category, of men who had suffered from concussion and blast effect who had been admitted as exhaustion cases though their troubles were essentially physical.[118]

Letourneau singled out the 5th Brigade as an example of how the system could be abused.

> I believe that the high total of these cases in 5 Brigade was partly due to lack of disciplinary action by Senior NCOs of the various battalions, and partly due to wrong diagnosis by Regimental Medical Officers.
>
> In his zeal to help the battalion, the RMO is often tempted to "unload" unsuitable personnel through medical channels by calling them "exhaustion", when, in effect these men should have been charged with cowardice.
>
> The greatest single proof of this is Capt Robert RMO of Regt de Maisonneuve. Capt Robert closely followed the classification of Exhaustion diagnoses in the early days of the Normandy campaign. As a result, his regiment had the highest exhaustion rate in the Division. He was

117. NA, RG 24, v.12,592, 11/4 FDS/1, Reports by Officers Commanding Medical Units, 4 Cdn Field Dressing Station, 1 Jul—30 Sep 44.
118. NA, RG 24, v.12,593, 11/18 Fd Amb/1, 18 Fd Amb, Quarterly Report, 30 Sep 44.

wounded and returned only 3 weeks ago. Since his return he has refused to recognize the condition, as a result of which few (diagnosed by other MOs) exhaustion cases have been suffered by this battalion. In fairness to other battalions, it must be stated that since Capt Robert's return, his battalion has not been engaged in the gruelling holding actions which produce true exhaustions.

Nevertheless, since RMOs have been warned not to "unload" through medical channels, the incidence has dropped somewhat.[119]

The number of exhaustion victims should thus be taken more as an indication of the severity of combat than as an accurate statistic of psychological casualties.

The army was not the only service to deal with the issue, the RCAF having formed fifteen bomber squadrons whose forays over Europe, many of which lasted all night against heavy flak and cannon-equipped fighters, placed aircrew under near-overwhelming physical and psychological pressure. As we have seen, what by 1941 was being called flying stress had been the subject of conjecture and research in Canada since the 1930s, if not before, the fifth meeting of the NRC's Associate Committee on Aviation Medical Research encapsulating work done up to the first years of the war. "Flying stress is the term commonly used for various psycho-neurotic manifestations of a degree which interferes with training or operations. The RAF Medical Branch had anticipated greater numbers of cases than have actually been admitted to hospital. There was a quite natural increase in numbers after both Dunkirk and the "Battle of Britain" when too few pilots were fighting too frequently and for too long a daily period."[120]

The committee pointed out that there was nothing to be done for those who, once in the air, discovered they had a phobic fear of flying, except to screen them out at enlistment. (The possibility is not so ridiculous as it sounds; in the late 1930s and early 1940s very few people flew, so would not know they suffered from chronic terror until they started training.) There were those, however, termed "traumatic", resulting from having experienced or witnessed a flying accident[121] or, once battle was joined, were in an aircraft that was shot up or shot down. Medically, these men were deserving of treatment but, operationally, might be hard to spare, especially with the extremely heavy casualties being experienced in Bomber Command in 1943 and 1944, when little more than half of aircrew could be expected to complete a tour of

119. NA, RG 24, v.12,593, 11/18 Fd Amb/1, 18 Fd Amb, Quarterly Report, 9 Sep 44.
120. NA, RG 24, v.5383, HQS 47-6-3, Proceedings of the Fifth Meeting of the Associate Committee on Aviation Medical Research, 18 Sep 41.
121. NA, RG 24, v.5383, HQS 47-6-3, Proceedings of the Fifth Meeting of the Associate Committee on Aviation Medical Research, 18 Sep 41.

30 sorties. Thus medical and hierarchical priorities clashed; squadron, base, and group commanders fearing that too-light a treatment of men refusing to fly would lead to an epidemic of "lack of moral fibre."

One example, taken from March 1944, was a member of Canada's 429 Squadron, as described almost 40 years later by Steve Puskas. In a sortie over the Ruhr the aircraft was attacked several times, including being caught in searchlights and "coned". After arrival, ground personnel mobbed the aircrew as they got out of the Halifax bomber.

> All the while, Wilf stood to one side, all by himself, and was very silent. We tried to involve him in our chatter, but to no avail. He informed us that this was it, and that was his last trip. I was sure he would change his mind after some sleep.
>
> During all the action, Wilf, a husky chap, had perspired profusely inside his electrically heated suit, which eventually caused the suit to short circuit, giving him some painful burns in his armpits and behind his knees. He was sure he'd been shot, when he felt the pain and felt something trickling down his side. Much to his relief, he discovered he was not holed, just burned. It had been perspiration trickling from his armpits, not blood.[122]

Next day Wilf told the station commander that he would no longer fly, and he was sent home as lacking in moral fibre, or LMF.

Puskas, in his relation four decades later, clearly admitted that "I have always felt ashamed of what the "organization" did to him. They could have been more understanding and compassionate instead of sending him home LMF. Everyone has a breaking point and the limit varies with each individual." The US, it was rumoured, treated such cases much differently. "The American air force had a "Flak House", a rest home, for those airmen who felt the strain and needed professional help. Not the RCAF. You were either in, fit to fly, or out. One or the other." For Wilf, it was the latter, even though his unwillingness to fly could be traced, according to Puskas, to a most harrowing experience. "Two weeks previously, we had ditched in the North Sea, at night, and with the wheels retracted. Wilf could not get by the tail wheel, positioned between him and the rest of the crew, and his ditching position. He frantically tore at his clothing to get by, and finally made it. We were on fire and almost out of control, so time was of the essence. I'm sure this was the beginning of his uneasy state of mind."[123]

Wilf was certainly a candidate for a stress-induced breakdown, but continued to fly on operations until he simply could not bear it any longer. His removal from the squadron as a discipline case may thus

122. Steve Puskas, "A Night on the Ruhr," *Airforce* (December, 1983), 12.
123. Steve Puskas, "A Night on the Ruhr," *Airforce* (December, 1983), 13.

seem unfair, but at least he was part of a small minority, Al English, in his seminal book *The Cream of the Crop* estimating that those who were diagnosed with psychological disorders outnumbered Lack of Moral Fibre cases 10 to 1. Further, even those handed over to disciplinary authorities could expect something of a second chance, the RCAF returning them to Canada where about 6 per cent were exonerated as suffering from stress-related ailments and 75 per cent were simply found "inefficient," allowing them to keep their badges and rank—and at least some of their dignity.[124]

Those deemed to suffer from some form of mental illness received therapy in accordance with long-established principles; as English relates, already by the end of the First World War "Treatment, the medical authorities of the belligerents agreed, should be simple and administered near the front lines to be most effective."[125] Also, "specialists concluded that the best treatment for combat stress was to talk about one's problems with a sympathetic MO and to look to simple medical remedies to relieve physical symptoms. For those who had been in combat for prolonged periods, rest while on leave away from the front completed the cure. Other, more complex regimes, including Freudian psychotherapy, showed little promise."[126] The RAF's (and thus the RCAF's) approach to psychological casualties was thus similar to that of First Canadian Army; so was the scope of the problem, English calculating that about one aircrew member in five within Bomber Command (and hence within 6 Group RCAF) was lost in that manner, a scale similar to Ist Canadian Corps in Italy and IInd Canadian Corps in northwest Europe.[127] The latter's battle exhaustion rate diminished, however, after American forces broke through the German lines near the end of July 1944, and the Canadian Army's battle turned into a pursuit in the last days of August.

If the army and air force faced similar challenges in dealing with psychological casualties, at least one RCAF unit also dealt with the physical ravages of war in much the same way as its army counterparts. This was No 52 (RCAF) Mobile Field Hospital, whose formation was part of the growing symbiosis (admittedly imperfect) that developed between airmen and soldiers in the latter part of the war. As 21st Army Group, of which First Canadian Army was a part, prepared to invade the continent in the final months of 1943, No 83 Group (RCAF) trained its 16 fighter, fighter-reconnaissance, and photo-reconnaissance squadrons

124. Allan D. English, *The Cream of the Crop: Canadian Aircrew, 1939-1945* (Montreal and Kingston, 1996), 155-162.
125. Al English, *The Cream of the Crop*, 62.
126. Al English, *The Cream of the Crop*, 63-64.
127. Al English, *The Cream of the Crop*, 100-101.

to support its ground-bound brethren in the campaign; and looking to provide medical care for that aerial formation, whose airfields would be located as close to the fighting as feasible, was the field hospital. In the months preceding the D-Day landings its staff underwent training that would have been familiar to its army counterparts, including security, small arms, chemical warfare defence, first aid in the field, the dangers of VD, treatment of shock, the use of field water supply equipment, the art of camouflage, and more.[128]

After D-Day the unit did not have long to wait before becoming part of the campaign, an Advanced Surgical Team (or AST) moving to the continent two days after the landings. Sited near an advanced landing strip, "On several occasions personnel were fired upon by German snipers in the adjoining field and the section was dive-bombed on at least two occasions," anti-personnel bombs being particularly dreaded by hospital staff. "Safari beds of patients and the operating theatre were completely dug in... Fortunately no casualties were suffered by hospital personnel. All patients treated were army and air force casualties from enemy action." The hospital's main body disembarked on the Canadian beaches on 18 June though "An air raid was in progress directly overhead as the vehicles drove off the ramp." It then proceeded inland. "The AST was contacted and on the 19th in the face of heavy driving rain the two sections joined and the first camp site was pitched on top of an exposed hill a quarter of a mile from Rivierre [sic], about 8 miles from Caen, and overlooking a large part of the battlefield of the British and Canadian Sector. Camp was pitched in the driving rain and slit trenches were dug through what seemed to be solid rock; all in all the circumstances were dismal, but the spirit of all personnel was high."[129]

In the weeks that followed surgery was a mix of tactical, where "On several occasions the surgical staff operated throughout heavy German air raids," and medical, penicillin being used as a matter of course. A problem that arose after the unit had been in Normandy about a month was the length of stay for each patient; while the army tried to move casualties out of front-line hospitals—either forwards or backwards—after a few days, 52 MFH held on to its charges for weeks in the hopes of returning them to their cockpits. Because "many of the patients were fighter pilots tuned to a fine pitch, an intensive programme of occupational therapy was inaugurated," including a library, various games, a photo club, movies shown weekly, and tools for various crafts, though "Perhaps the most difficult problem during this period was making

128. NA, RG 24, v.22,844, Operations Record Book, 52 Mobile Field Hospital, Oct 43 to Feb 44.
129. NA, RG 24, v.22,844, ORB 52 MFH, Entry for June 1944.

compo rations palatable for ill patients." Also, "Air evacuation during this period entailed long journeys (in length of time) from the MFH over rough an dusty roads, and frequently long waits at the airfield before loading on the aircraft. Several times aircraft for evacuation failed to arrive. The need for improved organization of air evacuation was obvious."[130]

In early August the hospital moved forward yet again—to an area laced with land mines, booby traps, and unburied bodies. In the course of the month "an acute Dysentery reached major epidemic proportions and was experienced by at least four out of five men," the strain predominating varying with locality. Sulfaguonidine, one of the sulfa drugs, proved a most useful therapeutic adjunct.

> Fortunately, few serious or prolonged cases were encountered. Most camp sites were in or adjoined apple orchards, in which apples rolled on the ground in thousands. Bodies of horses, cattle, sheep and men lay rotting and unburied over Normandy. Consequently, fly control was an impossibility. In addition dust rolled over the area in billowing clouds, penetrating everything and probably acted as an additional source of infection. At the MFH particular attention was paid to field hygiene, e.g. dish washing, enclosure of cooks and meat by mosquito netting, control of food handlers, etc, and though a number of cases of dysentery appeared the epidemic never reached extreme proportions. Unfortunately, DDT spray was not available during this period and Sulfaguonidine was in short supply, so that it could not be used prophylactically and not therapeutically in all cases.[131]

At the end of the month, as German forces began a general withdrawal, the hospital struck its tents and moved again, except for a skeleton medical staff left behind to look after men with abdominal wounds who could not travel. For 52 MFH, as for First Canadian Army, the Normandy campaign was over.

The battles of summer 1944 had been among the most trying in Canadian military history, but even after they ended Medical practitioners still had a lot on their hands, especially given the fluid nature of the fighting. As John Burwell Hillsman later related, "the casualties were light but those we were getting were in bad shape and a few arrived dead who should never have died at all." Priority was for the movement of ammunition, food, and fuel, medical units not being allowed to use the roads to get close to their patients. "The High Brass thought that by rushing troops and supplies up now they could end things in a hurry and save thousands of lives. They figured it worth the few we would

130. NA, RG 24, v.22,844, ORB 52 MFH, June and July 1944.
131. NA, RG 24, v.22,844, ORB 52 MFH, August 1944.

lose by delayed medical attention." We now know that they gambled wrong, but that is twenty-twenty hindsight, and the commanders of the time had to take risks if the war was to end anytime soon. Still, Hillsman faced one of the most challenging periods of his short operational career.

> The situation was difficult. We were the only Surgical Unit open to cover the Army moving forward. We had to handle all the casualties for at least twenty-four hours. I had no relief surgical team and no Transfusion Unit with me. We hadn't any blood or penicillin for the wounded. What's worse we hadn't an icebox to keep the blood in and it would only last twelve hours in the heat... We set up the canvas and just as we started to sterilize the instruments the first ambulance rolled in. For thirty-six hours we operated continuously without sleep or rest.[132]

When it was all over, "I slept like a drunken man."

In the three months of the Normandy Campaign, from 6 June to early September, 5000 Canadian soldiers died, compared to the 6000 who fell in the gruelling 21 months of the Mediterranean War. The great bulk of such casualties were among the long-suffering infantry, and the RCAMC lost only two per cent of its strength in every month of intense operations, and 3/4 of a per cent in normal periods.[133] Though there were still terrible battles ahead in both theatres, the opening scene in the liberation of north-west Europe can be taken as the climax of the history of the Canadian Army in the Second World War. After Dieppe, Sicily, southern Italy, and Normandy, the medical corps can be said to have completed its difficult education, and though it would continue to learn in the six months or more that remained in the conflict, it did so as an experienced organization—in both the medical and military realms.

---

132. John Burwell Hillsman, *Eleven Men and a Scalpel* (Winnipeg, 1948), 51.
133. NA, RG 24, v.6919, No 134.

Chapter Seven

Medicine in the Victory Campaign

By the autumn of 1944 there was little doubt as to how the war would end, though battle-scarred soldiers, second-tour aircrew, and old (though still in their 20s) sailors could be forgiven if they evidenced a certain skepticism as to *when* victory would come. (One should remember that there was still a conflict to fight against Japan.) The soldiers of IInd Canadian Corps, for example, were unaware of the nature of the campaign that awaited them in north-west Europe, but were no doubt experienced enough to know that it would not be easy and it would not be quick; allied plans, in fact, envisaged them opening the port of Antwerp to shipping, a task the Germans would oppose with all the resources they could muster. The largest port in north-west Europe, Antwerp fell to British forces in early September, but the city is not on the coast; rather, there is a long estuary leading down to the sea and this was still under control of German forces ensconced in various large islands, with Walcheren guarding access to shipping lanes. Clearing it resulted in a month-long operation that often saw Canadian soldiers fighting up to their waists in water.

One of the first battles of the campaign was an assault-water crossing by the 9th Infantry Brigade, with the support, among others, of 23 Field Ambulance. The medical plan was to have the unit's B Company cross the estuary with six loaded jeep ambulances and set up a casualty clearing post near the landing beach. By that time in the north-west European campaign amphibious vehicles were available, in the form of Alligators, Buffaloes, Terrapins, and others, and these would be used to evacuate casualties, over five miles of water, to the unit's field dressing station. From there a Motorized Ambulance Column (or MAC) would take the wounded 25 miles to Number 2 Canadian Casualty Clearing

Station, in Ghent. The operation opened on 9 October, but as so often happens the unit's well laid plans crumbled once battle was joined; B Company was immediately pinned down on the beach, where it remained for 48 hours, unable to set up its casualty clearing post because of German fire. It thus distributed its jeeps and stretcher-bearers among the regimental aid posts, casualties being taken directly to amphibious vehicles without benefit of intermediate treatment until the third day of the battle, when it became possible to begin evacuating as planned.[1]

As the Canadians slowly wrested the area from the enemy the temperature began to drop, so that casualties due to cold, such as frost bite, hypothermia, and immersion foot (which was not just a navy problem) began showing up at casualty clearing posts. Number 11 Field Ambulance, for one, reported that "In the advance along the Beveland Peninsula, the problem of supplying warmth to the wounded casualty arose. To meet this, each CCP was equipped with a coal burning box stove. Other methods of heating did not seem to be adequate... To protect the casualty from wind and exposure while in transit from the RAP to the CCP, Lieut M.T. Cooper devised a windbreak for the Jeep Ambulance,"[2] consisting of enough canvas to protect the patient's head, and perhaps his chest.

After the stressful months of the Normandy battles and the exhausting moves of the September pursuit the north-west European campaign was beginning to take its toll not only of infantry, but to a lesser extent of supporting arms as well, including medical units. As Hillsman wrote in his autobiographical account of the war, "One man started fainting at the sight of blood. I had to send him back. Another got quite surly and unco-operative. He was one of my best men and I tried to reason with him without too much success. I kept him, hoping he would straighten out. A third youngster began to talk and laugh with a hint of hysteria. The Corporal reported he had heard him sobbing in his sleep several times. He would have to be watched carefully."[3] Later, when warned that the FSU would be involved in an assault-water landing on the island of Walcheren, Hillsman decided to send the surly orderly back, but the hysterical case so begged to continue in his duties that the surgeon decided to retain him. He was taken out of the operating room for a while and given the task of sterilizing instruments, and he "carried on to the end of the war."[4]

1. NA, RG 24, v.12,593, 11/23 Fd Amb/1, 23 Fd Amb, Quarterly Report, 31 Dec 44
2. NA, RG 24, v.12,593, 11/11 Fd Amb/1, 11 Fd Amb, Quarterly Report, 31 Dec 44
3. John Burwell Hillsman, *Eleven Men and a Scalpel* (Winnipeg, 1948), 34
4. Ibid, 92

While the experiences of the previous four months or so were push-
ing some medical personnel over the edge, they also allowed others to
grow, such as a bald orderly whom Hillsman had had doubts about early
in the campaign.

> I walked into his dimly lit ward. Everything was quiet and efficient. His
> orderlies were going around adjusting nasal suctions and giving penicil-
> lin. I did not see him at first. Then the gleam of his bald head gave him
> away. I walked over. He was shaving a desperately ill case. I beckoned to
> him. We went outside. "Look here, Corporal, you are supposed to be in
> charge of this ward. Your job is supervising. What the devil's the idea of
> this barber business?" Well, Sir, it's a funny thing. Most of these boys
> think they are going to die. When I shave them, Sir, they figure I wouldn't
> be wasting my time on a dead man. They brighten up and seem to do
> better." I beat a hasty retreat. This man knew his job![5]

So did many others.

The campaign to clear the Scheldt estuary ended with an assault on
Walcheren by British commandos, preceded by a massive aerial bombardment. Several Canadian units would provide medical support, 17
Light Field Ambulance tasked with following 47 Commando and
establishing a Beach Dressing Station, holding casualties until 10 Field
Dressing Station and its attached surgical and transfusion units arrived
to form a Beach Surgical Centre. While the latter took care of resuscitation and surgery, the field ambulance would focus on evacuating those
casualties that were fit to be moved, by way of landing craft operated
by the Royal Navy.[6] Medical units began gathering the kit they would
need in the days preceding the battle, as Hillsman remembered.

> The problem of what equipment to carry on the assault was a difficult one.
> Our space in the Alligators was limited and all superfluous material had to
> be left behind. I had to prepare to handle casualties from two weeks of
> fighting during which time we would be cut off from all sources of supply.
> There were so many varying types of equipment that were essential. I had
> to list the surgical instruments necessary for any type of operation we could
> possibly encounter. I then had to estimate such variables as the quantity of
> anaesthetic, catgut sutures, gasoline for the generator, kerosene for the
> sterilizers and the amount of fresh drinking water for the wounded. What
> we could do for lights if the generator was knocked out and how we could
> maintain tents on sand in high winds had to be solved. The final problem
> was to distribute the equipment on two separate Alligators in such a man-
> ner that if one was lost we would still have enough equipment to operate.[7]

All was ready—or as ready as it could be—at the end of October.

5. John Burwell Hillsman, *Eleven Men and a Scalpel* (Winnipeg, 1948), 69
6. NA, RG 24, v.12,617, 11/17 Lt Fd Amb/1, Appx A to 17 Cdn Lt Fd Amb RCAMC Quarterly
    Report Ending 31 Dec 44
7. John Burwell Hillsman, *Eleven Men and a Scalpel* (Winnipeg, 1948), 94

On 1 November the 4th Special Service Brigade, made up of commandos, assaulted the beaches of Walcheren with 9 Field Surgical Unit serving as eyewitness as it waited in landing craft for its turn to land. In describing the operation, there was at first no hint of fear, rather "it was exciting and rather pleasant to sit on our craft and watch the show."[8] Going in 80 minutes after the commandos hit the beach, "The danger still seemed remote to the uninitiated, but when we came in close a stream of shells which were accurately trained on the beaches began to fall around us," fire lasting almost an hour and a half. Eventually locating a site large enough for an advanced surgical centre, the surgeons and staff nevertheless had no time to set up, focussing on helping the beach dressing station deal with the 150 casualties that had accumulated by nightfall, evacuating them in a landing craft.

It was two days before 9 FSU could put up its tents, a task performed "in a driving sandstorm." Ordered to move on the 4th, "The unit tore down, moved, set up and did six cases by 1900 hrs the same day. The set-up consisted of operating in the small operating theatre and nursing the patients in the small ward. There was enough for six patients comfortably and probably twice that number in various spots. The tent was erected and used for sterilising and resuscitation."[9] Operations and post-operative treatment were carried out in a small fortress, Walcheren having served as guardian of the mouth of the Scheldt for centuries. Interruptions due to enemy fire and weather meant that some casualties had waited some time before they could undergo surgery, including a commando with gas gangrene. Perhaps the most difficult victim to treat had an abdominal wound, which "probably should not have been touched," the resuscitation unit spending hours trying to get his blood pressure up, but "As soon as the abdomen was opened it was obvious that it was useless." As 9 FSU's commander explained, "When, on making the incision, the abdominal wall is entirely relaxed and only a little dark blood appears in the subcutaneous tissues, when the abdominal cavity [is] filled with old very dark blood which feels cool to the hand and when the viscers have lost all tone, one knows then that the patient is already dying."[10]

John Hillsman was with 8 FSU, which found itself in the midst of the maelstrom as its landing craft closed into the beach.

> We grounded with a grating jar and the Sergeant in charge of the Alligator yelled above the din. "Hold on! We're going off!" The Alligator

8. NA, RG 24, v.12,596, 11/9 FSU/1, Quarterly Report, Appendix 1
9. NA, RG 24, v.12,596, 11/9 FSU/1, Quarterly Report, Appendix 1
10. NA, RG 24, v.12,596, 11/9 FSU/1, Quarterly Report, Appendix 1

lurched down the ramp and into the gap. Fragments were shrieking overhead. Sand and water was blown by the continual explosions all over our equipment. An Alligator to our right hit a mine. It burst into flames and men poured over its sides. The wireless operator threw back his turret and started to climb out. His clothes were blazing. He got half out and fell back into the flames. I looked back. Our LCT had been hit and flashes of fire could be seen bursting through a heavy pall of smoke. I looked to the left. A bulldozer was hit and the driver was flung high in the air turning over and over as if in slow motion. A fragment banged into the tarpaulin above my head and I burrowed deep into the Alligator. I had seen enough.[11]

There would be more, however.

For after the landings, and while medical staff were setting up to deal with the inevitable heavy casualties to come, members of 10 Field Dressing Station became trapped in a dugout by exploding ammunition, some supply Alligators having been hit. Hillsman and a Captain Ptak were thus the only medical officers left, at least for a while, and so attempted to make their way to 10 FDS' site, where their services would be much needed.

We had to crawl two hundred yards on our bellies with the exploding ammunition shooting at us from one side and the Germans from the other. We finally reached the tent and found that the Staff Sergeant had organized a rescue team and was going down in that blazing mess and bringing out the survivors. One of the medicals went inside of an exploding Alligator to reach a wounded Commando. He was blown in two by a mortar bomb. For the next half hour we lay on our faces in the sand dressing wounds, stopping haemorrhages and splinting fractures. Constant explosions were blowing sand over us as we worked. Our heads were retracted down in our helmets until the edge of the damned things almost reached our shoulders. I never fully appreciated the advantages of a turtle until then.[12]

The proper place for a surgeon might well be near the front, but it was still possible to be too close to the fighting to carry out one's task, and like 9 FSU the 8th had to wait two days before it could properly begin work, when seven cases were selected for emergency surgery. Operating in a tent, which heavy wind threatened to carry away, sterilization was done with chemicals in bowls laid on the floor, lighting being provided by a single electric bulb which was replaced with acetylene torches when it failed; Hillsman had to crawl under the table in order to change sides. No doctor in Canada, whether in Toronto, Moose Jaw,

11.   John Burwell Hillsman, *Eleven Men and a Scalpel* (Winnipeg, 1948), 101
12.   John Burwell Hillsman, *Eleven Men and a Scalpel* (Winnipeg, 1948), 105

or in the country, ever worked under such conditions. The island's German garrison capitulated on the 8th.[13]

Given such experiences, it is not necessary to closely examine infantry operations to know that the Scheldt was a very difficult campaign. It was not, however, as stressful and traumatic as Normandy had been, and "The incidence of Exhaustion during this quarter was much less than during the previous quarter." According to 11 Field Ambulance's commander, "This I am sure was partly due to a more proper appreciation and treatment of the condition by the Medical Officers within the Division. A large percentage of patients with exhaustion were retained and treated in the Divisional Recovery Centres and only the severe cases were evacuated further."[14] The fact, however, that the last quarter of 1944 saw only a month's intense fighting, as opposed to three times longer in the Normandy campaign, may have gone further towards explaining the reduction in psychological casualties.

In fact, as hard as the Sheldt might have been on the common soldier operations in Italy at that time were no easier, and lasted longer. Waterways in the peninsula tended to run east-west, making them excellent sites for the Germans to set up defensive positions, resulting in what became called the Battle of the Rivers. This was a series of that most complex of military operations—the assault water crossing—which as we saw at Walcheren could bring support units like FSUs into the heart of the fighting. G.W.L. Nicholson, historian of the Italian campaign and of the Royal Canadian Army Medical Corps, later related how

> While the 1st Canadian Corps had benefited as a whole from its period of rest during November, by mid-December front-line units were again feeling the strain of contending with not only a stubborn enemy but the hostile weather that accentuated the misery of what was for many a day after day existence in far from adequate shelter. In the course of a tour of the 5th Armoured Division's forward area on December 17, Colonel Hunter, ADMS, found a noticeable increase in the rate of neuropsychiatric cases attributable to battle exhaustion, brought on apparently by a lack of decent sleep. Regimental MOs reported that it was not unusual for some battle casualties, in spite of the pain they were experiencing, to fall asleep while their wounds were being dressed. At the same time the Corps DDMS, now Brigadier H.M. Elder, was receiving reports of a sharp rise in the incidence of battle exhaustion in the units of the 1st Division.[15]

13. NA, RG 24, v.12,596, 11/8 FSU/1, Major Hillsman's and Capt Merkeley's Observations, 2 Nov 44
14. NA, RG 24, v.12,593, 11/11 Fd Amb/1, 11 Fd Amb, Quarterly Report, 31 Dec 44
15. G.W.L. Nicholson, *Seventy Years of Service* (Ottawa, 1977), 197

Lieutenant-General E.L.M. Burns, who lumped venereal disease, military crime, and psychiatric cases together as examples of preventable wastage (as had his predecessor Harry Crerar), had not however found any way to avoid losses due to battle exhaustion.[16] As for his troops, though the war only had four months to go it is perhaps understandable if they could not see the end of their ordeal from their muddy slit trenches.

After the Scheldt in north-west Europe and the Battle of the Rivers in Italy, policy makers at headquarters deemed the time right to determine how well the medical system was performing in its support of infantry and other combat units. Some 585 wounded Canadian soldiers, convalescing in base hospitals in England after being evacuated from both theatres, were questioned at length after their medical records were combed for information. The latter revealed that 36 per cent of surviving casualties had been injured by shell fire, 17 per cent by mortar bombs, 10 by rifles and other small arms, 7 by machine guns, five from aerial bombs, four had been evacuated due to organic or pathological disease, three suffered from blast, two from grenades, and one per cent each were withdrawn due to their own artillery or malaria. Such overall casualty rates varied when different theatres were compared, accidents and mines, for example, causing more losses in Italy than in north-west Europe (the different effects of mine warfare was particularly dramatic, such devices causing 19 per cent of losses in Italy but only two per cent in France and the Netherlands).[17]

As for the treatment they had received at the hands of medical personnel, a report prepared from the questionnaires claimed that

> Service by stretcher bearers or MOs was prompt. Three quarters of the men questioned received medical attention from stretcher bearers or from MOs within an hour after they were wounded. Artillery men received more prompt attention than Infantry or CAC [Canadian Armoured Corps]... Evacuation to Base Hospitals of troops questioned was also rapid: 85% of the sample reached their Base Hospitals within 2 days... Efficiency of stretcher bearers, Regimental MOs and Base Hospitals was considered satisfactory by from 83% to 90% of troops questioned... First Aid Training was considered adequate by 3 out of 4 men questioned.[18]

Of interest in discussing evacuation was the fact that only 5 per cent of injured tank crews had to be lifted out of their vehicles, the remainder either able to get out under their own power or being outside the tank when they were wounded.

---

16. Terry Copp and Bill McAndrew, *Battle Exhaustion* (Montreal and Toronto, 1990), 91
17. NA, RG 24, v.8127, NS 1287-2, Questionnaire of Wounded Soldiers
18. NA, RG 24, v.8127, NS 1287-2, Questionnaire of Wounded Soldiers

Of soldiers generally, one in four received medical attention from a stretcher bearer or medical officer within five minutes of being injured, though satisfaction differed according to theatre. "Opinion of casualties from the Mediterranean theatre was markedly less favorable than that of casualties from France on several points. They reported that they were longer in receiving attention from stretcher bearers, or MOs; that they were slower in being moved to Base Hospitals; that their treatment by stretcher bearers and at Base Hospitals was not as satisfactory, and that their First Aid Training had not been as adequate."[19] The sample of 585 soldiers included only 74 from the Mediterranean, however, so one had to be careful in making such comparisons. Generally speaking, though, there were few complaints about medical treatment either in the above survey or in first-hand accounts, and Canadian wounded certainly seemed to be doing better than the Germans', if 14th Field Ambulance was reporting accurately. "Comparison in speed of evacuation and adequate treatment between our own casualties and those of the enemy was possible in this quarter. Due to lack of supplies and delayed evacuation, the wounds of most of enemy casualties were almost invariably infected, while our own cases were clean. Some of the former showed B Welchii infection [a cause of gas gangrene], in addition to grossly purulent wounds and general toxic states."[20]

To treat such injuries, first aid grew in sophistication, amounting to more than just wrapping bandages and injecting morphia. Resuscitation with blood products, for example, was done as far forward as possible, sometimes in regimental aid posts, while further back, at advanced dressing stations, volunteers might be called upon for direct transfusions if stored products were not bringing a patient around. In one case, 18th Field Ambulance saw fit to enquire about such a case a week later, and was encouraged to discover that he was still alive.[21] However, as 5 Canadian Transfusion Unit admitted, ""Shock" continues to be a puzzling problem at times. Casualties in whom wounding appears not to be serious enough to cause death terminate fatally while others recover when according to all rules they should not. The above adds a facination [sic] to this work which might otherwise become a dull and monotonous routine of sticking needles into veins and watching blood pressures rise,"[22] though it is doubtful patients would have shared the doctor's perspective on the issue.

19. NA, RG 24, v.8127, NS 1287-2, Questionnaire of Wounded Soldiers
20. NA, RG 24, v.12,593, 11/14 Fd Amb/1, 14 Fd Amb, Quarterly Report, 31 Dec 44
21. NA, RG 24, v.12,593, 11/18 Fd Amb/1, 18 Fd Amb, Quarterly Report, 31 Dec 44
22. NA, RG 24, v.12,596, 11/5 Cdn Fd Transfusion Unit, Quarterly Report, 31 Dec 44

Thus as the last full year of the war neared its end many medical questions remained unresolved, including that of the proper place for a surgeon. Since Bethune's operations in China Canadian doctors had suggested that surgery be carried out close to the front, but as we saw at Walcheren the results could mean pinning down medical units so they were unable to work. It was thus understandable that 23 Field Ambulance, in its quarterly report ending 31 December 1944, related how "Considerable controversy still goes on over the siting of FSUs, who feel they should be further forward. There is much to be said for and against."[23] For the commander of 21 Field Dressing Station there was no doubt, and "It is felt that the divisional FDS could be very well employed as an ASC. The ideal situation would be to have Surgical Teams and a Transfusion Unit attached. Pre-operative and post-operative care could be adequately rendered by the FDS. This would push surgery and resuscitation farther forward. This is considered necessary,"[24] along with the attachment of nursing sisters to advanced surgical centres. As 5 Field Dressing Station reported, "It was found that the Nursing Orderlies under the guidance of the Nursing Sisters did a remarkably efficient job in the nursing of abdominal and chest cases and with intravenous therapy. It must be appreciated, however, that the presence of a Nursing Sister in the Ward makes a tremendous difference. It is hoped that the present policy of attaching four Nursing Sisters to the ASC will remain."[25]

From early November to the launching of Operation Veritable on 8 February, First Canadian Army essentially held the line along the Maas River, the intense operations of the previous half-year slackening somewhat, though raiding expeditions, patrols, and fire fights still caused casualties. (Hitler's Ardennes offensive of mid-December was halted before it approached the Canadian sector, and involved mainly American forces.) Medical personnel thus faced somewhat different challenges from previous months, as 14 Field Ambulance related. "Diphtheria and Pulmonary Tuberculosis made their appearance. The prevalence of the former is noted in Holland. Numerous skin conditions are also in evidence," including impetigo, a contagious ailment marked by pustules, and pediculosis, a lice infestation. "The last two diseases are considered due to contamination from civilians. Certainly it is noted that most of the children and many adults in Holland present skin infections. Whether this is due to dietary requirements cannot be proven, but this fact is probably the basis of the trouble. Due to exposure to wet and cold, the

23. NA, RG 24, v.12,593, 11/23 Fd Amb/1, 23 Fd Amb, Quarterly Report, 31 Dec 44
24. NA, RG 24, v.12,593, 11/21 Fd Dressing Stn/1, 21 FDS, Quarterly Report, 31 Dec 44
25. NA, RG 24, v.12,592, 11/5 FDS/1, Quarterly Report, 31 Dec 44

men of this Division have shown a greater incidence of upper respiratory infections. How severe they are is not known at this level."[26] That soldiers were being felled by disease harboured in the civilian population was cause for some concern, 18 Field Ambulance reporting that "Since the arrival of this unit in its present location 10 November 44, a foretaste of what we might expect to find in the occupation of Germany was experienced... Only 2 doctors were available in the whole area, including 4 villages ... with a population of approximately 10,000 people."[27] The unit thus set up clinics to deal with such conditions as scabies, impetigo, and lice. (The rate of 1 doctor per 5000 population can be compared with the situation in Canada, where it was 1 doctor per 1014.)

Not all medical institutions dealing with such problems were army organizations, No 52 (RCAF) Mobile Field Hospital continuing to operate on the continent in support of the air force. On 9 October, just as the Scheldt campaign was getting underway, the MFH moved to Eindhoven, where it would remain until the end of March. Compared to previous sites, and the facilities for many of its army counterparts, its new location was nothing short of luxurious; the building had been used by the Germans as a naval hospital. With a capacity of 320 patients the enemy had left bulky equipment behind when evacuating, so No 52 MFH might have thought about dropping the word "mobile" from its name. As for air evacuation, which had proven less than perfect in Normandy, a Canadian Air Evacuation Unit (CAEU) was located on the same airfield, close enough to elicit no complaint from the hospital. Their busiest day was 1 January 1945, when the Germans launched Operation *Bodenplatte*, an attack by hundreds of aircraft against allied airfields, as part of the general (by then failing) Ardennes offensive. As the Canadian hospital reported, "The new year started very badly. At approximately 0900 hrs, enemy aircraft attacked the aerodrome B.78 (as well as others in the area) causing considerable damage and casualties. 40 cases were admitted to this hospital, the majority of which were gunshot wounds and burns... CAEU personnel were occupied caring for wounded, applying first aid, and delivering casualties following the attack. No casualties evacuated by air. A Harrow aircraft used for evacuating wounded destroyed on ground." The Operations Record Book still managed to avoid an ironic tone when it immediately added that "8 Nursing Orderlies arrived from various units in the area to attend refresher course."[28]

---

26. NA, RG 24, v.12,593, 11/14 Fd Amb/1, 14 Fd Amb, Quarterly Report, 31 Dec 44
27. NA, RG 24, v.12,593, 11/18 Fd Amb/1, 18 Fd Amb, Quarterly Report, 31 Dec 44
28. NA, RG 24, v.22,844, ORB 52 MFH, 1 Jan 45

After *Bodenplatte* came a period of relative quiet, which itself came to an end with the Allied campaign to clear the Rhineland preparatory to a thrust into the heart of Germany. Beginning on 8 February, First Canadian Army's part in the offensive would evolve in two main operations, Veritable and Blockbuster, preparing the way for the crossing of the Rhine on 22 March. Medical installations removed all patients that could travel to make room for an expected thousand casualties a day, and evacuating the latter from the battlefield would be a major challenge, as the Canadians' advance would be through flooded lands in the first part of the operation, then through forests for the second. Thus some units, such as 10 FDS, set themselves up as Casualty Transfer Points, at which

> the value of breaking a long Ambulance journey for wounded men was clearly demonstrated. Battle casualties arrived in many cases completely fatigued after a two to three hour journey over bumpy roads...

> All dressings were checked and changed or reinforced where found necessary. Clothing was completely removed in many cases and in all cases where the trousers or shoes were wet. Blankets were straightened and stretcher pillows substituted for blankets. Soup and thin sandwiches were provided. It was found that as soon as these small comforts were provided the soldiers with painful wounds would fall off to sleep. On an average, cases were kept just over an hour...

> It was noticed that many cases that are "walking wounded' at an ASC rapidly deteriorate and are in reality, stretcher cases by the time they have spent up to two hours in the back of a lorry. At least twenty percent that arrived here as "walkers" were made stretcher cases.[29]

Further back in the evacuation stream, amphibious vehicles, such as the appropriately-named DUKW, carried casualties through flooded areas, "much faster than they would have if the long, rough roads had been used."[30]

Not only the nature of evacuation, but the types of wounds differed, 14 Field Ambulance reporting "that there appeared to be a larger percentage among wounded cases of walking and sitting type. This can be attributed to the type of enemy fire. Many wounds were caused by small arms fire. Another characteristic feature was the extent of casualties caused by mines. Many of those seen had traumatic amputations of the foot with considerable destruction of soft tissue as far up as the knee joint. Shock was usually severe in these cases."[31] No 11 Field also noted

---

29. NA, RG 24, v.12,592, 11/10 FDS/1, 10 Canadian Field Dressing Station, Quarterly Report, 1 January to 31 March, 1944
30. NA, RG 24, v.12,593, 11/23 Fd Amb/1, 23 Fd Amb, Quarterly Report, 31 Mar 45
31. NA, RG 24, v.12,593, 11/14 Fd Amb/1, 14 Fd Amb, Quarterly Report, 31 Mar 45

that there were more wounds to small arms fire, adding that the death rate among casualties was approaching 50 per cent, as opposed to the 33 per cent or so of previous campaigns,[32] a clear indication of the battle's ferocity.

Heavy casualties meant a lot of men in pain, and though as we have seen Canadian medical staff had been using morphia for some time, in the course of the Rhineland campaign they experimented with other methods—with sometimes near-catastrophic results. As 11 Field Ambulance reported, "Intravenous morphia by syrette, or solution by syringe was found to be the best method of relieving pain, and quietening apprehension. Chloroform was used once and succeeded in relieving pain, while a partial traumatic amputation was completed, but the casualty stopped breathing, and much time was consumed in bringing him around to a state safe for evacuation. Two Medical Officers in the ADS state that they have seen a similar respiratory spasm on 2 occasions when chloroform with morphine was used in an ADS on severe casualties."[33]

In dealing with shock the field ambulances and other units were on much firmer ground, mainly because if they erred it was on the side of caution. As 17 Light Field Ambulance explained, "There is little scope for specialized professional treatment of the wounded soldier in a Field Ambulance, and it is felt that the basic principle of treatment on this level is the assumption that every wounded soldier is a potential case of shock. The Medical Officer must use good judgement with good sound common sense and base his treatment on the fundamental principles of the treatment of shock."[34] As before, ambulance attendants were trained to give transfusions so wounded could be evacuated as soon as possible, almost always with plasma, as whole blood was still difficult to store for any length of time and tended to go to waste. Volunteers from within the medical units could still provide the life-giving fluid if necessary,[35] though resuscitation techniques also came to rely on coal stoves, as in the Scheldt, and other means of keeping patients warm.[36]

After resuscitation often came surgery, especially in a campaign "the like of which we in this division have never seen before,"[37] according to 22 Field Ambulance, which further insisted that "This operation certainly proved beyond any doubt the enormous value of having [an] ASC at ADS level." What were called P1 and P2 (P for priority) cases were thus treated soon after wounding, an important consideration

32. NA, RG 24, v.12,593, 11/11 Fd Amb/1, 11 Fd Amb, Quarterly Report, 10 Mar 45
33. NA, RG 24, v.12,593, 11/11 Fd Amb/1, 11 Fd Amb, Quarterly Report, 31 Mar 45
34. NA, RG 24, v.12,617, 11/17 Lt Fd Amb/1, Quarterly Report, 31 Mar 45
35. NA, RG 24, v.12,593, 11/18 Fd Amb/1, 18 Fd Amb, Quarterly Report, 31 Mar 45
36. NA, RG 24, v.12,593, 11/11 Fd Amb/1, 11 Fd Amb, Quarterly Report, 10 Mar 45
37. NA, RG 24, v.12,593, 11/22 Fd Amb/1, 22 Fd Amb, Quarterly Report, 31 Mar 45

when fighting in terrain which had been flooded by the enemy's destruction of dykes and embankments. Ensuring nursing sisters were available to work at the advanced surgical centres completed the lessons of the Normandy campaign, which seem to have been applied, in the main, in the Rhineland.[38] Surgeons, for example, generally seemed to be developing in their work, and according to the commander of 3 FSU,

> During the past quarter we have felt, more than ever before, how specialized our role as forward surgeons had become. Almost unconsciously we find ourselves thinking more and more of the wound itself—the type of missile, it's course and what it would hit or miss—the surgery itself being almost automatic and simple. It is surprising to find how accurate one may be and how canny one's decision in the thoraco-abdominal or glueto-abdominal wound, and yet there are surprises at every turn and one's best armament is an open mind. It is, in fact, the only way to remain sane![39]

With a mortality rate among serious cases of 6 per cent, it was perhaps an easy enough task, but fatality statistics varied from one FSU to another. Number 6 performed 66 operations in February with a single death, and 77 operations in March with 11 deaths, so that in 8 per cent of surgical interventions in this period the patient succumbed.[40] In 8 FSU, Hillsman noted that the unit treated its 1000th case in late March, but saw little cause for celebrating; rather, "It was appalling to think that nearly two hundred men had died under my knife in the last nine months."[41]

The main reason for high fatality rates was that men with abdominal injuries continued to have the lowest chances of survival, 19 per cent of them dying in 3 FSU,[42] and of those with combined chest and belly wounds, a third died. Complicating matters was a high incidence of respiratory infection, which was first reported while First Canadian Army was wintering on the Maas, aggravated by the physical exhaustion that followed heavy fighting.[43] One possible solution was to specialize, sending abdominal wound victims to a unit entirely devoted to their care, though 6 FTU later reported that the scheme was "open to sharp criticism," without providing details.[44] The organization chosen for such specialized work, 5 FDS, was more forthcoming, relating how, after moving to Bedburg on 22 February, "only severe penetrating wounds of the abdomen were sent to 5 Cdn FDS."

38.   NA, RG 24, v.12,596, 11/10 FSU/1, Quarterly Report, 31 Mar 45
39.   NA, RG 24, v.12,596, 11/3 FSU/1, Quarterly Report, 31 Mar 45
40.   NA, RG 24, v.12,596, 11/6 FSU/1, Quarterly Report, 31 Mar 45
41.   John Burwell Hillsman, *Eleven Men and a Scalpel* (Winnipeg, 1948), 129
42.   NA, RG 24, v.12,596, 11/3 FSU/1, Quarterly Report, 31 Mar 45
43.   NA, RG 24, v.12,578, 11/ 3 CCS/1, Quarterly Report, 31 Mar 45
44.   NA, RG 24 v.12,596, 11/6 FTU/1, Quarterly Report, 31 Mar 45

This was the first time that an attempt had been made to concentrate this type of casualty in one unit. It created certain problems in post-operative care and extra nursing sisters were attached bringing their number to fifteen. A dietician was also temporarily attached and her advice and guidance in our ward kitchen was invaluable. The nursing orderlies regulated penicillin drip and took complete charge of all gastric suctions and intravenous therapy. The manner in which they carried out these duties speaks highly for their training. The nursing sisters were thus freed to supervise treatments and to attend to the comfort of the patients. The presence of nursing sisters had a morale effect, which, I am convinced, contributed greatly to the eventual recovery of the wounded. To them it is further evidence that they are receiving everything possible in the way of surgical care.[45]

A mortality rate of 15 per cent was only a little better than before, but one must be reminded that such dry statistics did—in reality—represent lives saved.

As for those whose injuries were of the mind, 23 Field Ambulance reported that "The exhaustion cases were about normal in number," though there was a disturbing trend among them. "It is noted that a high percentage is occurring in soldiers who have either been evacuated before for exhaustion or have been previously wounded and returned to the front line."[46] Treatment was as far forward as possible, as we have seen, though avoiding having patients within the sound of the guns. In effect, each divisional field dressing station, with a psychologist in residence, took on those patients deemed to be quickly responsive to rest and analysis, only the more serious cases being sent to the Exhaustion Treatment Unit, which "has therefore taken on the role of a forward psychiatric hospital."[47]

There were disadvantages to the scheme, however; because psychological cases were first treated at an FDS, they arrived at the Treatment Unit in groups, sometimes overwhelming the staff there. Thus the personnel of another FDS, which was located nearby, had to be called upon, carrying out "a considerable proportion of the work, under the supervision of the psychiatrists." Other problems included the use of the word "exhaustion," which the Treatment Unit's commander insisted might imply to the patient that he was a "mental case", hence hindering his chances of recovery. More mundane difficulties included a lack of quarter-master stores and transport, as well as laundry facilities, the necessity for the latter brought home by the dirty and ragged condition

45. NA, RG 24, v.12,592, 11/5 FDS/1, Quarterly Report, 31 Mar 45
46. NA, RG 24, v.12,593, 11/23 Fd Amb/1, 23 Fd Amb, Quarterly Report, 31 Mar 45
47. NA, RG 24, v.12,593, 11/21 Fd Dressing Stn/1, 21 FDS, Quarterly Report, 31 Mar 45

of admitted soldiers. The commanding officer recommended the formation of a full-fledged hospital with three psychiatrists on staff and an internist with administrative training to run the place, as "It is felt that the psychiatrist has a full time job in diagnosis and treatment and should not have to add the job of administering the unit to his other work."[48]

The campaign ended when remnants of German divisions on the south bank of the Rhine withdrew across the river or surrendered. Meanwhile, in Italy, the arduous struggle continued much as it had for the previous year and a half, medical staff having to go to continuing great lengths to provide treatment for sick and wounded soldiers. Evacuation through rugged terrain posed the first major challenge, such as that following an attack by the 11th Infantry and 5th Armoured Brigades in January. The assault was a success, and the two formations advanced into enemy territory, but the main road leading back from the now-fluid front line was heavily shelled; so 24 Light Field Ambulance was instructed to set up a field dressing station near some marshes not far from Ravenna. The alternate route had not been used up to that time because both a culvert and bridge had been blown, the obstacle thus created only passable on foot; the Field Ambulance thus quickly converted itself into a field engineering unit, and managed to repair the bridge to the point where it was useable by stretcher parties. A (real) engineering company also provided a ferry service with assault boats. "Although the volume of casualties did not tax the capacity of the ADS, it is interesting to note that this medical ferry service evacuated an estimated 1500 civilian refugees and numerous dogs, bicycles and carts. Passage of larger animals was refused."[49]

Long lines of communications over mountains and rivers meant that surgeons had to carry out much work that would normally be put off until a wounded soldier was in a fit state to travel. Number 4 Casualty Clearing Station, for example, was 25 miles from the front in January and early February, responsible for third priority casualties, but it was still 100 to 400 miles from the nearest hospital, depending on how the campaign was going. So, it held on to "all battle casualties whom it was judged could be returned to Corps level within 3 weeks."[50] Some more seriously wounded made the trip to the CCS as well, "though most of them came down in rush periods when it was no doubt decided they would get quicker attention down the line than by waiting their turn at more forward units." The station did not mention how long it took to evacuate wounded through 25 miles of Italian countryside, but if the

48. NA, RG 24, v.12,593, 11/21 Fd Dressing Stn/1, 21 FDS, Quarterly Report, 31 Mar 45
49. NA, RG 24, v.12,593, 11/24 Fd Amb/1, 24 Fd Amb, Quarterly Report, 31 Mar 45
50. NA, RG 24, v.12,578, 11/ 4 CCS/1, Quarterly Report, Period ending 31 March 1945

experiences of 24 Light Field Ambulance, related above, are any indication, it was far from quick.

Thus whenever movement was involved, medical practitioners in the Italian campaign seemed to have had a more difficult time than their colleagues in north-west Europe, and the resulting need for forward treatment was not limited to physical wounds and injuries. In dealing with psychological casualties Lieutenant-Colonel A.M. Doyle, commenting on psychiatry in the Mediterranean theatre, insisted that "The practise of military neuropsychiatry must begin in the forward area. This is the only way that the Psychiatrist can become thoroughly acquainted with the life and work of the combat troops and so give intelligent advice and treatment."[51] As for the latter, practitioners in Italy continued to rely heavily on the Special Employment Companies, as "The single most effective way of handling these casualties is to put them at work quickly." Results were far from spectacular, however, as fewer than 20 per cent of such men could be returned to full combat duty after treatment, though many could still contribute to eventual victory in supporting roles. According to Doyle, a "Drastic weeding out of the unstable, the neurotic, the criminal, the inadequate, appears to be the only way in which Neuropsychiatric casualties are likely to be reduced. It must be accepted as a principle that a good army has to have good personnel and that there is no place in it for misfits."[52] Again, the concept that every soldier had a breaking point had not gained universal acceptance.

Combat casualties, either to body or mind, seem to have been in the minority, however, 24 Field Ambulance reporting that in the first three months of 1945 only 6 per cent of its patients had battle-related injuries, while a little over 81 per cent were sick.[53] Number 5 CCS noted that its medical specialist, among other tasks, investigated tuberculosis contacts.[54] In northwest Europe, with the Rhineland campaign over, the laboratories that investigated infectious diseases and other conditions noted that "by mid-March the troops were resting again and business picked up rapidly."[55] Worthy of mention was that "there are sufficient Typhoid Fever and Paratyphoid Fever carriers throughout liberated and enemy territory to be a Health Hazzard to our troops, if there is any

51. Lt-Col A.M. Doyle, "Psychiatry with the Canadian Army in Action in the CMF," *The Journal of the Canadian Medical Services* (January, 1946), 106
52. Lt-Col A.M. Doyle, "Psychiatry with the Canadian Army in Action in the CMF," *The Journal of the Canadian Medical Services* (January, 1946), 106
53. NA, RG 24, v.12,593, 11/24 Fd Amb/1, 24 Fd Amb, Quarterly Report, 31 Mar 45
54. NA, RG 24, v.12,578, 11/ 5 CCS/1, Quarterly Report, 31 Mar 45, Appx 9
55. NA, RG 24, v.12,621, 11/Mob Bact Lab/1, No 2 Cdn Mob Bact Lab, Quarterly Report, 31 Mar 45

laxity in maintaining a high state of Hygiene efficiency,"[56] though other dangers threatened unsuspecting liberators. As No 2 Mobile Hygiene Laboratory insisted, "It is believed timely that the troops be warned of the dangers involved in wantonly drinking seized preparations which may or may not be alcoholic beverages,"[57] and in April "Four deaths directly attributable to a failure to heed this advice, on the part of the troops, have come to our attention."

Laboratory work went much further than looking into the causes of disease outbreaks, some investigators carrying out basic scientific research. In Italy, for example, medical investigators continued to put penicillin to the test, their report becoming available in February 1945. John Hamilton, a member of the research laboratory, explained how "During the past ten months the wound infection team of the Research Laboratory has been investigating, first, the bacterial flora of wounds at Forward Surgical Centres, Lines of Communications and Base Hospitals and, secondly, the effect of intramuscular penicillin therapy, administered in the forward area, on these wounds. To date, approximately 1000 wounds have been examined, at various stages from a few hours to several weeks after wounding."[58] One interesting discovery was that 54 per cent of patients harboured bacterial strains that were resistant to the drug, which could "only be explained on the basis of insensitivity induced by previous penicillin therapy." Bacteria that survived an attack by the antibiotic reproduced into full strains able to resist treatment; only the development of antibiotics other than penicillin could control them, engendering a war of measure and counter-measure that has lasted to the present day and shows no signs of abating.

The Second World War in Europe was drawing to a close, though many soldiers may have been hard to convince since the fighting was as harsh as ever. In March 1945 Canada's Ist Corps left Italy to join IInd Corps, and that same month British and American forces, with some Canadian units, crossed the Rhine in force. First Canadian Army was given the task of liberating the Netherlands, which at times turned into a full-scale pursuit reminiscent of the break-out from Normandy. As G.W.L. Nicholson related, after 1 April "So rapid had been the advance that often an ADS was scarcely open before the brigade it was to serve was almost out of reach. Before April ended, No 14 Field Ambulance had had to move eleven times,"[59] while No 9 left a detailed report of how it coped with quickly-changing circumstances.

56. NA, RG 24, v.12,621, 11/2 Mob Hyg Lab/1, Monthly Report ending 31 Mar 45
57. NA, RG 24, v.12,621, 11/2 Mob Hyg Lab/1, Monthly Report ending 31 Mar 45
58. NA, MG 30, B85, Harris Papers, v.4, John Hamilton, Bacterial Flora of War Wounds and Penicillin Therapy, February 1945
59. G.W.L. Nicholson, *Seventy Years of Service* (Ottawa, 1977), 236

The short time of evacuation from the time of wounding to the time of admission to the ADSs accounted for the fairly good condition of many battle casualties. It was found, however, that there was an unusually high percentage of severe and dangerous casualties resulting from accurate small-arms fire as well as shell-fire. Whole blood was very useful in restoring exsanguinated patients to a condition where they could withstand the remainder of the journey to the surgical teams. Blood, plasma and glucose-saline is placed in a specially constructed box containing an electric light so that it is not too cold when administered. A special attachment to the stretcher to hold the bottle containing blood has been designed by one of our sergeants, and by the use of this, many casualties can be transfused at the same time when casualties are heavy.[60]

This one unit, at least, had learned well.

So had 17 Light Field Ambulance, which described the arsenal available to practitioners in their attempts to mitigate the ravages of the battlefield. "Medical treatment in the Fd Amb resolved itself on all occasions to a sound knowledge of first aid. Shock was treated using plasma, heat, fluids and morphine as required. Fractures were always splinted to the best of ability. Haemorrhage was controlled with available means—using tourniquets only as a last resort. Oxygen was administered where necessary. Sucking chest wounds were always sealed as efficiently as could be hoped for. Burns were treated with sulfanilamide cream dressings or normal saline dressings."[61] The aim was still to stabilize a wounded soldier and make him comfortable before evacuating him further down the line, but field ambulances seemed to have more in the way of resources and knowledge to do so than their brethren of previous conflicts—or even previous Second World War battles.

Surgery saw no changes in technique—or results—but the Netherlands added a new feature simply because of the pace of operations, 10 FSU's experiences being rather typical. "April has been the Unit's record month—six moves, eighty eight cases," it reported as it attempted to keep up with 4th Armoured Division driving its way through eastern Holland and north-western Germany. "All of our cases ranked high in priority, the bulk of them resulting from the battles of the Kusten Canal area. Ambulances carrying both incoming and evacuated casualties were obliged to negotiate extremely difficult road conditions—delays were inevitable. The severity of the wounding was the greatest we have yet encountered and exceeded that of our experience at Bedburg," where it had spent the month of March. "As a comparison of volume—at Bedburg the Unit operated on a total of 42 cases in 22

60. NA, RG 24, v.12,593, 11/9 Fd Amb/1, 9 Fd Amb, Quarterly Report, 31 Mar 45
61. NA, RG 24, v.12,617, 11/17 Lt Fd Amb/1, Quarterly Report, 1st April to 30 June 1945

days, of these 27 were abdominals or thoraco-abdominals; at Friesoythe the Unit operated on a total of 49 cases in 11 days, 29 of the cases being abdominal or thoraco-abdominal. There were 15 deaths during the month, the majority of these had sustained a degree of trauma precluding survival."[62] Conditions were primitive, buildings being used as operating wards having had their windows broken in the fighting, a situation that "did not facilitate rapid resuscitation and it is felt that in some instances operation was too long delayed on this account."

With the front semi-fluid and medical units moving about the country-side to find suitable locations from which to support their higher formations, certain procedures had to take a back seat to the demands of the moment. Proper accounting and statistical work, for example, suffered, so that when 3 CCS reported that "Traumatic chest cases presented most of the problems from our viewpoint" in the month of April, it was conveying no more than a general impression. "Unfortunately, the mortality rate of chest injuries in the field cannot be accurately calculated now as some cases were just dying or were dead on admission and often they were operated on by FSU teams and evacuated or died without the medical staff seeing the patient at all. In any future active theatre of war, this might be foreseen and a medical clerk be detailed to collect and correlate information on the spot."[63]

The pace of operations was also affecting air force medical units, the Canadian Air Evacuation Section relating its tales of woe in a detailed report. Arriving at airfield B108 on 7 April, it faced several obstacles before its operations could get off the ground (if the author can be allowed such an expression). "The runway at B108 was unserviceable until late afternoon 10 April, 1945, and no casualties were evacuated until then. At this airfield communications were extremely poor. It was impossible to ascertain either the number of aircraft arriving for casualties, or their times of arrival. Bids for aircraft were submitted daily, but requirements were seldom met." Moving to another airfield, B114, the unit found that operations had been complicated by a decision to move recently-liberated prisoners-of-war back to England by air. Though the will to get these men home as soon as possible was laudatory, problems arose when pilots reported they could not evacuate casualties because their orders explicitly limited them to transporting freed prisoners.[64]

For No 52 Mobile Field Hospital, of which the CAES was a part, the final moves in the campaign brought mixed blessings. "For the first time since landing on the Continent, at B100, No 52 MFH was situated

62. NA, RG 24, v.12,596, 11/10 FSU/1, Surgical Report, Apr 45
63. NA, RG 24, v.12,578, 11/ 3 CCS/1, Quarterly Report, 1 Apr 45 to 30 Jun 45
64. NA, RG 24, v.22,844, ORG 52 MFH, Apr 45, Remarks on and Discussion of Statistics

within the confines of an airfield," which as an RCAF unit it only thought appropriate. However, "This airfield was in the midst of one of the heavily mined belts of the so-called Siegfried Line. An attempt was made to find a suitable site near the airfield. A captain from an Army Bomb Disposal Unit accompanied the Recce Party on this search. Several suitable sites were found but were abandoned because de-mining would have required a minimum of two weeks. Hence the hospital was eventually located within the confines of the airfield near its CAES, and the Dakota landing strip."

Then the war, for Canadians in northwest Europe at least, ended; German forces in the Netherlands surrendered on 4 May, with the Third Reich as a whole giving up the fight on the 7th. By then some 35,000 people had served in the Royal Canadian Army Medical Corps, of whom over 3600 were nursing sisters; a total of 107 practitioners died. The nature of the fighting and medical developments like the treatment of shock made for a reduction in the death rate from 114 Canadians of every 1000 wounded in the First World War to 66 in the Second; sanitation and the war against the microbe reduced the number of fatalities to disease from 22 per 1000 soldiers in the Boer War to 0.9 per 1000 in 1939-45.[65] With war's end, however, one type of casualty actually grew in importance, 12 Light Field Ambulance reporting that VD rates had increased from 9 per cent of all admissions to 14, and "This increase becomes more noticeable since the cessation of hostilities."[66]

The word "cessation" was not entirely accurate, though, as there was still a war to fight against Japan, a task which, with the exception of the disaster at Hong Kong, Canada left mainly in the hands of the navy. Thus the latter, even while it concentrated on the timely arrival of convoys across the North Atlantic in a merciless and gruelling anti-U-boat war, prepared for operations in the Pacific. For medical personnel, that meant investigating the equipment and supplies they would need for a variety of climates, the war having been fought in such far-flung places as the equatorial jungles of New Guinea and the frozen islands of the Aleutians. At the second meeting of the joint services to discuss the issue of medical supplies on 10 July 1944 (the first meeting had been the week before), "The general opinion seemed to be that tropicalization of medical equipment and supplies was well advanced in the United States who had a large reserve of equipment and supplies, some of which might be made available to Canada, if proper steps were taken to obtain it... With regard to medical equipment and supplies for tem-

65. G.W.L. Nicholson, *Seventy Years of Service* (Ottawa, 1977), 252
66. NA, RG 24, v.12,617, 11/12 Lt Fd Amb/1, Quarterly Report, 30 Jun 45

perate zones, it was felt that the existing medical equipment and supplies would be satisfactory."[67]

Though the North Atlantic could certainly not be described as having
a warm climate, Canadian researchers had begun looking into problems
posed by heat long before ships were sent to the Pacific. In early 1943
medical officers recorded the wet and dry temperatures of the hotter
parts of a sample ship as well as the temperatures and pulse rates of
naval ratings. Noting that "We ... wish it understood that no attempt
is being made to carry a banner likely to stir up sentiment in favour of
shorter hours, more pay or air-conditioning," they carried out their
work in the vicinity of Trinidad and in Port of Spain. Their report read
in part that "the only unusual occurrence was a slight increase in pulse
rate," and that "Aside from the fact that it is "damn hot" at times in
No 1 stokehold and the galley, the heat and humidity with the present
system of ventilation seem to have no harmful effects on the robust and
physically fit stoker or galley worker. However the ventilation could be
improved. This is especially true in the stokers' large mess where the ports
are near water level and closed tightly most of the day... As can be seen
from the Table a stoker would be more comfortable in a detention
cell,"[68] though whether sailors were purposely breaking the rules to get
temporary relief in the brig is doubtful.

Naval staff officers could also look to the experiences of other navies
to determine the effect of heat on sailors' health, such as a report by
Surgeon-Captain R.W. Mussen of the Royal Navy.

> Before the United States entered the war, it was realized that difficulties
> would arise concerning ventilation and high temperatures on board
> warships. It was realized that since the last war there had been an enor-
> mous increase in horsepower and sources of wild heat and a correspond-
> ing increase in equipment and the personnel to operate it. It was seen
> that with the danger of air and submarine attack, ships would have to be
> closed tighter than in older vessels, with doors and hatches closed down
> when the ship went to sea, and a complete closing down of the ven-
> tilating system in action. All the heat produced inside the ship had to be
> removed by ventilation or by transmission through the hull, and when
> the sea temperature and outside air temperature rose above 75 ˚ effective,
> the transmission loss became negligible and ventilation was entirely
> responsible for removing heat from the ship.[69]

The US Navy, for its part, had carried out substantial tests, finding that
"an effective temperature of 90 is the limit for health of persons engaging

67. NA, RG 24, v.8134, NSC 1288-2, Dir Naval Stores to DWT, 10 Jul 44
68. Surg-Lt A.L. Chambers, "Observations on Body Heat in Engine Room," *Canadian Medical Association Journal* (March, 1943), 214
69. NA, RG 24, v.8134, NSS 1288-7, Surgeon Captain R.W. Mussen RN to MDG Adm, 3 Aug 44

in light activity. It was found, however, that in engine rooms where a high velocity of cool air was available to personnel, effective temperatures of 94 could be stood without detriment." A Royal Navy report warned nevertheless that "Climactic conditions make it impossible for a given number of men to accomplish the same amount of work in the tropics as they could in the temperate area."[70]

Another issue arising from operations in many parts of the Pacific was that "Disease incidence is greatly increased. Possibly a 20% wastage is due to illness alone," making prevention a major challenge.[71] Given the experiences of allied forces, it seemed that good care could keep the hospitalization rate down to ten days per person per year (it was nine in the RCN generally), with a loss to the total establishment of 2-15 per cent, but poor health management could triple such figures. "Surgeon Captain Critchley's report on Royal Naval ships and establishments visited in Africa, India and Ceylon, puts the malaria morbidity at a possible 25%. Furthermore, he warns that we must be prepared for the possibility of malaria spreading, under Japanese occupation, into places like Singapore and some Pacific Islands, previously free from malaria."[72] Though for most Canadians their western ocean no doubt conjured up scenes of blue lagoons and islands of paradise, reality was somewhat less idyllic.

The first ship to begin making its way to the Far East was HMCS *Uganda*, a cruiser recently-acquired from the British which left Belfast on its way to war at the end of 1944. The duties and concerns of a surgeon on such a vessel, in this case Surgeon-Commander R.K. Thompson, were encapsulated in one of the first reports of its medical department. (PMO means Principal Medical Officer, in this case Thompson himself.)

> The general health of the ships company was good during the month of December. The ship left refit yards and proceeded to working up exercises by the middle of the month. It was noticeable that the attitude of the ships company improved as soon as the ship left the refit yard, where the presence of dockyard matey's and the constant turmoil and dirt offered no incentive to cleanliness of ship or person, or to orderliness of mind. It was considered by the PMO that the ordinary rating could not see progress, and the fruits of his labours were sour during periods of dockyard refit. This plus the lack of healthy and varied recreation was to a large degree responsible for the high incidence of exposure to, and development of, venereal disease, and infestations of scabies and pediculosis pubis.[73]

---

70. NA, RG 24, v.8134, NSS 1288-7, Disease Incidence in Far East, Oct 44
71. NA, RG 24, v.8134, NSS 1288-7, Disease Incidence in Far East, Oct 44
72. Ibid
73. NA, RG 24, v.11,732, CS 153-15-18, Report of Medical Department HMCS Uganda, December 1944

The reference to "orderliness of mind" is of interest here, as the ship's surgeon was also responsible for dealing with psychological injuries, and as *Uganda* left for war service the doctor reported that "The morale of the ship is good and is improving. This is going to be of vital importance in keeping the psychiatric casualties to a minimum. Several cases have arisen who could not be retained as useful ratings. Several have been seen who show evidence of instability, which is apt to become more marked under difficult conditions which may exist in the Pacific. Unfortunately the two weeks in December during which PMO was in the ship gave no time to make a systematic or even cursory survey from a psychiatric point of view."[74]

The cruiser's complement had a perhaps more prosaic view of health and illness aboard the cruiser, A. Murray Rogerson, for example, writing in his diary how "Athlete's foot ran rampant throughout the ship. It was impossible to control and we would cut everything possible away from our shoes to let the air circulate around our feet, and ankles. Some had it so bad they would spend half an hour at times in the Sick Bay with the Sick Bay "tiffy" pulling dead skin away."[75] That was in February 1945; by April, when *Uganda* had joined the British Pacific Fleet and prepared to support operations to capture Okinawa, Rogerson was complaining that "Conditions were so bad with water rationed and lack of refrigeration to carry fresh foods, I developed bad boils on the legs. The Medical Officer was to be seen around ship with a skin rash which he was unable to clear for himself—so there was little hope for the crew's problems."[76] He may have had a point, writing three weeks later that "Life is grim as ever. Treating boils all over legs."

HMCS *Ontario*, Canada's second and last Second World War cruiser, did not leave European waters until the Japanese war was almost over, but can still serve as an example of the kinds of medical challenges posed by 900 men living and working in close quarters. From commissioning on 26 April, 1945, to the end of June, its sick bay treated 68 patients, the largest group, of 16, for tonsillitis and related illnesses; the next largest, of seven men each, suffered from pneumonia and minor injuries respectively. In the same period 694 sailors were treated at sick parade, while there were also "several minor epidemics of food poisoning. On June 10th, there was a major epidemic of diarrhoea involving more than 600 of the ship's company. This was attributed to faulty handling of meat in the main galley in that it was cooked at 0300, cooled and put

74. NA, RG 24, v.11,732, CS 153-15-18, Report of Medical Department HMCS Uganda, December 1944
75. DHist, Biog, Rogerson, A. Murray Rogerson Diary, Footnote to 19-21 Feb 45
76. Ibid, Footnote to 7 Apr 45

through the meat grinder by hand at 0500 and allowed to stand in the warm galley until 1100 when it was warmed and served. Steps were taken to correct such practises and with the co-operation of the supply department a more satisfactory method of dealing with meat in bulk was worked out."[77] With what little free time they had after dealing with such crises, the medical staff gave first aid lectures and demonstrations to the ship's company.

Like an army in camp, a ship at dock faces a constant—and often losing—battle against venereal disease. Aboard *Ontario*, prophylaxis consisted of a free issue of condoms and the administering of two grams of sulphathiazole (one of the sulpha drugs developed since 1935) to anyone who might become exposed to the disease. "At first an effort was made to take the names of those who applied for sulphathiazole for the purpose of assessing results but it was soon found that this discouraged ratings from coming for prophylaxis and this practise was discontinued."[78] By this stage in the war penicillin was in much wider use, and it had been found to be effective against both gonorrhea and syphilis, the ship's surgeon reporting that he had achieved "good results" in fifteen cases of the former. He also related, however, that six men were under weekly or twice weekly treatment for syphilis, suggesting that older methods for dealing with the disease were still in vogue.

The whole purpose behind looking after the health of sailors was so they would be up to the stresses—physical and emotional—of operations; for with the acquisition of larger warships and the decision to send them to the Pacific the RCN moved into a realm of naval warfare that differed greatly from the convoy battles of the North Atlantic. When a cruiser went into action, unlike smaller vessels it was expected not only to inflict punishment but to absorb it as well, and though only one of Canada's larger ships, HMCS *Uganda*, fired its guns in anger, when it did so its medical organization was designed to deal with dozens of wounded without interfering with operations. Its first encounter with Japanese forces was on 13 April 1945, when kamikaze attacked the British Pacific Fleet of which *Uganda* was a part, and in the months that followed air attack would be the main threat to the vessel's existence—as well as to sailors' life and limb.

In preparing for action the ship's medical personnel, consisting of a surgeon commander (an internist in civilian life), a surgeon lieutenant-commander (previously a surgeon), a surgeon lieutenant (once an expert

---

77. NA, RG 24, v.11,731, CS 153-10-18, Health Report on HMCS Ontario Covering Period from Commissioning to June 30th, 1945
78. NA, RG 24, v.11,731, CS 153-10-18, Health Report on HMCS Ontario Covering Period from Commissioning to June 30th, 1945

in public health), a sick berth chief petty officer (registered nurse), a sick berth petty officer, a leading SBA (X-ray technician) and three SBAs,[79] decentralized their work so their entire operation could not be disrupted by a single bomb, torpedo, or kamikaze strike. An Emergency Operating Station (EOS) was set up, as far as possible from the sick bay since they both served similar purposes in battle; it was to accommodate two per cent of the ship's company sitting and another two per cent lying down. Naturally, it had to be accessible to stretchers, as "great harm is done to wounded men, by carrying them through a series of narrow passages and man holes, and up and down ladders to the treatment centre."[80] Several First Aid Posts, or FAPs, were also to be provided, located near action stations such as gun turrets and anti-aircraft weaponry, taking advantage of such spaces as bathrooms, recreation centres, the captain's quarters, wide lobbies, and other areas that were not used during action. In keeping with the goal of decentralization the principal medical officer was not allocated to a particular location, running the sick bay, EOS, and FAPs being left to subordinates. His role was to move to where he was needed most.

Once engaged with the enemy, casualties occurring near FAPs were to be dealt with immediately in those posts, while sailors falling in less accessible areas were to be put under cover, first-aid being administered by comrades. In a language reminiscent of the Duke of Wellington's peninsular campaign, instructions suggested that "If opportunity offers, sorties are made from the FAPs to render more skilled assistance and supervise moving of serious cases."[81] Also, whenever possible stretcher cases were to be moved from what cover their friends had evacuated them to to FAPs, though, interestingly, instructions insisted that "No attempt should be made to take personnel to the EOS during action except under the instructions of a medical officer."

The reason for the latter injunction was that the sick bay and EOS were to be used as operating theatres and thus were not to be crowded with casualties who did not require surgery. After action ceased medical officers would determine where more permanent stations were to be set up, for though "The sick bay or EOS may be available ... allowance must be made for the possibility of these being damaged."[82] As for priorities, "The immediate work after action will be resuscitation, which will occupy a considerable time. Arrangements should be made for anti-shock treatment," such as transfusions of dried serum or whole blood

79. S.T. Richards, *Operation Sick Bay* (West Vancouver, 1994), 117
80. NA, RG 24, v.11,706, NB 1854-1, "Medical Organization for Action'
81. Ibid
82. Ibid

and the provision of hot liquids, many patients having to wait some time before they were deemed fit for surgery. Thankfully, the system in *Uganda* was never put to its ultimate test, no kamikaze getting close enough to the ship to cause serious damage or casualties. Medical practitioners, of course, were unaware of the vessel's eventual good fortune, so they drilled and practised and trained in order to be prepared—they could hope—for the worst.

Uganda was in Esquimalt when the atomic bombs were dropped on Hiroshima and Nagasaki and the Empire of Japan surrendered, all in the eight days leading up to 14 August 1945. The last Canadian naval mission in the theatre was thus left to the auxiliary cruiser *Prince Robert*, which soon after the Japanese surrender picked up the survivors of the Hong Kong debacle. They had not fared well, prison facilities in Hong Kong and Japan ranging from uncomfortable camps of neglect to dens of horror. The reasons for this are still rather obscure, for though the "Code of Bushido" has often been suggested as the cause, prisoners of war not being considered fit to live, the *Hagakure*, or *Book of the Samurai*, makes no mention of the treatment of captured soldiers, though it does refer to the proper procedure for surrendering a castle.[83] Furthermore, in previous conflicts Japanese officials had treated prisoners of war rather well; as Jonathan Vance has pointed out in *Objects of Concern*, during their confrontation with the Russians in 1904-05 "the Japanese evidently took pride in the extent to which they observed the Hague Convention, a fact borne out by contemporary Japanese literature on the conflict," while President Theodore Roosevelt suggested that the Japanese Army's treatment of its captives demonstrated that "the most reckless indifference to death and the most formidable fighting capacity can be combined with a scrupulous compliance with all the modern ideas as regards the proper treatment of prisoners."[84]

Medical neglect in the Second World War was, however, a documented fact, the ordeal beginning on Christmas Day, 1941, when 1686 Canadians fell into the hands of the enemy, at first being confined in Hong Kong's North Point Camp. "This was a period of rapid deterioration of health," Doctors J.N. Crawford and J.A.G. Reid later wrote, with "A diet grossly deficient in animal protein, animal fat, and caloric content, and with the B-complex exhibiting the most spectacular inadequacy with respect to vitamins. The change from the Canadian army rations to the prisoner regime was very abrupt."[85] Major Gordon Gray, RCAMC,

83. Yamamoto Tsunetomo, *Hagakure: The Book of the Samurai* (Tokyo, 1983), 140

84. Jonathan Vance, *Objects of Concern: Canadian Prisoners of War through the Twentieth Century* (Vancouver, 1994), 21

85. NA, MG 31, J7, Sneath Papers, v.2, Military Medicine, Nutritional Disease Affecting Canadian Troops Held Prisoner of War by the Japanese, Apr 47

would remain in Hong Kong for the rest of the war, but the first few months were decidedly the worst. "North Point camp was a bad spot," he related in a later interview. "It was overcrowded. That's where we began to have a lot of dysentery. We had very little to treat them with. That's one of the terrible things about being a doctor in that situation. We knew there were just tons of sulpha drugs in Central Medical Stores in Hong Kong, but it appeared later the Japanese moved this stuff out of there for their own use."[86] Such appropriation of allied supplies was a consequence of the Japanese Army's logistical system being inadequate to stand up to the pressures of a modern conflict. According to Albert E. Cowdrey, in his history of American medicine in the Second World War, "The imperial high command had launched its great push for empire with no realistic attempt to calculate the supply requirements of its forces or the amount of shipping that would be needed to nourish and sustain them."[87] In the Philippines, for example, supplies of quinine, available from the nearby Dutch East Indies, ran out because only sufficient quantities were on hand for the *expected* one-month duration of the campaign.

In Hong Kong, severe rationing could only make a bad situation worse, with a daily food intake in the first months of captivity of about 900 calories per soldier, "totally insufficient for men averaging 170 pounds."[88] Then, even these meagre supplies were cut as collective punishment for an escape attempt, the reduction remaining in force from July to November, 1942. As William Allister, a POW who related his experiences in *Where Life and Death Hold Hands*, described,

> Malnutrition began to take its toll. More men died. We seemed marked for the seven plagues of Egypt. A disease called pellagra brought open, running pus sores to many parts of the mouth and body. One of the curses produced red, swollen testicles, dubbed "strawberry balls." Another turned them into huge melon-sized monstrosities called "Hong Kong balls." Wet and dry beri-beri stymied the medics. Men developed "electric feet"—painful nerve shocks in the toes that continued relentlessly day and night. This curse attacked those with large feet most... It progressed in stages. First came the pain-filled sleepless nights, which produced exhaustion and lack of appetite. In time, at the middle stage, the misery gradually drove men mad. They could neither eat nor sleep. Finally they wasted away and died.[89]

86. Daniel G. Dancocks, *In Enemy Hands: Canadian Prisoners of War, 1939-1945* (Edmonton, 1983), 230

87. Albert E. Cowdrey, *Fighting for Life: American Military Medicine in World War II* (New York, 1994), 42

88. Patricia Roy et al, *Mutual Hostages: Canadians and Japanese during the Second World War* (Toronto, 1990), 71

89. William Allister, *Where Life and Death Hold Hands* (Toronto, 1989), 65-66

During this period the Canadians remained on Hong Kong island, where they had surrendered, but in September 1942, at about the time when rations were reestablished to their normal—if meagre—levels, they prepared to move to the mainland, to Sham Shui Po.

There, Captain J.A.G. Reid, RCAMC, faced his first major challenge, as

> just before we left we got a few cases of diphtheria. In any adult group you have some carriers, the membranes in the mouth and throat had gone down and the diphtheria became virulent in some throats and they passed it on to others. We got a few cases and tried to send them out to the Dunen Road Military Hospital but the Japanese wouldn't let them go, so we took them over with us, took them in the same crowded boat and when we got into Sham Shui Po it became epidemic. We had thirteen hundred men in the camp; we had over 500 cases of diphtheria. This time we had no anti-toxin. Finally they brought in some, some of our own and some Japanese. They had our medical supplies that they had picked up and I remember one night after we got the antitoxin we had to go into the long ward among the men with diphtheria and we had only a small amount of antitoxin and we had to use it where it would do the most good. We would say this one is too late, this one will, this one wont [sic]; just playing God in a way you don't want to play God anymore, signing life and death warrants. We found that a very small dose would tip one of these dipths over onto the safe side. A little over a thousand units was sufficient with very bad cases a little more. We had dipth penis, dipth scrotum, dipth throat and noses, all kinds, every conceivable thing you can imagine as far as diphtheria went.[90]

William Allister later reported how "The death toll rose ominously. At first makeshift coffins were built of odd boards. Burying parties left each day for the graveyard nearby. As deaths increased there were no boards left and the corpses were carried on stretchers and laid unprotected in their graves. Thirty-one Canadians died in October," the death toll to diphtheria eventually reaching 50.[91]

In February 1943 some 500 Canadians were moved to Japan (the first of 1184), to work in ship yards and coal mines, with Captain Reid accompanying them as MO and officer commanding. Though it seems that rations were better there they were reduced in the summer of 1943, as Reid later related.

> The first ration cut was in July and August another and September another and their weight went down, down, down, like that. All this time I was protesting and warning them what the next winter would be, they always

90. DHist 593.(D17), Notes from Interview with Captain J.A.G. Reid, 31 Oct 45, 13
91. William Allister, *Where Life and Death Hold Hands*, 73

said it was an order from the top and that was one of the reasons they said nothing could be done about it. Because of this—conservation—we had this bad time next winter—the worst of all, 1943-44—a great deal of pneumonia. The men were malnourished with very little resistance. That winter we lost eleven cases of pneumonia and three cases of other things, fourteen deaths this winter we are coming to—twenty-three for the whole two and a half years. That was the very worst time.[92]

Even the best times, however, were marked by general ill health among the prisoners, though a 4.5 per cent fatality rate was only slightly higher than among Canadians in German prison camps, making Reid's group the most fortunate of those to fall into Japanese hands.

Others suffered far more, and the authors of a post-war report presented a case study, a rifleman who by the spring of 1943 had lost 20 per cent of his body weight, with an apparent age of 50 years though he had been born in 1913. "His skin is dry and rough, loose and inelastic, and subcutaneous fat is absent... There are cracks at the corners of his mouth... He has a deep ulcer on the calf of the left leg. His tongue is sore, smooth, and very red at the margins and tip... Two teeth are chipped from biting on pebbles in his rice, and several other teeth are grossly carious so that it is difficult for him to chew his food properly."[93] There was more, as

> He complains that he cannot read ordinary print but he can make out the newspaper headlines... He complains of a sensation of constriction, like a band, around his chest... He has a mild, dry, unproductive cough but his chest is clear to clinical examination... He states that both lower extremities are numb from mid-thigh level to the toes... The toenails are brittle and markedly thickened. The right toe is deformed, where a tropic ulcer has healed... He states that he staggers when trying to walk in the dark but manages moderately well in the daylight. Two months earlier his feet were very painful but this has been greatly relieved since the numbness has supervened. He also has some numbness of his hands, particularly of the fingertips. This makes him clumsy, so that he has trouble trying to roll a cigarette.[94]

William Allister's symptoms were far less severe; five feet nine inches tall before the war, he returned at five foot seven and a half. Of his comrades, he noted telegraphically: "Grant seriously ill in hospital; Newfie in the loony bin; Tony having a lung removed; Bob, too, having a lung removed in a Montreal hospital, and facing a painful divorce.

92. DHist 593.(D17), Notes from Interview with Captain J.A.G. Reid, 31 Oct 45, 82
93. NA, MG 31, J7, Sneath Papers, v.2, Military Medicine, Nutritional Disease Affecting Canadian Troops Held Prisoner of War by the Japanese, Apr 47
94. NA, MG 31, J7, Sneath Papers, v.2, Military Medicine, Nutritional Disease Affecting Canadian Troops Held Prisoner of War by the Japanese, Apr 47

Blacky, like many others, was to die of heart disease in the coming years."[95] All returned veterans suffered from avitaminosis, their life expectancy 10 to 15 years less than the Canadian national average; a medical study completed in 1963 found their death rate to be 23 per cent higher than other veterans. Of the less fortunate, 128 died in the Hong Kong camps of Sham Shui Po and North Point (50 of them victims of diphtheria), with four more executed for an escape attempt, while 136 lost their lives in Japan, in all a 16 per cent fatality rate.[96] Among those not part of Reid's group, over one in five died.

With the return of the Hong Kong prisoners the Second World War was indeed over, except for those suffering permanent physical or psychological damage. For doctors, nurses, and some NCOs (especially among sick berth attendants in the latter case), returning to a non-military life was eased to some extent by the nature of their work in the armed services—essentially applying civilian techniques to the illnesses and injuries of soldiers, sailors, and airmen, including psychological casualties. For most NCOs and lower ranks, who had learned their trades only after joining up, coming back to Canada represented an important departure from the life and work they had come to know. For both groups, the main difference between military medicine and what was practised in the cities, towns, and countryside back home was not in its technical aspects but in its tactical realm. The mass casualties of the battlefield, where soldiers fell in numbers rarely seen back home (except for mining catastrophes, hotel fires, and similar disasters) were the result of human ingenuity applied to the military science of large-scale destruction. It was this aspect of military medicine that most contrasted it with peacetime practice—in Montreal, Moncton, or Mattawa, no one was trying to kill you as you followed your vocation.

95. William Allister, *Where Life and Death Hold Hands*, 229, 236
96. Carl Vincent, *No Reason Why: The Canadian Hong Kong Tragedy, an Examination* (Stittsville, 1981), 214; Daniel G. Dancocks, *In Enemy Hands: Canadian Prisoners of War, 1939-1945* (Toronto, 1983), 246, 248

Chapter Eight

Post-war, Cold War, and Peacekeeping

The period that followed the Second World War was different from that following the First in one very important respect—Canada did not return completely to peaceful pursuits. Soviet manoeuvring in eastern Europe, the Korean War, the threat of nuclear holocaust, and the country's attempts to forge a place for itself in the world—as a so-called middle power—meant that its military establishment, though seriously reduced in strength when compared with its peak in 1944, was substantially stronger than it had been in the 1920s and 1930s. As we shall see, the history of the medical corps was thus far more than the development of theory and the training of small units at summer camp, but involved fighting a war in Korea, preparing to fight a full-scale conflict in Europe, looking into the medical consequences of nuclear catastrophe, and sending individuals and units to far-flung corners of the globe on observer, peacekeeping, or other missions. The post-war era was thus the most active peacetime period in the history of Canadian military medical practice.

The immediate need, obvious long before the war was over, was to rehabilitate as many as possible of those who had been disabled in some fashion as a result of their service; in the same way that the medical profession tried to return wounded soldiers to the front with minimum delay, it also sought to make them active contributors to Canada's economy. By spring 1946 there were some 22,000 in-patients in veterans' hospitals (which of course does not include those being treated as out-patients).[1] In preparing them for jobs or careers, medical practitioners had the help—though they may not have seen it that way—of various veterans' groups, one example being the War Amputees. As related by Doctor Langdale Kelham, who with others carried out an investigatory

---

1. G.W.L. Nicholson, *Seventy Years of Service* (Ottawa, 1977), 253.

tour of Canada and the US before the war ended, "Canadians who have lost a limb in the last War have formed themselves into a very powerful Club widely known as "The Amps', whose activities are partly political and partly social. A representative of the Club meets every amputee as he lands from a hospital ship, keeps an eye on him during treatment, visits his relatives and discusses with them the man's future, and then when the amputee has been satisfactorily fitted with a limb, arranges employment for him."[2] According to a March 1944 conference on amputations held by the NRC's Subcommittee on Surgery, when the issue of rehabilitation came up, "In a brief discussion on this subject it was pointed out that in Canada the amputees are better re-established than are any other class of disabled veterans,"[3] though their patients may not have been in complete agreement.

Another example of post-war rehabilitation attempts was the difficult case of the psychological casualty, who does not seem to have had an organization similar to the War Amps to turn to. There was, however, interest in the problem, the NRC's Associate Committee on Army Medical Research issuing grants for work in the area, it being estimated in early 1944 that, already, 15,000 men had been discharged from the army with psychiatric disabilities. One who looked into the matter was Colonel J.D. Griffin, who with an NRC grant funded social workers so they could interview 500 ex-servicemen.

> The appraisal of civilian readjustment was made by personal visits. In all cases an attempt was made to interview the man himself. Members of his immediate family were also interviewed and in many cases contact was made with his employer. An effort was made to gather all pertinent information concerning the status of his health, social and emotional adjustment prior to Army service. Special study was also made of any family patterns of illness or emotional instability. The Social Worker interviewed the family in an effort to get a detailed life history of the ex-soldier. Particular attention was paid to the incidence of neurotic traits in childhood, difficulties in school, extracurricular activities of the man, his work history, the interpersonal relationships in the home as well as his social interests and contacts outside the home. Similar detailed information was obtained with respect to his post discharge adjustment...

> Most were cases of neurosis of civilian origin. They should probably never have been admitted to the Army. Slightly less than half the men examined after discharge were feeling worse than before enlistment.[4]

2. NA, RG 24, v.12,574, 11/Amputations/1, Report on a Visit of Dr Langdale Kelham, et al, to Canada and America in February 1944.
3. RG 24, v.8129, NS 1287-3-1, Proceedings of the Twelfth Meeting of the Subcommittee on Surgery, 16 Mar 44.
4. NA, RG 24, v.312, file 6, History of the Associate Committee on Army Medical Research, 1942-1946, 67-68.

As it had since the First World War, the psychiatric profession insisted that proper screening was the best way to avoid such casualties, though how such testing could be made effective is a problem that remains unresolved to this day.

Rehabilitation was thus a tricky business, and after a few short years was left in the hands of civilian agencies such as the Department of Veterans' Affairs, National Defence focussing on the harsh business of fighting another war. In doing so, the period immediately following the victory of 1945 brought few changes to Canada's medical doctrine, though a 1947 report of the Canadian Defence Medical Association stated that "Employment of Medical Units with Airborne and Assault Formations and in the Arctic will be the subject of special communi-cations."[5] While such issues were being discussed at the deliberate pace one would expect in peacetime, North Korean divisions invaded their southern neighbour in June, 1950, the United States began sending formations from Japan to the peninsula, and Canada, an American ally and itself concerned about the expansion of Soviet influence, found itself at war yet again.

Given the belief prevalent among politicians and military leaders that the Korean war was a deliberate communist diversion, permanent force units were retained in Canada for service on the main front, in Europe, those to be sent to the Far East to be made up of volunteers from civilian life (including many veterans of the 1939-45 conflict). Thus 25 Field Ambulance, which received verbal notice to form a Service Force Field Ambulance on 8 August, decided its immediate training policy would be to have veterans undergo four weeks of general military indoc-trination, a refresher as it were, while untrained recruits would require a ten week course; subsequent specialist training would take until 1 November. Potential medics learned how the corps was organized, the chain of evacuation, anatomy and physiology, the human skeleton, the circulatory system, how to control haemorrhage, the various types of wounds and fractures, the use of various bandages, how to test water supplies, control insect-borne diseases, and more.[6]

In November the unit, along with most of the Canadian contingent, moved to Fort Lewis to continue to learn its trade, though by early January it was evident such would not be easy. "Training since arrival has been practically non existent. The main reasons for this anomalous situation being: (a) lack of vehicles (b) lack of canvas (c) heavy Camp commitments. A small fraction of the unit, a total of some sixty bodies

---

5. NA, MG 28, I157, Canadian Defence Medical Association, v.15, DMA, RCAMC Tactical Doctrine, 1 Nov 47.
6. NA, RG 24, v.18,386, 25 Cdn Fd Amb, 8 Aug, 12, 30 Aug 50.

plod on with repetitious basic training and basic Corps subjects... It was intended to have a series of 2 day exercises followed by exercises of from 6-10 days duration, with special emphasis on night operations, but due to above shortages it has been impossible to attempt even a one day exercise."[7] The field ambulance was so busy supporting other units' training, running sick parade and an ambulance service, that it had no time for its own, though the following month the situation was slightly brighter. "At last some small progress can be seen in training. This is mostly due to Major Anderson's efforts. There have been a number of compass marches, both by day and night, and one section exercise (Paregoric). The latter cannot be claimed as a success but it served to show the deplorable state to which we have sunk. It is hoped to have a similar exercise weekly."[8]

The Canadian contingent moved to Pusan in May 1951, by which time US-led United Nations forces had made substantial progress against the North Koreans. It having been decided that a Common-wealth Division would be formed of British, Canadian, and Australian formations, the issue of creating an FDS came up. "A Field Dressing Station is capable of providing a firm base for the operations of Surgical Teams and Transfusion Teams and thus providing what is, in effect, a small hospital for the definitive care of wounded soldiers,"[9] after these had been given first aid at regimental aid posts, then evacuated and given further treatment by field ambulances. Eventually Canadian medical personnel would be available at all stages of a sick or wounded soldier's progress, from first aid to hospitalization in Japan, those serving near the front spending a year in theatre, like the units they supported, while others, stationed in Japan for example, might serve longer periods.

Many of the medical problems these men and women faced would have been familiar to their colleagues of previous wars. For example, as in 1914-1916 many of the volunteers of 1950-1953 managed to pass physicals even though they might not be up to the harsh task of soldiering, and the Canadian Section at the British Commonwealth Hospital in Japan used its war diary to bring the problem to the atten-tion of its superiors in Ottawa. "We would like to enter a plea for more careful screening of personnel on Ex-Canada drafts. During the month of July we have had occasion to recategorize another recent arrival in this theatre who had had a nephrectomy [removal of a kidney] per-formed previously. There have been several arrivals with long-standing histories of bronchitis or asthma—one of whom was on embarkation

---

7. NA, RG 24, v.18,386, 25 Cdn Fd Amb, Jan 51, Appx 4.
8. NA, RG 24, v.18,386, 25 Cdn Fd Amb, Feb 51, Appx 5.
9. NA, MG 31, J7, Sneath Papers, v.3, Papers Circulated to Members, No 87.

leave within a week of discharge from hospital in Canada—diagnosis: Acute Bronchitis with Asthma."[10]

For veterans the terrain of Korea might have reminded them of Italy, as would the malaria; prevalent in both peninsulas at the time, as a problem however it never reached the scope in 1950-53 as it had in Sicily ten years earlier. Paludrine seemed successful in preventing the disease, though "following the rotation of the Canadian Brigade in 1952, over 1000 cases of malaria were reported during the next several months in Canada."[11] Treatment with the drugs of the day, however, mainly primaquine plus quinine or chloroquin, was on the whole successful, and there were few recurrences. Still, though the 1953 rotation's incidence of the disease was only a fifth as severe as the first outbreak it was never completely eradicated, Canadian doctors in Japan complaining that "Development of malaria among personnel arriving from Korea still constitutes somewhat of a problem and the reason still appears to be failure to adhere rigidly to the daily intake of Paludrine. It is felt that serious consideration should be given to the possibility of administering a three day course of Chloroquine in therapeutic doses, to all Canadian Personnel returning from Korea,'[12] before they were sent home.

A previously unknown disease, haemorrhagic fever, posed far more of a challenge. It was first described by the Japanese in 1939 and consisted of horrific symptoms, including "capillary permeability,' meaning blood vessels leaked, as well as general haemorrhaging and kidney damage, some cases needing treatment for shock because of internal blood loss.

> The cause of the disease has been difficult to determine but is now generally considered to be a virus with the vector a chigger mite associated with rodents. Preventive measures have been directed to the eradication of rodents and the impregnation of clothing with miticidal and repellant materials. The treatment is non-specific consisting chiefly of carefully controlled physiological support. Cases travelled poorly by road so helicopter evacuation was used when feasible and was felt to reduce haemorrhage and shock. It was found best to centralize such cases for the benefit of experience in evaluation and therapy. The mortality rate among United Nations troops was 5% to 7%.[13]

The Canadian Section in Japan noted in June 1952 that the incubation period could be as high as 35 days. "It is quite conceivable therefore, that servicemen returning to Canada on rotation, may develop their initial symptoms on board ship or, in the case of those travelling

---

10. NA, RG 24, v.18,383, Cdn Sect Britcom Gen Hosp, Jul 52, Appx 4.
11. NA, MG 31, J7, Sneath Papers, v.3, Papers Circulated to Members, No 87.
12. NA, RG 24, v.18,383, Cdn Sect Britcom Gen Hosp, Jul 52, Appx 4.
13. NA, MG 31, J7, Sneath Papers, v.3, Papers Circulated to Members, No 87.

by air, after their return to Canada,'[14] forcing medical officers, as well as family physicians back home, to be extra vigilant. It was unknown whether the restoration of kidney function in a victim meant he or she could return to duty so no chances were taken, recovered victims being sent back to Canada.[15] (According to Barry E. Zimmerman and David J. Zimmerman, in *Killer Germs: Microbes and Diseases that Threaten Humanity*, the cause of the disease was not discovered until 1976, and named Hantaan, for a river in Korea, hence hantavirus. Its vector is a field mouse, and the disease can spread when the virus in its urine becomes airborne. A 1993 outbreak in the midwestern US struck 40, of whom 25 died.)[16]

Other conditions that had proved problematic in previous wars were of far less significance in Korea, such as venereal disease, which became much easier to treat with the advent of penicillin, removing the need to keep afflicted soldiers in hospital for convalescence.[17] Frostbite, and its related condition trench foot, was far less prevalent than on the western front or in Italy, not because of any break-through in drug therapy, but because much more was known about human physiology in low temperatures, so the necessary preventive measures could be taken. As 25 Canadian Field Transfusion Team reported from its parent unit, the 8055th Mobile Army Surgical Hospital (or MASH), in November 1951 no Canadians suffered from the condition, though it forced the hospitalization of a few American and British soldiers.[18]

The main medical challenge was thus posed by those who fell in battle, whether in the many small offensives that punctuated the war or the endless skirmishing that came to characterize it. Any man wounded at the front could expect rapid treatment, at least according to a report by Major B.D. Jaffey of the RCAMC. "Casualties receive first aid as soon as stretcher bearers can reach them. The application of shell dressings, splints and the administration of morphine is done where they lie. On reaching a friendly outpost, the battalion Cpl stretcher bearer is normally available to render first aid and supervise the onward evacuation. At company level, the company Medical Assistant quickly checks the casualty and supervises the evacuation to jeep head level. Here a team consisting of an RCASC or regimental driver and an RCAMC medical assistant return the casualty to the RAP by jeep ambulance."[19] At the

14. NA, RG 24, v.18,383, Cdn Sect, Brit Com Hosp, Jun 52, Appx 4.
15. NA, RG 24, v.18,383, Cdn Sect, Brit Com Hosp, Jan 52, Appx 7.
16. Barry E. Zimmerman and David J. Zimmerman, *Killer Germs: Microbes and Diseases that Threaten Humanity* (Chicago, 1996), 142-145.
17. NA, MG 31, J7, Sneath Papers, v.3, Papers Circulated to Members, No 87.
18. NA, RG 24, v.18,398, No 25 Canadian Field Transfusion Team, 30 Nov 51.
19. NA, RG 24, v.18,385, 37 Cdn Fd Amb, Sep 52, Appx 3N, Maj B.D. Jaffey RCAMC, Casualty Evacuation in Korea, 30 Sep 52.

regimental aid post, "the casualty's injuries are assessed by the Regimental Medical Officer, further treatment is provided and documentation is initiated. Serious cases receive anti shock therapy and helicopter evacuation direct to one of the MASHs by passing the Field Ambulance entirely." In less severe cases, evacuation was carried out by road in 3/4-ton ambulances to casualty clearing posts and advanced dressing stations. "Helicopter evacuation facilities are available at both CCP and ADS levels,"[20] though air evacuation will be discussed in greater detail later.

Just behind the front line were the 242 all ranks of the field ambulance, organized into a headquarters, which set up an advanced dressing station, and three sections, each of which ran casualty clearing posts further forward. Each of the latter was essentially self-sufficient in ambulance vehicles while "Medical equipment at the CCPs is sufficient for all first aid procedures and for some resuscitation. At the ADS there is equipment sufficient to carry out emergency surgery and all resuscitation measures."[21] The role of the field ambulance as a whole remained essentially unchanged from the Second World War, consisting in the rapid collection of sick and wounded, rendering first aid to casualties, preparing and classifying them for further treatment, and completing the necessary documentation.

One should not, however, exaggerate the smoothness with which a wounded soldier could be carried to a safe place for medical treatment. "Due to the poor road conditions and often times the forward routes being under enemy observation and within range of enemy mortars and shelling, the ambulance team must run the gauntlet of enemy fire during daylight hours or travel without lights after dark in order to reach company jeep head levels. They must return via the same route at low speeds (5 mph) depending on the severity of injuries sustained by the casualty,"[22] presuming vehicles could negotiate the harsh Korean topography. For, "On occasion, the hilly terrain and the location of company headquarters platoons and outposts anywhere up to two miles beyond jeep head level necessitates the carry by stretcher of wounded that distance uphill and doundale [sic], through slit trenches and above ground until jeep head level is reached. Normally the greatest time loss encountered in casualty evacuation is found to be this needful long carriage of wounded back to where the ambulance is waiting. Once embarked, only a fraction of the time is required to return the wounded to RAP level."[23]

20. *Ibid.*
21. NA, RG 24, v.18,393, 38 Fd Amb, Dec 52, Appx 3.
22. NA, RG 24, v.18,385, 37 Cdn Fd Amb, Sep 52, Appx 3N, Maj B.D. Jaffey RCAMC, Casualty Evacuation in Korea, 30 Sep 52.
23. *Ibid.*

For a time, the medical system underwent no severe tests; after the offensives and counter-offensives of the first year of the conflict the military situation took on some of the characteristics of siege warfare, so that field ambulance CCPs did not have to treat casualties *en masse* as they had in Italy or north-west Europe. An exception was October 1952, which turned into a busy month for No 1 Casualty Clearing Post of 37 Field Ambulance, ending in three nights of non-stop casualty evacuation. Of the 65 victims treated, two groups were from the Royal Canadian Regiment, one from a patrol and the other the result of an enemy attack, while a third group came from Princess Patricia's Canadian Light Infantry, which had encountered the enemy during a patrol and suffered losses in the ensuing fire fight. It was perhaps indicative of the nature of the fighting, where being on the defensive meant creating a target, that 50 casualties were caused by a Chinese attack on 23 October, including 14 killed and 21 missing.[24] December was more typical, however, with 13 wounded being treated by the CCP and 30 by the advanced dressing station,[25] though even supposedly quiet periods could require complex evacuation procedures. To avoid areas being routinely shelled by the enemy, for a while wounded of the Royal 22e Régiment were moved to their RAPs, then by a roundabout route through the 60th Indian Field Ambulance before arriving at 37 Canadian Field Ambulance.[26]

As in the First World War units and formations rotated through the front line, and when they were in reserve field ambulances became far less concerned with evacuation and first aid than with other matters. In July 1952, for example, 37 Field Ambulance set up shop as an ADS, sick bay, and urology clinic. The first ran sick parades for nearby units, the second received patients from the Commonwealth Division to take some of the load off the field dressing station, and the third examined personnel being sent back to Canada or on leave while also handling those with VD.[27] It could also treat civilians, as the field ambulance reported in February 1953.

> Koreans from the neighbouring villages attend for medical assistance. An afternoon clinic has accordingly been organized and is held in the ADS department. Lack of interpreters has interfered with the progress of the clinic. The recent acquisition of another interpreter during the afternoons is clearing it satisfactorily at the present time. Three hundred civilians have attended up to date. The majority of them are women and children.

24. NA, RG 24, v.18,385, 37 Cdn Fd Amb, Oct 52, Appx 3J.
25. NA, RG 24, v.18,385, 37 Cdn Fd Amb, Dec 52, Appx 7.
26. NA, RG 24, v.18,385, 37 Cdn Fd Amb, Sep 52, Appx 3.
27. NA, RG 24, v.18,384, 37 Cdn Fd Amb, Jul 52, Appx 10.

Respiratory and dermatological lesions are most commonly encountered. Pulmonary tuberculosis presents a problem due to the complete lack of facilities for hospital or sanatorium care for this type of patient in Korea.[28]

A doctor or nurse on the Maas in the winter of 1944-45 would quite likely have reported in similar terms.

To understand the nature of field ambulance operations in the Korean War, it might be best to trace the experiences of one such unit, such as 38 Field Ambulance, which performed its work in the last months before the cease-fire of July 1953. In May it was in reserve, but still close enough to the fighting to get involved when the Chinese attacked the Royal Canadian Regiment, sending up ambulances and medical assistants to deal with casualties. Later that same month it treated people injured by American F-84 Thunder Jets after they accidentally attacked UN positions, evacuating an American and a Korean by helicopter, sending two Koreans to 25 Field Dressing Station, and returning two more to duty. Another emergency came up in the early morning of 9 June, when Captain H. Gaist, the medical officer for the 2nd Battalion of the Royal Australian Regiment, called for help. Captain J.J. Glynn made his way forward with extra plasma, and "In fifteen minutes four badly wounded men were given intravenous plasma by Capt JJ Glynn while Capt H Gaist went out into the company positions to attend to the casualties there. At first light four casualties having been resuscitated sufficiently were evacuated by helicopter and on enquiries throughout the week are believed to be all doing well."[29] The next month was a now-familiar routine of running a 125-bed hospital, a medical inspection room for sick parades, and a VD clinic, with one section evacuating casualties from 25 Canadian Infantry Brigade at the front. There was also time for lectures, such as one by Major R. Pillsbury of 43 MASH on resuscitation, and even some sports.

The knowledge and resources a field ambulance could bring to bear are exemplified by a single case of 10 July 1953, as described in the unit's war diary.

> The Corporal Medical Assistant on duty received a call from a Royal Engineer unit nearby stating that one of their men was very near death and for us to despatch an ambulance, medical assistant and to have a medical officer and a padre standing by. Before our ambulance could reach the gate a call was received stating that they could not wait for the ambulance but were sending the patient directly here. The medical officer on duty, not knowing the religion of the patient, summoned both the Roman Catholic and Protestant Padres. As an added precaution

28. NA, RG 24, v.18,386, 37 Cdn Fd Amb, Feb 52, Appx 12.
29. NA, RG 24, v.18,393, 38 Fd Amb, 3 May 53.

another medical officer was despatched to the ADS in case his services proved necessary. The dental officer reported as well in case he could be of any assistance. All the medical assistants were alerted examining trays, splints, etc, made ready for instant use. The Dispenser was routed out of bed to provide plasma and to make available any extra drugs or equipment which might be found necessary.

The guard at the gate was alerted to direct the vehicle directly to the ADS.

The clerks were standing by with the necessary papers for documentation. Altogether there were about 25 or 30 people involved in preparation for the reception of the patient.

Then, a 2 $^{1/2}$ ton vehicle came roaring through the gate, followed by a jeep containing Lieutenant-Colonel J.D. Galloway, the commanding officer of 38th Field Ambulance, and Captain G.A. Vanner. On being informed at the gate of the emergency, the CO immediately proceeded to the Advanced Dressing Station.

When the vehicle pulled up at the ADS a medical officer and two medical assistants rushed out, placed the patient on a stretcher and hurried him into the examining room.

It did not take much of an examination to determine that the patient was pretty well out but from intoxicating beverages, and any pain he was in was caused by a distended bladder.

A short walk up and down took care of the bladder trouble and a couple of cups of coffee soon brought him to life again and in a matter of minutes he was returned to his unit, the emergency ended.[30]

Whether the field ambulance received any official congratulations for this piece of work is unknown.

Had the unnamed sapper required further attention, moving him deeper into the medical system, to a field dressing station or hospital, might have been carried out by a Motorized Ambulance Column, No 38 MAC of the Royal Canadian Army Service Corps transporting almost 7000 patients its first year in theatre.[31] It was not an easy task, the terrain rearwards of the front being no different from that around the trenches, as Major B.D. Jaffey of the RCAMC explained.

The evacuation of sick and wounded in Korea has created many problems for the Medical Services... Korea is a very rugged and picturesque country interspersed by valleys which run between the many hills which make up the geographical terrain. The majority of roads in the forward areas are class III roads and the main supply routes are class II roads. There are not class I roads beyond the country's capital Seoul. In addition

30. NA, RG 24, v.18,393, 38 Fd Amb, 10 Jul 53.
31. NA, RG 24, v.18,393, War Diary, 38 Cdn Mac RCASC, 4 May 1951 to 30 Apr 1952.

seasonal variations make the maintenance of roads a most difficult feat. During mid-summer when the rainy season is present, many roads are washed away or become quagmires of mud necessitating the use of alternative routes.[32]

One of the largest such rivers was the Imjin, which as it wound its way from east to west sometimes formed the front line, sometimes created an obstacle not far to the Canadians' rear. No 38 Field Ambulance thus reported that

> Some system for the evacuation of casualties over the Imjin River is most necessary in case the bridges are washed away or rendered impassable during the rainy season. In this connection a demonstration of the evacuation of casualties by cable over the Imjin at Pintail Bridge was held at 1130 hours. The Engineers had the cables up and operating with two cable cars. One car was a two-tiered structure built to hold two stretchers and the other was a single platform which would hold one stretcher case or two men sitting. Cars travel from side to side in just over two minutes.
>
> Loads were carried while we watched and then the ADMS, Lt-Col Galloway and Capt Vanner went across to check on the ease of on-loading and off-loading and see if the ride was smooth. No discomfort was felt on the journey,[33]

but the cease-fire intervened before the cableway could be put to use.

One means of evacuation that has been much popularized in film and on television has been the helicopter, which by the outbreak of the Korean War had been of interest to Canada's armed services for some time. As early as 1945 Squadron Leader W.C. Gibson was reporting on an article in Popular Science "containing pictures of the helicopter built by Stanley Hiller and which I saw in Berkeley California in November."[34] He thought it might be of use in rescue work in British Columbia, and though his suggestion was shelved for the time being, the rotary aircraft saw much use in the hilly terrain of Korea. It was not, however, a simple matter of putting a helicopter down just anywhere, as 38 Field Ambulance could attest. Deciding in July 1952 that evacuation by road in its area of responsibility would be too difficult, the unit decided it would have to rely on aircraft, and infantry battalions were instructed to immediately institute reconnaissances to locate suitable landing sites, but these had to be flat and free of obstructions such as trees or tall hills.[35]

Helicopter evacuation soon took on romantic overtones nonetheless, one FDS describing how "There is no finer sight than that of a Helicopter

32. NA, RG 24, v.18,385, 37 Cdn Fd Amb, Sep 52, Appx 3N, Maj B.D. Jaffey RCAMC, Casualty Evacuation in Korea, 30 Sep 52.
33. NA, RG 24, v.18,393, 38 Fd Amb, 16 Jul 53.
34. NA, RG 24, v.5393, HQS 60-1-46, S/L W.C. Gibson to PMO Western Air Command, 4 Jan 45.
35. NA, RG 24, v.18,384, 37 Cdn Fd Amb, Jul 52, Appx 9.

coming up a Korean valley to evacuate a seriously wounded or injured soldier. It is a dramatic scene, and one that many of those in Korea will remember, especially those whose lives have been saved by this rapid, comfortable mode of transportation."[36] But one must not be carried away; such aircraft were extremely vulnerable to ground fire, so their use was as much a tactical as a medical decision. Add to that the fact that they could only fly in daylight and clear weather, and their limitations become obvious. Even the FDS quoted above pointed out "that choppers needed for other work, such as recce and rescuing downed pilots, especially in busy periods. Thus its role is limited, and can only serve as an adjunct to motor ambulances."[37] As a result, from 1 July 1951 to 29 February 1952, only 31 Canadians were transported in this manner.

In many cases, the purpose of these varied evacuation procedures was to procure timely surgery, though not necessarily by Canadian hands. As Brigadier K.A. Hunter and Colonel J.E. Andrew explained, "As there was only one Canadian Field Surgical Team in Korea, and in the early days it was based on an American Mobile Surgical Hospital (MASH), part of the initial or forward surgery was performed by American and to some extent by Norwegian surgeons. As soon as it was possible such of our casualties were returned to Canadian channels. Further hospitalization and surgery, as required, was carried out at the British Commonwealth Hospital in Kure, Japan, where there was a Canadian Section."[38] The surgical team in question operated as an integral part of the 8055th Mobile Army Surgical Hospital, Captain T.A. McLennan rotating shifts with an American anaesthetist while Major G.G. Lippert worked a similar schedule with an American surgeon.[39]

In many ways, aside from the tents and dirt roads, a MASH was very much like a civilian surgical section in North America or Europe, including regular lectures to keep up with recent developments in the field; for example, in early 1952 Mclennan spoke on the use of cocaine in anaesthesia. Other subjects were far less likely to be discussed back home, however, such as the speaker who followed. "Dr Pollard, Specialist Metabolism from Cornell University spoke to the doctors at 8055th MASH concerning the vital importance of proper and controlled alimentation for repatriated PsOW. He classified PsOW into three groups for oral rehabilitation depending on their physical condition,"[40] a reminder of the difficult circumstances prevailing in Chinese

---

36. NA, RG 24, v.18,396, 25 Cdn FDS, Aug 52, Appx 9.
37. NA, RG 24, v.18,396, 25 Cdn FDS, Aug 52, Appx 9.
38. NA, MG 31, J7, Sneath Papers, v.3, Papers Circulated to Members, No 87.
39. NA, RG 24, v.18,398, No 25 Cdn Field Surgical Team, 31 Jan 52.
40. NA, RG 24, v.18,398, No 25 Cdn FTS, 2 Feb 52.

prison camps. Of more immediate application was a course offered a few months later on vascular operations, the Canadian FST's war diary exclaiming that "It was evident that Arterial Surgery had progressed greatly since the last war."[41]

For some challenges lectures or short courses were insufficient and more elaborate research was required. One of these was a sometimes fatal kidney condition called nephron nephrosis, which was studied in detail at the 11th Evacuation Hospital (US) in the summer of 1952. As 25 Canadian Field Surgical Team reported, "Although this field has many implications in civilian medicine, the need for further study in Korea was obvious. Current resuscitative measures and surgical facilities have greatly increased the survival rate even since the end of World War II. However, there are still quite a number of patients whom, although they would survive the initial surgical procedure develop the syndrome of lower Nephron Nephrosis, and probably die within the following five to ten days."[42] The condition was thus a serious one, and affected 50 to 60 patients in the six months prior to the study, and "A good proportion of these may have been saved had special facilities been available for more elaborate blood chemistry studies."[43] The syndrome could develop from wounding or haemorrhagic fever, and through the month of July 28 such cases were flown to the 11th Evac, of whom 18 died. All showed improvement in kidney function, however, after treatment with dialysis or drugs, so success seemed to be mainly a matter of getting to the patient in time.

As for the actual practice of surgery, unfortunately No 25 Canadian Field Surgical Team has left us with few details concerning its daily operations, except for the shift work mentioned above. War diary entries tend towards the cryptic, such as one for July 1952 which simply states that "Work during the month had been quite heavy, mostly due to American casualties due to considerable activity in their sector."[44] More details are available concerning issues of organization, especially when in August 1952 the FST ceased its work with the 8055th MASH and became attached to 25 Field Dressing Station in order to have as much surgery as possible done in Korea to lower the number of soldiers being evacuated out of the Commonwealth Division.[45] The impetus for the arrangement had come from the hospital in Japan, which in June 1952 noted that "The fact that no CCS

41. NA, RG 24, v.18,398, No 25 Cdn Field Surgical Team, 25 Jun 52.
42. NA, RG 24, v.18,398, No 25 Cdn Field Surgical Team, Jul 52, Appx 2.
43. *Ibid.*
44. NA, RG 24, v.18,398, No 25 Cdn Field Surgical Team, 7 Jul 52.
45. NA, RG 24, v.18,398, No 25 Cdn Field Surgical Team, Aug 52.

or Hospital is stationed in Korea has led to an increasing number of evacuations from the field to this unit. Since, by such evacuation, personnel are lost to the operational units for a minimum of three weeks, and often for as long as two months, it is felt that a serious consideration should be given to making use of American medical and surgical installations and specialist [sic] to a greater extent than is the practice at present,'[46] instead of sending patients to Kure.

The soldiers in question suffered from such conditions as dyspepsia, peptic ulcer, and low back pain, or required therapeutic circumcision, none of which required the facilities of a rearward city-based hospital.

> The manpower wastage in the past year, due to evacuation of such patients has been enormous and it is felt by all components of this hospital, that steps must be taken to eliminate it. The psychological factors, too, are most important, and this is reflected in the gradual increase in such admissions during the past few months. It is recommended, therefore, that the investigation of all such cases be completed in Korea, at least to the point where there is definite proof that the individuals can serve no longer in any capacity in the field, or that prolonged *treatment* is required...

> Out of some 160 war wounds admitted during the past fortnight, fully 30% were of an extremely minor nature, requiring merely delayed primary closure and a few days convalescence. In the absence of a Commonwealth CCS or hospital on the spot, it is felt that consideration might be given to employing the Field Surgical Team for such cases, since evacuation, here again, means loss of a trained soldier, to the unit concerned, for several weeks.[47]

To the same end, the FST requested that nurses be made part of the establishment, two having been attached for the first few days of October to assist in surgery on a duodenal ulcer patient. In a comment reminiscent of similar demands in the Second World War, the unit reported how "The nursing sisters greatly facilitated the post operative care of these patients and it is felt that if four or five could be attached hear [sic] for such purposes as well as operating room and ward supervisor it would help to provide better post operative care."[48] In the spring of 1953, it was decided to employ nursing sisters with 25 FDS, of which the Field Surgical Team was a part.

The Field Dressing Station to which the FST was attached had itself been originally established to deal with minor sick and injured from the Commonwealth Division so it would not be necessary to evacuate them

---

46. NA, RG 24, v.18,383, Cdn Sect, Brit Com Hosp, Jun 52, Appx 4.
47. NA, RG 24, v.18,383, Cdn Sect, Brit Com Hosp, Jun 52, Appx 4.
48. NA, RG 24, v.18,398, No 25 Cdn Field Surgical Team, Oct 52.

to Japan; with 200 beds, its mandate was to hold any patient who required 14 days or less hospitalization before being returned to his unit (or RTUd in military parlance). As for routine, September 1951 was a busy month with 710 admissions and 32 operations, including eight circumcisions. The national make-up of the formation it supported was evident in the British, Canadian, New Zealand, Australian, and Indian patients that passed through its wards, with 97 psychiatric casualties forming the largest group, 94 dermatological patients coming a close second.[49] There were also times of higher stress, especially in the latter months of 1951 when the Chinese launched a minor offensive; on 4 October a telephone request came from 121 Evacuation Hospital for ambulances, and they were despatched eight minutes later; by midnight, a little over two hours after the request was received, the FDS had received 17 stretcher cases and 15 walking wounded. The month as a whole saw a marked increase in admissions, especially of battle wounds, as the only other hospital unit in the Seoul area, the above-mentioned 121 Evac, filled up with patients. November saw the inflow reach its peak, and "It is noted that there is a noticeable increase in psychiatric cases,' a sure sign that fighting at the front was increasing in intensity, as was the number of men with shell wounds. With the coming of a Korean winter, there was also a noticeable increase in burn cases as soldiers used oil and gasoline in improvised stoves to keep warm and cook food, though in December the fighting diminished dramatically and most patients were found to be suffering from respiratory ailments.[50]

In the 18 months that followed work at the FDS mirrored events at the front, with May 1952 perhaps being fairly typical of a quiet period. One man was "admitted to hospital, diagnosis post traumatic syndrome,' one of the first times battle exhaustion was referred to by that term. Two others arrived suffering from haemorrhagic fever and were immediately placed on helicopters for transport to the 8228th MASH, which specialized in treating the disease. Circumcision continued to be the most common surgical procedure carried out, though ingrown toenails topped the list the following month. Gunshot wounds did not form the largest group requiring surgery until October, and then again in November, as fighting went through another of its periodic peak phases.[51] Breaking up the routine was the odd medical anomaly, such as a situation that developed in May 1953 when the FDS found that

49. NA, RG 24, v.18,395, 25 Cdn FDS, Aug 51, Appx V, Sep 51, Appx 6.
50. NA, RG 24, v.18,395, 25 Cdn FDS, V, 4 Oct 51; Oct 51, Appx 5; Nov 51, Appx 5; Dec 51, Appx 5.
51. NA, RG 24, v.18,395, 25 Cdn FDS, 4 May 52; 31 May; May 52, Appx 5; Jun 52, Appx 5; Oct 52, Appx 5; Nov 52, Appx 5.

There has been an increase in the number of [psychiatric] cases this month (70 compared with 53 last month). The recent heavy fighting in the sector is without doubt responsible in part for this increase in patients, but it has been noted that referrals from positions of relative safety such as base and rear divisional areas, have increased proportionally with those from front line fighting positions. Fighting, although heavy, has been mostly sporadic and instances of units being engaged with the enemy or under shelling or mortar fire for prolonged periods of time are relatively rare and in consequence only 2 cases of battle exhaustion are reported. Most of the other cases from the battle area were found to be acute reactions to battle stress by immature and poorly motivated individuals.[52]

Heavy fighting was held accountable for the continuing influx of psychiatric cases the following month, and then again in July, just as the cease-fire approached. "A large proportion of the patients came from combat areas but once again none of them conformed to classical "battle fatigue" and usually the man was found to be of poor psychological structure and inadequate motivation, or of the childish immature type... Correlating the increased front line psychiatric casualties with the decreasing activity we can assume that tension in the minds of the men must have been higher and the fear of being killed just at the last moment "greater"."[53] The approaching end to the war thus added stresses of its own.

Whether near the beginning of the conflict, or near its end, treatment of psychological cases was pretty much the same, as explained by Brigadier K.A. Hunter and Colonel J.E. Andrew. "During the period of active hostilities in Korea the Divisional Psychiatrist for the 1st Commonwealth Division was being supplied by the RCAMC. This officer was stationed at the Field Dressing Station where he maintained a small ward for observation cases and short term treatment. The general policy of treatment as close to the front as possible was being maintained" to avoid what was called "gain through illness," or a reinforcement of depression resulting from guilt. Furthermore, "The Psychiatrist visited regularly the Field Ambulance where the patients were sent. Those with slight or no disability were returned directly to duty. Cases of more severe disability were treated at the Field Dressing Station for short term psychotherapy and sedation with the majority either being returned to their units or employed in rear areas in Korea." There was obviously no sense of crisis, as "Psychoneurosis occurred at the rate of

52. NA, RG 24, v.18,395, 25 Cdn FDS, May 53, Appx 5.
53. NA, RG 24, v.18,395, 25 Cdn FDS, Jul 52, Appx 5.
54. NA, MG 31, J7, Sneath Papers, v.3, Papers Circulated to Members, No 87.

two per thousand per annum; this is the rate to be expected in any comparable group of people." In fact, "Battle exhaustion did not occur to any great extent due, it is felt, to the nature of the fighting in which battles were of short duration and the fatigue factor was not operative." With fewer cases than in previous campaigns, the divisional psychiatrist was available for other work, and "Psychiatric consultation was frequently requested in the case of soldiers accused of breaches of discipline. These cases were examined and if no medical disability was present, were returned to their units for administrative disposal,"[54] i.e, punishment in accordance with military law.

For many casualties, whether physical or psychological, the first step on the trip home was the Canadian Section at the British Commonwealth Hospital in Kure, Japan, set up in June 1951 with an establishment of 11 officers, three sergeants, and 17 rank and file.[55] In a typically quiet month, such as February 1952, battle casualties were rarely seen in Kure, most patients consisting of what was called "cold" surgery, such as hernias, varicose veins, and internal knee derangements.[56] As for infectious diseases, in June 1953 the hospital reported that "Medical admissions continue to conform to established patterns of morbidity for this theatre. Parasitic infestations are not as prevalent as would be thought judging by the universal native incidence. This speaks well of the indoctrination of the troops and the practical sanitation and food management within the Service. The incidence of Venereal disease is lower than six months ago. Several factors are responsible among which are close supervision of drafts and a decreased tendency to promiscuity among the established troops."[57] Or perhaps soldiers were just being more careful when they were "promiscuous".

If for any reason (VD not being one of them) it was decided to evacuate a casualty further back than Japan, the sick or wounded soldier in question might find himself in the hands of RCAF personnel. By the time war broke out in Korea the service had 13 flight nurses qualified, and many were attached to the US Air Force as it flew casualties from Japan to San Francisco. In one operation during the summer of 1951 Canadian patients who had been flown to Tacoma, Washington, were then taken up by a converted Dakota air ambulance of No 435 Squadron, which carried them to Edmonton and other centres where the Department of Veterans' Affairs ran hospitals. The plane was equipped with oxygen systems, litters, and litter holders as well as the normal pharmacopoeia and equipment of a city ambulance, and was staffed

55. NA, RG 24, v.18,383, Cdn Sect, Brit Com Hospital, Jul 51, Appx 1, Appx 2.
56. NA, RG 24, v.18,383, Cdn Sect, Brit Com Hosp, Feb 52, Appx 4.
57. NA, RG 24, v.18,384, Cdn Sect Britcom Gen Hosp, Jun 53, Appx 3.

with a nurse who had undergone a nine-week course on air evacuation followed by 21 weeks of on the job training with transport aircraft of the United States Air Force.[58] Though the system was reminiscent of previous air evacuation schemes in the Mediterranean and north-west Europe during the Second World War, it was not until Korea that Canada became a routine terminus.

The Royal Canadian Navy, as it had in previous conflicts, fought a war much removed from the army and air force, though in the realm of medical matters little had changed since the campaign in the North Atlantic. Doctors were even fewer and far between, however, the navy having to compete with the other two services and Canada as a whole, placing it at a distinct disadvantage as few medical practitioners were prepared to go to sea for months at a time when there were so many more pleasant alternatives; furthermore, the war against the North Koreans and the Chinese somehow failed to capture the public imagination in the same way as the crusade against the Nazis. In any event, recruits with the necessary medical skills were sufficiently rare that when one presented himself, in the words of RCN historian Edward C. Meyers "He was pounced upon with the swiftness of an eighteenth-century press gang."[59]

This explains why a complete impostor, Ferdinand Demara, could join Canada's naval service as a surgeon with the stolen credentials of a Doctor Joseph Cyr of New Brunswick. As had his predecessors in the Second World War, however, he found that his duties aboard HMCS *Cayuga* were mainly routine, made up of steam burns, cuts and rashes, and various other similar complaints. He was also fortunate in having Petty Officer Robert Hotchin as his assistant, whose medical education was not much short of that of a general practitioner ashore. Still, the doppelganger, as Cyr, handled even the more stressful aspects of the job well. "The ship's records show Demara to have performed several operations during a two-month period" as *Cayuga* supported South Korean amphibious raids against the North, "ranging from the amputation of a gangrenous foot to the removal of bullets from arms and elsewhere. He operated quickly and efficiently, and gave no one any reason to question his talents as a surgeon."[60]

His moment of glory came in September 1951. After a raid by South Korean commandos, called Salamanders, on the 7th, three were left seriously wounded and by the 10th were close to death.

---

58. G.W.L. Nicholson, *Canada's Nursing Sisters* (Ottawa), 214.
59. Edward C. Meyers, *Thunder in the Morning Calm: The Royal Canadian NAvy in Korea, 1950-1953* (St Catharines, 1992), 168.
60. Edward C. Meyers, *Thunder in the Morning Calm*, 170.

Demara took one look and made a snap decision. He ordered the startled Hotchin to bring his surgical equipment to the upper deck at once. He quickly explained that he felt at least one would die while awaiting his turn in the sick bay. By treating all three at once, he might be able to pull them through. Demara did an admirable job. The worst of the three would surely have died had treatment not been swift and expert. By the time he had finished he had collapsed the lung and removed a bullet from the man with the chest wound while successfully treating the other two as well. Demara had indeed saved the three men, but the greatest feat was the work he did on the chest wound. While the collapse of a lung might have been accomplished by any qualified medical assistant, Demara had known exactly what to do and how to do it.[61]

The result, however, was publicity, exposure by the real Doctor Cyr, and a quiet dismissal from the RCN—or almost. For, some three decades later, Demara attended a reunion of *Cayuga*'s complement, where "he was greeted with warmth by those who had known him as a friend and shipmate twenty-eight years before. The welcome made it obvious that Demara had made no enemies aboard *Cayuga*. By all accounts he enjoyed the party."[62]

With the signing of the cease-fire in July 1953 it was time to take stock, some 309 Canadians having been killed (all but 15 in the infantry) and a further 1202 wounded or injured (over 93 per cent of them infantry).[63] For the RCAMC an important statistic was the reduction in the fatality rate among recovered wounded from 66 per 1000 in the Second World War to 34. How much of that was due to the lower intensity of the fighting, with no Dieppe, Ortona, or Normandy to overwhelm the medical system with casualties, is unknown. According to Brigadier Hunter and Colonel Andrew, "Surgical practices in the management of wounds were much as they were in 1945. The same adequate debridements and the "no suture" techniques were employed. Plentiful antibiotics might improve results but were no substitute for thorough, early, initial surgery." Thus, "The improvement in mortality rates in Korea was due to a number of factors: helicopter evacuation, armoured vests, more abundant and varied antibiotics and improvement in resuscitation and the treatment of impending or established renal shut-down."[64] But the number of Canadian soldiers evacuated by helicopter was no more than a handful, and those suffering from haemorrhagic fever would not have added many more; perhaps the nature of the fighting was the more important explanation, even if not noted by Hunter and Andrew.

---

61. Edward C. Meyers, *Thunder in the Morning Calm*, 172.
62. Edward C. Meyers, *Thunder in the Morning Calm*, 176.
63. Herbert Fairlie Wood, *Strange Battleground* (Ottawa, 1966), 257-258.
64. NA, MG 31, J7, Sneath Papers, v.3, Papers Circulated to Members, No 87.

Since the initial invasion by North Korean divisions was seen as the opening move in a general offensive by the Soviet Union and its allies, Canada in the early 1950s prepared for war on the home front, the Soviets having tested an atomic bomb in 1949. Civil Defence, however, was not at the time a responsibility of the three services, as the Chief of the General Staff, General Charles Foulkes, made clear in September 1950. According to his Canadian Army Policy Statement No 65, the tasks of the armed forces in case of a nuclear attack or natural catastrophe would be limited to organizing their own local protection, assisting civil authorities to prepare plans, and providing reserves "*in a secondary role*," the latter underlined in the original. Such reserves could be used to reconnoitre damaged areas, help to clear debris, carry out elementary rescue operations, as well as assist to restore communications and public services.[65]

This might seem rather harsh, but the military of 1950 had to face two very difficult truths: first, it had a limited budget and could not create the kind of large standing army a massive aid to civil power would have required; second, in case of nuclear war it would suffer casualties sufficient to overwhelm its own treatment system. As a medical report that predated Foulkes' policy statement explained,

> The occasional accidental case of acute ionizing irradiation illness and the thousands of cases that would occur after an atomic bomb explosion present two entirely different problems. This is so because military casualties present a unique medical problem in which the primary object- ive is the return of men to duty so as to maintain the fighting strength at a maximum. This is accomplished by caring for the less seriously injured first and returning them to duty. Those that have a reasonable chance of salvage are attended next, and the fatally injured are given palliative treatment as soon as practical,[66]

if they had not succumbed to their injuries first. If officialdom was to be believed, such policies were nothing new, military practitioners for centuries having had as their primary institutional concern the return of soldiers to duty, though we have seen how patient care often insinuated its way to the top of the priority list. In any case, from a purely organizational perspective "The critical problem is the quick, accurate segregation of casualties into three categories on the basis of the amount of radiation received... Without segregation and reassurance to those that have a chance for survival, panic and utter chaos can be anticipated.

---

65. NA, RG 29, v.654, C102-3-2B, Charles Foulkes, CGS, Canadian Army Policy Statement No 65 (DMO & P) Participation of the Armed Forces in Civil Defence, 27 Sep 50.
66. NA, RG 29, v.674, 108-1-12, Acute Total Body Radiation Illness, Its Role in Atomic Warfare and Its Influence on the Future Practice of Military Medicine.

With segregation and reassurance a large group can be salvaged to carry on essential work."[67]

Based on the horrific experiences of Hiroshima and Nagasaki, the three categories referred to above seemed straight-forward enough when explained in terms of symptoms. As Brigadier A. Sachs suggested, first were "Those receiving a lethal dose of radiation. In such cases, severe vomiting and diarrhoea came on within 1 to 3 hours and fever and marked wasting developed within one week, by the end of which time the majority had died, though some survived for as long as two weeks." Second were "Those receiving a large, but not necessarily lethal, dose. The onset of symptoms was delayed until the end of the second week after exposure. These consisted of loss of appetite and malaise, diarrhoea and some wasting, and loss of the hair. Recovery largely depended on good nursing." Third were the most fortunate, "Those receiving a low dose. Symptoms of the above type were present to a slight degree after the second week or were entirely absent." Proper testing could help sort out the living from the dying, as "An examination of the blood of casualties by counting the different types of blood cells gives a fair indication of the severity of the illness and a check on its progress."[68]

Compared with the known effectiveness of the atomic bomb, other weapons of mass destruction were far less worrisome; Brigadier Sachs referred to biological warfare as "one for which the most extravagant and unrealistic claims have been made." The fact was that modern society had been developing weapons against bacterial agents since the nineteenth century, so "Defensive measures against biological warfare agents must be based on the fundamental principles of public health for preventing the spread of disease." Chemical agents were not much different, gas warfare producing nothing like the fears of the post-First World War era, as seen in H.G. Wells novels, though defence against nerve gasses, which could be absorbed through the skin, would require substantial preparation. A substance called atropine could be used as an antidote, but it had to be administered immediately, leading Sachs to muse on the possibility of issuing self-injection syringes on a massive scale.[69]

If efficiency was to be measured in terms of killed and injured, how-ever, the atomic bomb was well ahead of its rivals and was easier to "deliver" than either biological agents or canisters filled with poison gas. One problem medical practitioners would face would be the lack

67. *Ibid.*
68. NA, MG 31, J7, Sneath Papers, v.3, Papers Circulated to Members, No 20.
69. NA, MG 31, J7, Sneath Papers, v.3, Papers Circulated to Members, No 20.

of blood products sufficient to transfuse the massive casualties a nuclear strike would cause, though one step towards a solution was born of the Korean experience; there, No 25 Canadian Field Surgical Team reported how two doctors lectured on the use of Dextran, a product which drew fluid into the bloodstream and hence could be used to fight shock. In effect, it made limited quantities of plasma go further.

> Although Dextran has been used in Sweden for several years it is only during the past two years that American investigators have been especially interested in it's use. Their interest was aroused mainly because of the ever increasing possibility of a large scale war in which case adequate supplies of plasma and whole blood would not be available. This would be especially true in event of a large number of casualties from Atomic explosion or any disaster causing extensive burns or body trauma. In addition the pooled plasma which is in current useage has been found to be responsible for homologous jaundice in 5-15 percent of cases. An incidence as high as 20 percent had been reported by some observers.[70]

(As a footnote, one might mention that in the Second World War it was whole blood that was associated with such problems and plasma that proved to be the proper substitute.)

By the mid-fifties the military establishment was more formally integrated with civil defence, Foulkes' policy on the matter having altered substantially over time. At a series of map exercises held in January 1955, for example, the Director-General Medical Services noted how his staff would be investigating three problems: the first was the medical plan to support a corps deployed for atomic attack; the second concerned the arrangements necessary to handle the "mass instantaneous casualties" following such an attack; the third focussed on "The action to be taken by the Command Medical Officer, Central Command, following an atomic attack on Toronto," Central Command being essentially responsible for the Province of Ontario.[71] In addition to such exercises, a Mobile Defence Corps was formed, at least on paper, and procedures developed for its deployment. In the purely medical sphere were Ambulance Companies of the MDC, broken down into sections for rescue and evacuation work; personnel were warned, however, that the latter would be particularly difficult following an atomic exchange, and "It is possible that after a nuclear attack there may be a certain period during which rescue operations as such (i.e. extrication of casualties from damaged buildings) will be possible only to a very limited extent due to the degree of radioactive contamination in the badly damaged areas;

---

70. NA, RG 24, v.18,398, No 25 Cdn Field Surgical Team, Jul 52, Appx 1.
71. NA, RG 29, v.659, 106-2-1, DGMS to Worthington, CD Coord, 12 Jan 55.

all available forces would then have to be concentrated on the evacuation of casualties from the slightly damaged outer periphery."[72]

Such difficult decisions were left in the hands of civilian authorities, and the Ambulance Company "must fit in with the civilian organisation operating in the area. The Company would deploy its three platoons, and each of them would establish an Ambulance Loading Point (ALP) or report to a civilian loading point already in being." As for actually picking the injured out of the rubble, "Casualties will be recovered from the "places of rescue" to ALPs by stretcher bearer parties. These parties will be controlled by and led by the stretcher bearer parties of the Ambulance Company, if the Company is working with its own Battalion, otherwise this part of the evacuation will be entirely civilian. The MDC Ambulance Section stretcher bearers will all have received advanced first aid training, and will thus be able to carry out any additional first aid necessary." It was at the Ambulance Loading Point that triage would be carried out, casualties being divided into four groups: those who required no further treatment and could be directed to a safe area; those who needed light treatment at a nearby field hospital; those requiring evacuation to a more sophisticated hospital facility; and those who needed immediate skilled treatment before they could be moved.[73]

Though map exercises and staff papers may have a certain rational and logical (and hence over-optimistic) tone to them, Canada's military leadership was not incognizant of the fact that nuclear holocaust meant overwhelming casualties. A staff college precis of May 1960 compared the situation to that of a First World War offensive, when ten CCSs handled 13,000 wounded in a single day.[74] As a paper from the US Army Medical School put it, "For the first time a country at war may visit upon its enemies thousands or millions of casualties—all generated simultaneously—so that necessarily a great disparity will exist between numbers of wounded and numbers of professional personnel available for treatment."[75] To make matters worse, a nuclear exchange could occur before mobilization had taken place, further diminishing the pool of qualified medical personnel to help deal with the disaster. As a result, the mortality rate among wounded, which in the US experience had been 2.4 per cent in Korea, was likely to resemble that of the Crimea, or around 17 per cent. Thus "Care of mass casualties must be based on

72. NA, RG 29, v.654, 102-3-2, Operational and Deployment Procedures for the Rescue Battalions of the Mobile Defence Corps (Provisional), 22 Dec 55.

73. NA, RG 29, v.654, 102-3-2, Operational and Deployment Procedures for the Rescue Battalions of the Mobile Defence Corps (Provisional), 22 Dec 55.

74. G.W.L. Nicholson, *Seventy Years of Service* (Ottawa, 1977), 288.

75. NA, MG 31, J7, Sneath Papers, v.3, Papers Circulated to Members, No 24.

the proposition that we must do the greatest good for the largest number at the right time and in the right place. The key to this type of treatment is sorting."[76]

As if theory was not pessimistic enough, practice proved worse, or at least the kind of practice one experienced on manoeuvres. For example, when in April 1959 Exercise Post Haste put various units through their paces the critique that followed made it obvious there was much room for improvement. Vehicles not in use were parked in areas that had been deemed contaminated for exercise purposes, including ambulances waiting for casualties; worse, there had been too much emphasis on paper-work, and "Casualty registration seemed to hold up the evacuation of casualties. We, in Civil Defence, teach these procedures; however in the face of radioactivity and the large number of casualties to be processed, it is questionable whether we can really afford the people to register or hold up the evacuation." As for basic techniques, some rescuers waited around for stretchers instead of using doors or boards, while those attempting to lower injured from upper floors did not seem to know how to lash them to stretchers properly.[77] Other criticism included such comments as "Very seldom were jacks used to raise collapsed walls or floors. Instead valuable time was wasted clearing the rubble and then hacking through floors," and "Some methods of casualty handling could have been improved viz tugging and pulling injured casualties is not conducive to their recovery." Organizing available personnel to achieve the greatest possible efficiency, which meant saving as many people as possible, was also a problem, and "On many occasions rescue men stood around waiting before being required e.g. waiting at the bottom of a building while a casualty was being treated or lashed onto a stretcher. These men could have been doing other jobs only being pulled off the job when they were actually required."[78] Preparing for nuclear war thus required as much time as training for a conventional conflict, even accepting that losses would be extremely high regardless of effort.

Canada's preparations were not limited to civil defence, but included sending a brigade to Europe, part of the British Army of the Rhine poised to defend West Germany against Soviet invasion. In support of the Canadian contingent was 27 Field Ambulance, formed in May 1951 and redesignated 79 Field Ambulance in September. In the years that followed it spent much of its time training, practising setting up and running regimental aid posts, casualty clearing posts, and advanced

---

76. NA, MG 31, J7, Sneath Papers, v.3, Papers Circulated to Members, No 24.
77. NA, RG 29, v.659, 106-2-1, H.E. Brown Brig 2 CIBG to J. Wallace Canadian CD College, 10 Mar 59.
78. NA, RG 29, v.659, 106-2-1, H.E. Brown Brig 2 CIBG to J. Wallace Canadian CD College, 10 Mar 59.

dressing stations, while rehearsing such manoeuvres as river crossings and withdrawals. Its experiences were thus not much different from those of permanent force medical units in Canada, though the presence of Soviet forces nearby must have added a certain sense of realism and immediacy to its training.[79] It was also on familiar ground, and in taking care of the ills and injuries of the Canadian brigade the field ambulance could rely on two world wars' experience with the climate and diseases of the region.

The same could not be said for many of the observer and peace-keeping missions Canadians contributed to from the late forties on; for the government of the time, whether Liberal or Conservative, saw the country's role as being more than an ally of the US, but also a factor in reducing regional tensions before they could escalate into major conflict. One of the first such missions to generate voluminous discussion about health issues followed the 1954 truce between France and nationalist Vietnamese which set up the International Commission of Control and Supervision to keep an eye on the erstwhile protagonists. Canada agreed to be a member, but sending soldiers to Indochina was far more than a matter of transportation. As G.W.L. Nicholson relates, "It was a task carried out in an environment and climate which combined to furnish the greatest test of preventive medicine that the Corps had ever been called upon to face."[80]

The ICCS was to operate in the old French colonies of Indochina, which included North Vietnam, Laos, and Cambodia, with a subsidiary headquarters in the South Vietnamese city of Saigon. "In general all these countries had one thing in common—a very low standard of hygiene," and a 1937 report listed malaria as the most important health threat, with enteric (i.e. intestinal) diseases following close behind. "The grim inventory included epidemics of cholera, with a high incidence among the natives of leprosy, beriberi, typhoid fever, trachoma, pneumonia, and yaws. Injuries caused by heat "were not to be dismissed lightly," and other noteworthy ailments included diseases of the skin, typhus fever, dengue fever, relapsing fever, filariasis, and infection with flukes and various helminths," the last three very unpleasant parasites for the human body to play host to. The Canadian Army's Deputy Director-General Medical Services travelled to Vietnam in August 1954 to conduct a medical reconnaissance, so that his superior, Brigadier Hunter, could plan for the difficult task ahead.[81]

79. NA, RG 24, v.18,389, 27 Cdn Fd Amb, 5 May 51; Jul 51, Appx 29; 19 Jun 51; Jun 51, Appx 13; Aug 51, Appx 9; Sep 51, Appx 1.
80. G.W.L. Nicholson, *Seventy Years of Service* (Ottawa, 1977), 274.
81. G.W.L. Nicholson, *Seventy Years of Service* (Ottawa, 1977), 274.

Thus, as in the wars of the nineteenth century, in peacekeeping operations preventing disease became the prime task of the military medical practitioner. When Canadian forces were sent to the Middle East in 1956 to supervise a truce between Egyptian and Israeli forces, they were accompanied by eight medical officers and 42 other ranks for exactly that purpose. Upper respiratory infections, gastro-enteritis, and skin diseases were their most important challenges, while immunization against polio was a high priority.[82] By the time a Canadian signals unit went to the Congo in 1960 dealing with tropical illnesses had thus become somewhat routine, and "the RCAMC placed emphasis on education, a close surveillance of the environment to determine possible sources of trouble, early diagnosis, and treatment of sickness and early evacuation."[83] Immunization before departure was now standard practice, and troops received comprehensive instructions on how to avoid malaria and gastro-enteritis.

The post-Second World War was thus not a return to the post-First World War, when military medical practitioners had engaged in no overseas operations. Like the interwar period, however, Canadian doctors, nurses, and medical assistants prepared to render support to their comrades in a conventional war, and looking back on the previous century dry statistics seemed to indicate that they had known increasing levels of success in doing so. Injured soldiers were surviving their traumas in ever-larger numbers, the fatality rate in hospital dropping from about 20 per cent in the Crimea to 10-12 per cent in the First World War to 6 per cent in the Second World War and 2-4 per cent in Korea. But, according to a paper prepared by the Medical Joint Training Centre, such numbers did not tell the entire story, as "too many deaths do occur *before* hospitals are reached and this remains a problem. There has been a fairly constant ratio in the battle of—one killed in action to three wounded. The "killed in action" includes immediate deaths and those that die before reaching medical installations. Many of these latter cases might have been saved by more effective first aid and evacuation facilities." Adding to the challenge was the way armed conflict had evolved in the middle part of the twentieth century, as "Marked changes in the methods of waging war have created more complex problems, which require development of new approaches to these problems. It has been estimated in a future war that 70% of casualties due to atomic weapons will be extremity wounds and thermal burns. To this must be added the ever-constant threat of radiation effects."[84]

82. G.W.L. Nicholson, *Seventy Years of Service* (Ottawa, 1977), 279.
83. G.W.L. Nicholson, *Seventy Years of Service* (Ottawa, 1977), 281.
84. NA, MG 31, J7, v.2, Military Medicine, Medical Joint Training Centre, Gen 1, 23 Oct 57.

Perhaps the best example of the medical difficulties posed by a military expedition in modern war was the Canadian contingent slotted for Norway in the early 1970s. Its role was to ensure a general Soviet invasion of western Europe would not easily be able to use a northern axis of advance, though the brigade would not have available the kind of resources formations on the main front in Germany could take for granted. Medical support would be the responsibility of 1 Field Ambulance, formed on 1 July 1970 at Canadian Forces Base Gagetown, and though not yet apprised of the deployment plan, or even of the composition of the force, the unit could immediately tell from the climate it would be working in what some of its equipment requirements would be. All-terrain ambulances would be needed, as would heaters for hospital tents, while at or near the front toboggans towed by snowmobiles might serve the dual purpose of moving supplies and evacuating casualties.[85]

Should the Canadian group actually engage Soviet forces, losses were expected to be on the order of 14 per cent per month in heavy periods, 6-8 per cent when fighting was moderate, and 3.5 per cent when static. These could change dramatically, however, given the lack of anti-aircraft weapons within the NATO contingent, the dearth of armoured fighting vehicles, and the fact that Soviet forces across the way could use nuclear and chemical weapons. Though hospitals would be available, "Because it is inevitable that evacuation will be completely stopped frequently in Northern Norway, the feasibility of a forward emergency surgical capability and holding capability within 1 Field Ambulance should be studied."[86] Also to be considered were the enemy's tactics, so that Canadians should expect

> A concentrated hard-hitting land-air battering that keeps our troops with their heads down for most of the time. There is a good possibility of contaminated casualties. There is excellent possibility of fragmentation injuries from shrapnel and rock fragments.
>
> If we are in position for any length of time, one can expect foot problems in the damp spring, frostbite and exposure in the winter, snow-blindness, and psychiatric problems from isolation and lack of entertainment. With the distance involved and the soviet air-sea menace, reinforcements are extremely unlikely unless it is a phoney war situation,[87]

recalling the early part of the 1939-45 European War when both sides avoided launching an offensive. In Norway, getting casualties to the Unit Medical Station (UMS) would be a nightmare. "The precarious road

---

85. NA, RG 24, Acc 84-85/167, Box 46, 2245-1/2, JR. Rail to Distribution List, 28 Apr 72.
86. NA, RG 24, Acc 84-85/167, Box 46, 2245-1/2, JR. Rail to Distribution List, 28 Apr 72.
87. NA, RG 24, Acc 84-85/167, Box 46, 2245-1/2, Unit CAST Briefing, 1 Fd Amb, 1973.

situation with spring flooding, winter darkness, avalanches, narrow, winding roads which increase time and distance, will all contribute to difficulties in evacuation, not to mention likelihood of vehicle accidents and mechanical breakdowns."[88] As for air evacuation, "Helicopter service will be unreliable at best with the terrain and weather conditions. For all these reasons it seems possible that we will depend more than customary on litter carrying on foot—and that requires good physical conditioning beforehand."[89]

Treatment would not be much easier.

> Because the Norwegian civilian and military medical facilities will be strained to their utmost, our field hospital will be tasked with handling more patients and more types of treatments than they are designed to undertake. This places a responsibility on the field ambulance for a high degree of sorting skill such that only casualties who really need hospital care are evacuated back to that level. The remainder will require treatment by our MOs at the evac platoon and treatment platoon levels—all the more so when we consider how precarious our ability to move patients will be with the crowded, twisted, infrequent and heavily bombed roads in poor weather conditions.
>
> The field ambulance holding policy may be for more extended periods than we are accustomed to living with. Medical resupply may be reasonably good, as it can be air-transported and dropped if necessary. Vehicle resupply is somewhat more difficult.[90]

The need to provide medical treatment as far forward as possible had generated some debate in the Second World War, especially where nursing services, psychotherapy, and surgery were concerned. If Canadians were to fight a war in Norway, however, there would be no choice in the matter.

Having determined to some degree the kind of conditions they would be operating in—in essence, hell after it froze over—staff officers looked to the type of training medical staff would need. It was certainly comprehensive, including as it did the handling of nuclear casualties, fragmentation injuries, and those falling to cold and damp. They would also need the ability to diagnose the early signs of depression while learning to drive in atrocious weather conditions on bad roads; other skills included winter survival and camouflage, the latter particularly critical given Soviet air superiority. Physical conditioning was also important, as was learning the proper care of patients over longer periods than field ambulance personnel were used to, including feeding,

88. *Ibid.*
89. *Ibid.*
90. NA, RG 24, Acc 84-85/167, Box 46, 2245-1/2, Unit CAST Briefing, 1 Fd Amb, 1973.

bathing, and latrine systems, as well as providing medical care in dug-in facilities.

Thankfully, though unknown to those attempting to predict the course of a war in Norway against the Soviet Union, such an event was not to come to pass, the USSR collapsing in the early days of the 1990s. Medical practitioners would thus practise their training elsewhere, and in the 1970s the most likely type of operation to call for their attention on a large scale was humanitarian relief. One example was an earthquake in Italy in 1976; another was a series of volcanic eruptions to strike the Caribbean Island of St Vincent in April 1979. As 2 Field Ambulance noted in an after-action report, the latter tragedy "necessitated the evacuation of 15-20,000 people to the southern part of the Island. These people were situated in some 60-70 refugee camps," and the unit sent a thirteen-member medical team to render aid. An Orders Group was held at 23:00 on 14 April, where those chosen to go were told their role was to "treat and hold casualties," "assist with any public health problems," and "evaluate the medical situation and report back to the Surgeon General's office, NDHQ within 24 hours after arrival." Deploying to Ottawa from Petawawa, its equipment included a cargo truck with trailer, an ambulance, tentage, blankets, water purification tablets, a generator, and Herman Nelson heater, all of it loaded into a C-130 cargo aircraft. It arrived at its destination on the 16th.[91]

The detachment soon met with a Dr Liverpool, the coordinator for the island's Emergency Medical Committee, as well as several members of Kingstown General Hospital. Potential problems were divided into types, accute difficulties being identified as gastroenteritis, scabies, and conjunctivitis, public health challenges including water and food handling, among others, and some chronic conditions to look out for being hypertension, diabetes, cardiac problems, parasitic infections, and dental diseases. At one point in this early period of liaison, a local professor of medecine recommended "at this stage to do faecal screening for parasites on 20,000 people, which is an endemic problem in this area,' but according to the unit's report, "Fortunately, sense prevailed and this scheme was abandoned. With such extreme views it was somewhat difficult for a medical newcomer to fully appraise the situation. It was decided that we should provide a mobile medical clinic to those areas where the need was greatest."[92]

Such deployments having been extremely rare until the 1970s, lessons learned were many. One concerned rations, which at the time consisted

---

91. DHH, Annual Historical Reports, 2104, Operation Abalone, Post Operation Report, nd.
92. DHH, Annual Historical Reports, 2104, Operation Abalone, Post Operation Report, nd.

of canned and dried goods in a package called an Individual Ration Pack, or IRP for short. "These menus were found to be similar in make-up and were felt to supply too heavy a meal for tropical climates. In the tropics, the calorie intake required per day/per man is approximately 2000 calories, the menus supplied a minimum of 5000 calories," perhaps doing more harm than good. Another food item, powdered milk, was deemed useful in its absence, cattle in the island suffering from Brucellosis, but no doubt such conclusions were reached unaware that most inhabitants of the region are lactose intolerant. Practitioners were on firmer ground in the realm of public health, however, a Master-Corporal Naylor proving "extremely useful in inspecting and advising on health measures within the evacuation centres, namely, over 60 centres providing food and shelter for 15-20,000 people. These reports dealt essentially with sewage disposal, food handling, and garbage disposal. These recommendations were passed on to the Central Medical Committee for further action." When it came to providing clinical medical care, the detachment basically filled in the gaps "in an otherwise normally functioning medical clinic system. Our mobility and speed of mobilization proved to be an asset." Finally, the lessons-learned column was completed with a note on sunburn, which with heat stroke and heat exhaustion could incapacitate even the most fit soldier; a period of acclimation was necessary.[93]

Following humanitarian relief operations to Italy (Operation Dolomite) and St Vincent (Operation Abalone), it began to seem evident to the Surgeon-General that the Canadian Forces Medical Service, or CFMS,

> will become increasingly involved in humanitarian operations in the future. These operations may take place anywhere in the world, including Canada. The CFMS may provide the only CF component (as in the case of St Vincent) or may constitute a part of a larger task force (as in the case of Italy). The involvement may range from the provision of a complete unit, such as 1 Canadian Field Hospital, a sub-unit, such as the treatment company of a field ambulance or a team specially tailored for an operation. Certainly, the specific nature of the medical support to be provided will seldom be the same for any two operations. It should also be noted that, in addition to providing humanitarian support, the CFMS element may have the additional task of dispensing medical care for all components of a CF task force.[94]

Such a state of affairs would demand the utmost in flexibility, since "The fact that each operation will inevitably have its own different set

93. DHH, Annual Historical Reports, 2104, Operation Abalone, Post Operation Report, nd.
94. NA, RG 24, v22,864, 3350-04, Op Handle (Thailand), Surgeon-General to Distribution, 25 Sep 79.

of circumstances makes it impossible to prepare detailed contingency plans to be used at the headquarters and unit level." A check list might help, though the one provided by the Surgeon-General ran some seventeen pages.[95]

If supporting combat operations against the Soviet Union never came to pass, and if large-scale humanitarian relief missions were somewhat rare, providing medical practitioners for the Armed Forces' own exercises was an entirely different matter, if perhaps less challenging. One large series of manoeuvres, called Rendez-Vous 83, ellicited the comment that "The medical operations for RV83, for the most part, were within the projected and planned workloads," any problems that came up tending to be of an administrative or logistical nature. For example, "At the start of the exercise units with pers on restricted duty, many of whom had come to RV83 on restricted duty, were still with units. At the time manoeuvre started units tried to pawn their unfit pers into the med system... Units must retain responsibility for their unfit pers or a Div transient/holding org should be formed to administer these pers." Also, though patient care was of a high standard, equipment sometimes left something to be desired. "The heating of the hospital deserves special mention since the Herman Nelson heaters are not only inadequate but pose a definite hazard. There [sic] were not designed for the role in which we use them for the prolonged hours of running. They require constant maint[enance] and, at times, pumped positively harmful fumes into the hospital. They are noisy and certainly make auscultation of patients difficult. They should be withdrawn from use and replaced."[96]

When focussing on its own training the Medical Service had greater control, and like other branches usually started small, with individual indoctrination, and then worked itself up to manoeuvres with full units. One such was 1 Field Ambulance's Exercise Rapier Thrust 84, which ended with a phase called "Bring "Em Back Alive"," rehearsing the evacuation of patients in a high intensity conventional conflict. Later, the unit participated in Exercise Frosty Warrior, evacuating a total of thirteen simulated casualties, though it still had to support the exercise as a whole, seeing a total of 411 patients while conducting an aggressive programme of preventive medicine, so that the field ambulance did not conduct as much of its own training as it would have liked. Furthermore, some casualties could have been prevented within participating

95. NA, RG 24, v22,864, 3350-04, Op Handle (Thailand), Surgeon-General to Distribution, 25 Sep 79.
96. DHH, Annual Historical Reports, 2103, RV 83 Div Med Coy Post Exercise Report, 13 Jul 84 (possibly 83).

units, the Brigade Surgeon noting that "An indepth analysis of med stats reveals that not all Commanders understand the seriousness and possible consequences of even primary frostbite. While our soldiers are well trained and can carry out most tasks without injuries, their susceptibility to weather-related injuries increases directly with their state of fatigue, dehydration and nourishment. Supervisors at all levels must be reminded continuously to pay special attention to the safety of their troops."[97] Like trench foot in the First World War, and like heat exhaustion in the tropics, frostbite could only be prevented with utmost diligence on the part of all concerned.

The Canadian Forces Medical Service also had a role to play, of course, so in the 1970s and 1980s they trained not only to practise medicine, but to do so under harsh circumstances. Exercise Starlight Mukluk, for example, involving 2 Field Ambulance from 16 to 19 January, 1989, "reaffirmed valuable knowledge and skills required for survival in extreme cold weather conditions," including "personal clothing and equipment," "bivouac and tent routine," "showshoeing and skiing," "navigation and march discipline," "rabbit snares," "nutrition and food preparation," "importance of keeping morale up," "importance of being physically fit," and "treating the sick and injured under extreme cold weather conditions,"[98] thus combining medical with military with survival operations. At another temperature extreme, medical practitioners with the Canadian Airborne Regiment reported after deployment to Texas in 1985 that units must "have abundant sunscreen of SPF8 or better and order the troops to use it," and that "each man should have goggles for windy days," and "abundant medication for chapped lips." No doubt giving pause to its readers was the report's admonition that there was a need for "more recent literature on desert operations, especially that related to treatment of snake-bites..."[99]

In the end, it was perhaps individual indoctrination rather than unit training that was more likely to be applied on operations. As the 1980s neared their end Canada's peacekeeping commitment expanded from a handful of missions to over a dozen, one task for field ambulances being to bring soldiers' first aid skills up to par before departure for overseas. In 1989, for instance, "2 Field Ambulance assisted a number of units during pre and post deployment phases of United Nations operations, inlcuding Op Snowgoose—Royal Canadian Dragoons Cyprus peacekeeping tour; Op Matador—89 Logistics Unit Namibia;

---

97. DHH, Annual Historical Reports, 2103, Post Exercise Report—Rapier Thrust 84, 20 Feb 84 (possibly 85).
98. DHH, Annual Historical Reports, 2104, For Year 1989.
99. NA, RG 24, v22,855, 3350-1, Part 78.01, 2 Fd Amb to Distribution, 19 Jun 85.

Op Sultan—Honduras peacekeeping tour; and Op Hugo a hurricane relief effort."[100] More elaborate operations involved actually sending medical practitioners overseas, such as support for Operation Vagabond, the peacekeeping mission that followed the cease-fire between Iran and Iraq in 1989. As the post-mission report noted, "Medical support to Operation Vagabond involved the provision of medical care to approximately 500 troops deployed along the 1200 km border between Iran and Iraq. The unit deployed into countries which have hostile environments; very hot and dry climates and many endemic tropical and unusual diseases. Living conditions vary from modern urban air-conditioned buildings to concrete block bunkers built into the side of a hill. The cultural differences in hygiene standards increased the importance of preventive medicine. Sanitation and ablution facilities also varied from modern to almost non-existent. Food and water sources were of unknown quality. There was a risk of chemical weapon injuries" from persistent agents that had been used during the war. "The spartan living and working conditions, the unstable political climate, family separation and boredom all combined to create stresses not normally experienced in Canada."[101]

A total of 36 medical practitioners were deployed, and though initial planning was something of a problem due to lack of information about the area, "The provision of care went smoothly and without any significant problems. This was certainly made easier by the support from the host nations. The host nation army medical care systems are fairly advanced. For future operations into less advanced countries more second-line support in terms of xray and lab need to be considered." Not unexpectedly, "Testing of water was a continual requirement. In some locations local would test clear one day and contaminated the next. For this reason bottle water was used in these locations throughout the tour." Other, similar challenges included food, where "we continually saw sides of meat piled high in the back of small pick-up trucks driving along the highway in 35 or 40 C temperatures"; as well, "Rats and insects were also a problem initially but were quickly brought under control," though "It is important that the supplies required to combat these problems are amongst the earliest supplies in theatre." Then, as if to remind medical practitioners that some challenges were neverending. "Malaria was of interest in both countries," though at least "There was good support from the leadership of the unit and appropriate precautions supported. A "pill day" was instituted under the supervision of the

---

100. DHH, Annual Historical Reports, 2104, For Year 1989.
101. NA, RG 24, v22,864, 3350-OV, Part 88.01, Dir Med Ops and Trg to CDS, 29 Mar 89.

troop commander to ensure the malaria chemophyloxis was followed."[102]

The Canadian Forces took on an increasing number of peacekeeping
tasks in the years that followed, so that in 1992 2 Field Ambulance found
itself supporting four different operations. For Operation Record, setting
out the boundary between Iraq and Kuwait, the unit provided first aid
and CPR training to two 45-member contingents as well as two medical
assistants for the operation itself. For Operation Harmony, in Croatia,
two medical practitioners went overseas, one to the 3rd Battalion, Royal
22e Régiment and the other to 4 Combat Engineer Regiment. For Operation Marquis, in Cambodia, it trained 200 peacekeepers in first aid and
CPR and provided two medical assistants. Finally, for Operation Deli-
verance, in Somalia, 2 Field Ambulance sent twenty of its members to
accompany the Canadian Airborne Regiment.[103] Another unit, 1 Field
Ambulance, reported that "Without question the most significant events
in 1992 were the deployment of fifteen Medical Assistants ... to the
United Nations Peacekeeping Operations—Operation Harmony in the
former Yugoslavia. These personnel provided medical support to the 3rd
Princess Patricia Canadian Light Infantry Battalion, 1 Combat Engineer
Regiment, and the Canadian Contingent Support Group, National
Medical Liaison Team. The field operating skills of our personnel were
critical to the sucess of the operation. This underscores the absolute necessity of maintaining a cadre of personnel who have both medical skills and
field operations training."[104] It was a lesson as old as the century.

The ultimate test of the Canadian Forces Medical Service ability to
absorb such lessons came in late 1990 and early 1991, following Iraq's
invasion and annexation of Kuwait. The United States and its allies
began to assemble a coalition which, with a mandate from the United
Nations, prepared to eject Iraqi forces from their recent conquests, preparations to do so including the stockpiling of materials in Saudi Arabia
and its neighbours, the movement of troops and equipment to the
theatre, and a blockade of Iraq's economic activity. The Canadian contribution in the early months of the operation was mainly in the form
of naval forces attempting to ensure the enemy could not acquire arms
or other materials and goods, with CF-18s arriving later to take part in
aerial operations against Iraqi forces. Though Canada would not provide
ground forces in formation-size, allies, especially the British, expected
heavy casualties and therefore requested Canadian medical support in
the form of a field hospital.

---

102. NA, RG 24, v22,864, 3350-OV, Part 88.01, Dir Med Ops and Trg to CDS, 29 Mar 89.
103. DHH, Annual Historical Reports, 2104, For Year 1992.
104. DHH, Annual Historical Reports, 2103, For Year 1992.

The Cold War and possible conflict with the Soviet Union notwith-standing, the country's armed services were hard-pressed meeting the British request; 1 Field Surgical Hospital was small, with only 60 beds, and there were only nine surgeons and the same number of anaethestists within the regular forces. "With one blow," wrote Canada's official historians of the conflict, organizing a field hospital "drained the Canadian military medical system."[105] Still, coincidentally just a few hours before the launch of Desert Storm, the attack against Iraqi forces, Minister of Defence Bill McNight announced the deployment of the 100-bed 1 Canadian Field Hospital (1 CFH) to the theatre to enable "the coalition to provide more adequately for the Geneva Convention's requirements for the treatment of captured war wounded."[106] What was called Operation Scalpel would first involve gathering 536 all-ranks as well as 247 vehicles and trailers from across the country and concen-trating them at CFB Petawawa. Then, "Personnel had to be prepared with courses and exercises covering the use of weapons, NBC defence materiel, and field medical procedures, which some people had not used since basic training. The radiologists, nurses, and doctors had to renew their familiarity with the arrangement of the modular tents for triage of the wounded and their systematic progression from one treatment tent to the next under combat conditions."[107]

Meanwhile, the hospital's 1st Advanced Surgical Group made its way to the front, where it joined a British medical unit. "The new arrivals were integrated into the 33 Field Hospital rotation teams and inserted into the day and night shifts. The modest numbers of injured were mostly due to traffic accidents, because of the large convoys from Jubayl to the west, which were in full progress. There were also victims of weapons accidents, some of which had tragic results."[108] After this ini-tial period of indoctrination, they then joined 32 Field Hospital, where "Tents were erected for accommodation and an operating room. In front of the operating room was a common triage room and a "resus-citation" room, and behind it there was a post-operative recovery room... From there, the patient would be returned to the British hospital,"[109] the Canadians in effect acting as part of an integrated medical ins-titution, beginning 13 February. Just outside artillery range of the front lines, they were later joined by the 2nd Advanced Surgical Group which arrived on the 18th. "Soldiers suffered from accidents, traumas, burns,

105. Jean Morin and Richard Gimblett, *Operation Friction 1990-1991: The Canadian Forces in the Persian Gulf* (Toronto, 1997), 217.
106. *Ibid*, 220.
107. *Ibid*, 221.
108. *Ibid*, 222.
109. *Ibid*, 223.

fractures, and lacerations. They arrived by road and air evacuation from 1 Division... Considerable experience was gained from the first cases, especially in triage and resuscitation..."[110]

When the remainder of 1 Canadian Field Hospital arrived in late February, ready to begin work on the 25th, it was a substantial organization divided into a headquarters and three companies: service, infantry, and treatment, the latter forming its operational hub. It was itself organized into five platoons, one for surgery (made up essentially of the two Advanced Surgical Groups), one for resuscitation, another to deal with clinical issues (pharmacy, laboratory, and radiology), yet another to run the ward, and the last incorporating the operating room, intensive care nurses, and bedside workers. Though never swamped like its predecessors of other wars, it did not lack for work, and as the official historians relate, "By 26 February the advancing British Division was discovering more and more wounded, mostly Iraqi survivors of the preparatory bombings for the ground attack. They were dirty and emaciated, with wounds several days old and unattended, already subject to suppurating infections. Given enough first-aid treatment to keep them alive, they were evacuated in large numbers by ambulance and helicopter to Coalition hospitals,"[111] the technology applied in trying to save them proving as advanced as that used to inflict their wounds in the first place.

Procedures to deal with the Iraqi injured were straight-forward.

> Patients were sent to the resuscitation sections of the two hospitals according to a priority system. As soon as they arrived, they were stripped of their soiled clothes, searched by the guards, examined by the doctor on duty, and sent for medical or nursing care. Some needed radiology, laboratory work, or examination by a specialist or surgeon. Most of the wounded had not eaten for several days, and some had been unconscious or only semiconscious for a long time. Selected Kuwaitis acted as interpreters... Surgery was performed on about 10 percent of them. The rest were bandaged, cleaned, sewn up, and plastered. In most cases, these simple measures, accompanied by good meals, were enough to restore their strength, so that they could be sent under escort to the British prisoner-of-war camp, where other medical personnel would conduct secondary, follow-up care. A small number were evacuated to the third- or fourth-line American or British hospitals.[112]

One particularly dramatic example was a soldier who arrived at the hospital on 1 March, the day after fighting stopped. (1 CFH ceased operations on the 3rd.)

110. *Ibid*, 226.
111. *Ibid*, 229.
112. *Ibid*, 229.

He had received shell fragments to his head, his nose had been almost completely blown off by an explosion, his right arm was considerably lacerated and infected, and his whole right side was riddled with holes from shell fragments. Surgeons Lieutenant-Colonel Ian Anderson and Major Barry Armstrong and orthopaedic surgeon Major Charles Buckley, assisted by an otorhino-laryngologist from 32 Field Hospital, spent nine hours cleaning and suturing his wounds to save him. They even opened his cranium to take out metal and bone fragments, which had penetrated up to three centimetres into the right and left frontal lobes of his brain. The patient was conscious and lucid before the operation, however, despite an infection which had had five days to spread. He had been left for dead by his fellows at the bottom of a trench and was discovered when British troops inspected the ground. Few believed that he would pull through, but the surgeons noted in their diagnosis that the patient had resisted his wounds extremely well, perhaps because of the nighttime cold, which had retarded the putrefaction of the wounds.[113]

Buckley saw him a few days later, and deemed him to be on the road to recovery. It should be noted here, however, that in more pressing circumstances his arm would have been amputated, a procedure that had never been completely superceded.

In a sense, then, military medical work of the latter 20th century had much in common with that of two hundred years or so before. Operations in Norway—which by plan or good fortune never came to pass—would force practitioners to ply their craft in abysmal battlefield conditions, while as we have seen peacekeeping missions forced an emphasis on hygiene and vaccination (the latter reminiscent of the fight against smallpox in the early 1800s). Throughout, Canadian medical practitioners adopted an aggressive approach towards injury and disease, what detractors of western medicine refer to as "heroic', but one which is wholly appropriate to a military organization. Within the culture of which a Canadian Forces doctor, nurse, or medical assistant is a part, death is not a natural process to be accepted, but an enemy to be faced and—whenever possible—defeated. To some, that is wrong-minded; to others, that is noble; to the historian, it is simply a characteristic of the society to which military medical practitioners belong.

---

113. *Ibid*, 230.

Appendix

A Note on Military Medical Organization and Terminology

It is characteristic of a military organization that as it evolves it tends to operate according to procedures that are a mix of the logical and the archaic, and though the author has attempted to explain these issues as they have appeared in the text, a separate appendix was deemed appropriate so the reader would have a constant point of reference.

Perhaps the best way to come to terms with organization and terminology is through a brief study of the chain of evacuation. In the Canadian context, the first step in treating a soldier has usually been within his or her own unit. Wounded were gathered from the battlefield by pre-assigned stretcher bearers or made their own way to a Battalion Aid Post or Regimental Aid Post (more recently Unit Medical Station or UMS). Those who fell ill in quiet periods would report to Sick Parade, which could be run by a Stretcher Bearer (later a Medical Assistant) or other medical practitioner (in the early days the latter may well have been the regimental Surgeon). Thus within the unit itself, an infantry battalion for example, there was already a medical system in place, with a Surgeon (or later, Medical Officer) in charge.

The expression "surgeon" requires some explanation, as historically it has had two distinct meanings. First, it could refer to a specialization, to that individual who carried out surgery; the surgeon in a Field Surgical Unit would fit that definition. But the expression could also have a much wider meaning, dating back centuries, and simply refer to the individual responsible for a unit's health. A regimental Surgeon of the nineteenth century would fit this definition, but so would a ship's Surgeon of the Second World War or a Flight Surgeon of the 1960s. More recently the expression "Medical Officer" has come to replace that of "Surgeon" in the Canadian Forces Medical Service (except as regards those whose specialization is surgery).

Next in the chain of evacuation was a variety of dressing stations, such as the Advanced Dressing Station (ADS) and Main Dressing Station (MDS), as well as the Casualty Clearing Post (CCP), all of which were parts of the Field

Ambulance (Fd Amb). The latter was thus not concentrated in one particular place but had various sections operating between the battlefield and rear areas. In general terms, the field ambulance provided two services: it treated the wounded and sick in the dressing stations and clearing posts noted above; and it was responsible for transporting patients from the Regimental Aid Posts (or equivalent) to the dressing stations and clearing posts, and then further to the rear. It should be noted here that the Field Dressing Station (FDS) that appeared in the latter part of the Second World War was an independent unit and not part of a field ambulance. Nor was it alone, the Field Transfusion Unit (FTU) and Field Surgical Unit (FSU) being similarly autonomous, though it was not unusual for these to work together in an Advanced Surgical Centre (ASC), itself independent of the Casualty Clearing Station discussed below. (In Korea the FTU became a Transfusion Team while the FSU became a Surgical Team; by the 1991 Gulf War the latter had again transmuted, becoming the Advanced Surgical Group.)

Behind the lines were, depending on the era, the Casualty Clearing Station and various types of hospital. For most of the period covered by this study the Casualty Clearing Station was the first place where a soldier could receive surgery - it was also the closest medical facility to the front lines where nursing sisters were posted. From the turn of the twentieth century the latter had officer rank and were responsible for the monitoring and care of patients before, during, and after surgery, while doctors and surgeons specialized in providing specific treatment. The expression nursing "sister" dates from the nineteenth century and was designed to distinguish trained military nurses from the untrained relatives and friends that had previously taken on such tasks (the Catholic Sisters of Charity may have been a model for the secular nursing sisters.) The Casualty Clearing Station was thus, in effect, a hospital, though further to the rear were facilities formally identified as such, variously classified as Stationary Hospitals, General Hospitals, or according to specialization; for example, the West Cliff Canadian Eye and Ear Hospital. These were run essentially along the lines of civilian facilities of the time.

Military medical organization and terminology has thus been characterized by much fluidity, but it is hoped the above may help the reader understand such arcana.

To summarize, in alphabetical order:

Advanced Dressing Station (ADS): that part of a Field Ambulance responsible for treating wounded or ill soldiers. Usually operated between the Regimental Aid Post and the Main Dressing Station in the chain of evacuation.

Advanced Surgical Centre (ASC): a combination of a Field Dressing Station, a Field Surgical Unit, and a Field Transfusion Unit. Usually operated between the Regimental Aid Post and the Casualty Clearing Station or hospital in the chain of evacuation.

Battalion Aid Post: within a unit such as an infantry battalion, often where soldiers first received treatment for their wounds or illnesses.

Casualty Clearing Post (CCP): part of a Field Ambulance responsible for the treatment of wounded or ill soldiers. Usually operated between the Regimental Aid Post and the Casualty Clearing Station.

Casualty Clearing Station (CCS): in effect, a hospital where soldiers could be operated on surgically and otherwise treated and held for short-term convalescence. Usually to the rear of Regimental Aid Posts, Field Ambulance units, Field Dressing Stations, and Advanced Surgical Centres.

Field Ambulance (Fd Amb): a unit responsible for evacuating patients from Regimental Aid Posts, treating them at Casualty Clearing Posts, Advanced Dressing Stations, and/or Main Dressing Stations before further evacuating them to Casualty Clearing Stations or hospitals.

Field Dressing Station (FDS): an independent unit responsible for treating wounded or ill soldiers. Usually operated between the Regimental Aid Post and the Casualty Clearing Station or hospital. Sometimes combined with a Field Surgical Unit and a Field Transfusion Unit to form an Advanced Surgical Centre.

Field Surgical Unit (FSU): an independent unit responsible for conducting surgery on wounded soldiers. Usually operated between the Regimental Aid Post and the Casualty Clearing Station or hospital in the chain of evacuation. Sometimes combined with a Field Dressing Station and a Field Transfusion Unit to form an Advanced Surgical Centre.

Field Transfusion Unit (FTU): an independent unit responsible for resuscitating wounded soldiers. Usually operated between the Regimental Aid Post and the Casualty Clearing Station or hospital in the chain of evacuation. Sometimes combined with a Field Surgical Unit and a Field Dressing Station to form an Advanced Surgical Centre.

General Hospital: like its civilian equivalent, a facility where soldiers could be treated and held for convalescence.

Main Dressing Station (MDS): that part of a Field Ambulance responsible for treating wounded or ill soldiers. Usually between an Advanced Dressing Station and a Casualty Clearing Station in the chain of evacuation.

Medical Assistant (MedA): a soldier or non-commissioned officer specialized in the treatment of wounds and illness.

Medical Officer (MO): generally, an individual with a medical degree who is also a serving officer in the armed services.

Nursing Sisters: since the 1970s simply referred to as 'nurses,' accredited practitioners responsible for general care of patients. From mid-nineteenth century were referred to as 'sisters' as the model for their work was provided by Catholic nuns.

Regimental Aid Post (RAP): same as the Battalion Aid Post.

Sick Parade: usually held in the morning, where soldiers who feel ill present themselves for diagnosis and possible treatment.

Stationary Hospital: like its civilian equivalent, a facility where soldiers could be treated and held for convalescence.

Surgeon: either a specialist who performs surgery or simply a medical officer in a unit (army and air force) or ship (navy).

Unit Medical Station (UMS): successor to the Regimental Aid Post.

As a final summary, then, the chain of evacuation, depending on the period being studied, could run from the battlefield to the battalion aid post to the field ambulance to the hospital,

or from the battlefield to the regimental aid post to the advanced dressing station to the main dressing station to the casualty clearing station to hospital

or from the battlefield to the regimental aid post to the advanced surgical centre to hospital

or from the unit medical station to the field ambulance to hospital.

Other combinations were possible, while nodes in the system could of course be bypassed depending on circumstances and the availability of such means of transportation as the helicopter.

Other abbreviations

ADMS, Assistant Director Medical Services
AMC, Army Medical Corps
AMO, Administrative Medical Officer
AMS, Army Medical Service
AST, Advanced Surgical Team
BEF, British Expeditionary Force
CAMC, Canadian Army Medical Corps
CF, Canadian Forces
CFMS, Canadian Forces Medical Service
CEF, Canadian Expeditionary Force
CO, Commanding Officer
DDMS, Deputy Director Medical Services
DGMS, Director General Medical Services

DMO, District Medical Officer

EOS, Emergency Operating Station

FAP, First Aid Post

HMCS, His or Her Majesty's Canadian Ship

HMS, His or Her Majesty's Ship

GP, General Practitioner

LMF, Lacking in Moral Fibre

MAC, Motorized Ambulance Column

MAO, Medical Associate Officer

MASH, Mobile Army Surgical Hospital

MD, Military District

MDC, Mobile Defence Corps

MFH, Mobile Field Hospital

NATO, North Atlantic Treaty Organization

NCO, Non-Commissioned Officer

NDHQ, National Defence Headquarters

NO, Nursing Orderly

NRC, National Research Council

OC, Officer Commanding

OR, Other Rank

PAMC, Permanent Army Medical Corps

PMO, Principal Medical Officer

POW, Prisoner of War

RAF, Royal Air Force

RCAF, Royal Canadian Air Force

RCAMC, Royal Canadian Army Medical Corps

RCN, Royal Canadian Navy

RMO, Regimental Medical Officer

RN, Royal Navy

RTU, Returned to Unit

SBA, Sick Berth Attendant

SEC, Special Employment Company

UN, United Nations

Index

S | **AGMV** Marquis

MEMBER OF THE SCABRINI GROUP

Quebec, Canada
2001